EAT TO CLIMB

EAT TO CLIMB

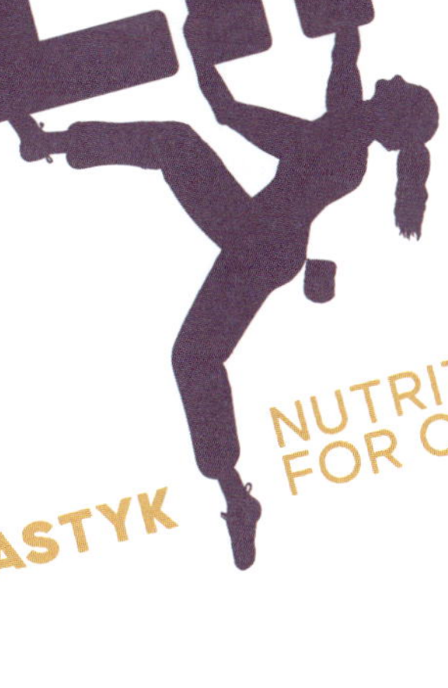

NUTRITION FOR CLIMBERS

MINA LESLIE-WUJASTYK

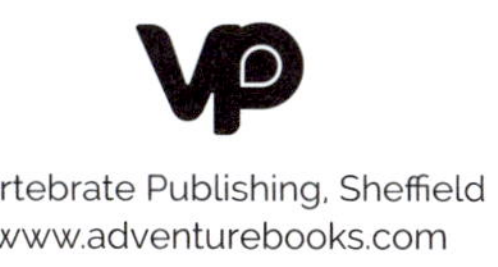

Vertebrate Publishing, Sheffield
www.adventurebooks.com

EAT TO CLIMB
MINA LESLIE-WUJASTYK

First published in 2025 by Vertebrate Publishing.

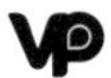
VERTEBRATE PUBLISHING
Omega Court, 352 Cemetery Road, Sheffield S11 8FT, United Kingdom.
www.adventurebooks.com

Front cover design by Jane Beagley. Illustration by Vicky Frost.
Back cover: the author on *Green Mamba*, Rocklands, South Africa. © Nick Brown.
Food photography by Colin Perkins. *www.colinperkinsphotography.co.uk*
Other photography as credited.
Illustrations by Vicky Frost.

A CIP catalogue record for this book is available from the British Library.

ISBN: 978-1-83981-272-9 (Paperback)
ISBN: 978-1-83981-273-6 (Ebook)
ISBN: 978-1-83981-274-3 (Audiobook)

10 9 8 7 6 5 4 3 2 1

Vertebrate Publishing is committed to printing on paper from sustainable sources.

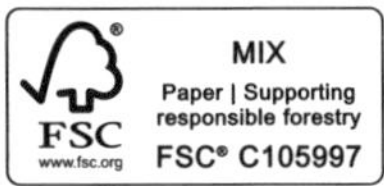

Printed and bound in Slovenia by Latitude Press.

CONTENTS

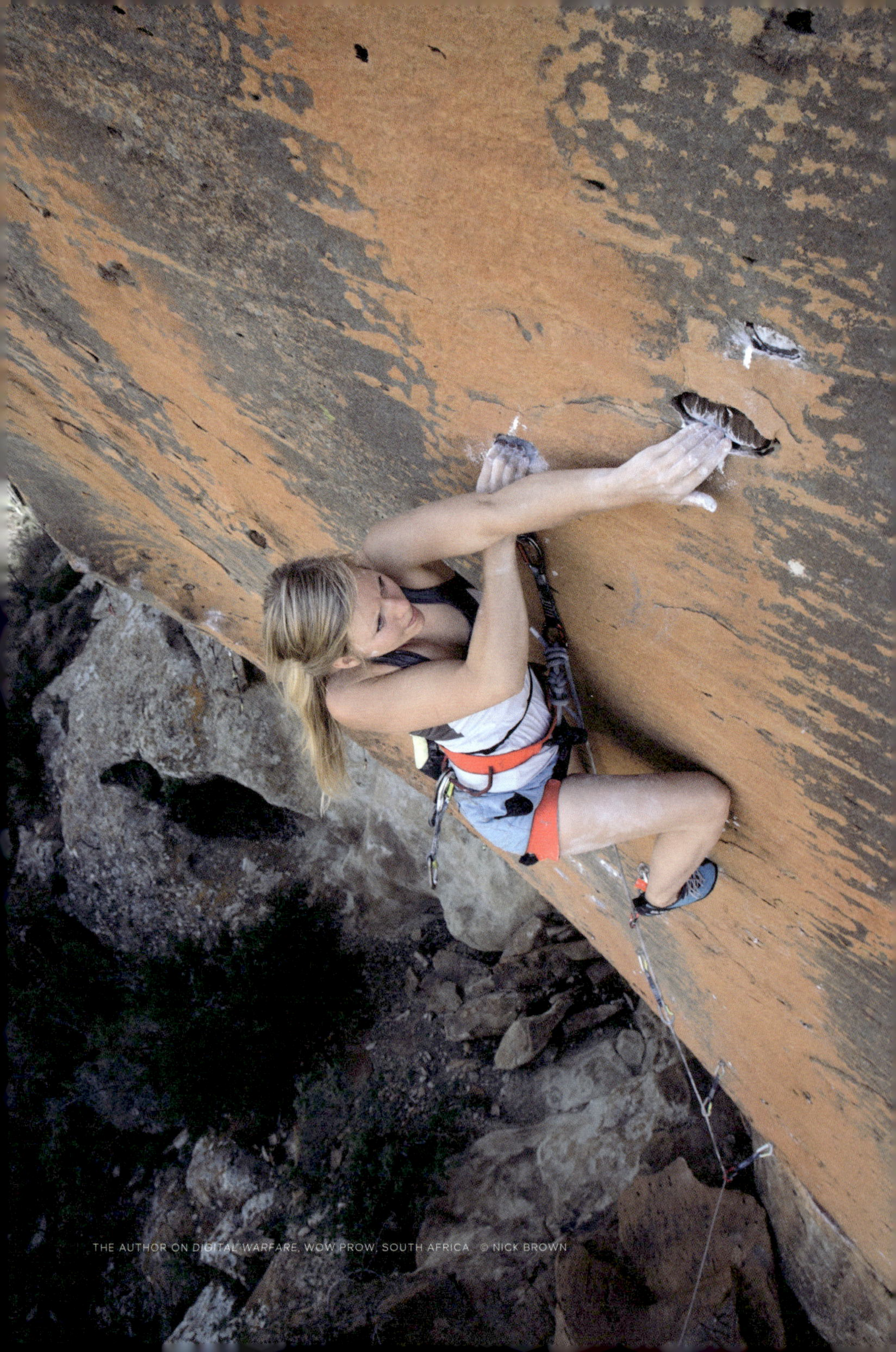

THE AUTHOR ON DIGITAL WARFARE, WOW PROW, SOUTH AFRICA © NICK BROWN

A WORD FROM THE AUTHOR

I don't really believe in prescriptive meal or nutrition plans per se; for many of us, tight instructions on what to eat can be counter-productive. While, in the short term, a plan may feel like it solves a problem or gives us an answer to a question, it will not give us the tools to support our body in the long run through life's inevitable changes. There needs to be more understanding, depth and nuance.

Early on in my nutrition studies I was introduced to **principles** and **methods** as two ways of understanding and implementing what we know about nutrition. Understanding the key **principles** that underpin evidence-based nutrition knowledge is, in my opinion, the best starting point. That is why this book has an educational feel. I want you to understand the *why* of what I advise you to do. I want you to understand the basic principles and the evidence that supports these principles, so that you have the confidence and the reference points to trust in your personal process.

There are many **methods** to choose from. You might be vegan, you might have an allergy, you might not like certain foods, you may love or hate cooking, you may have lots of time or be very time poor, and, of course, culturally there are many diverse ways of eating, cooking and enjoying food. Climbing disciplines and ways of training for climbing also vary and may require different methods. There is a method that will work optimally for each of us, but, although these may look very different, they should all connect back to the **principles** of evidence-based sports nutrition. This way of thinking gives you options, flexibility and – most importantly – informed autonomy over your choices.

The aim of this book is to serve as a platform for expanding your knowledge base; a core nutrition text for climbers. A book that will give you a long-lasting understanding of nutrition principles for climbing as well as plenty of tools and methods that you can use to support yourself in your climbing – and non-climbing – life. It will help you to navigate the plethora of nutrition fads out there and to be confident in the decisions *you* make for *your* body.

* * *

Now, a bit about me, about where my knowledge comes from and where my scope of practice lies. My undergraduate degree was in physiotherapy, but a few years later I studied a foundational course to become certified as a nutritionist, followed by a further two years in the postgraduate study of sports nutrition under the International Olympic Committee. Alongside this, I certified as an intuitive eating counsellor. I have worked solo and also supported clients with nutrition services at Lattice Training, and in 2024, I published my first paper in the *Journal of Science in Sport and Exercise* which focused on nutrition for female climbers.[1]

However, I am not a *medical* professional and as such cannot expand information in this book to include any medical situations where nutrition plays a role; this would be the role of a dietitian. My area is very defined within **sports nutrition**. If you have overlapping needs – for example, you are a climber but also diabetic, or you have irritable bowel syndrome – I recommend you consult a dietitian.

My knowledge of nutritional science has

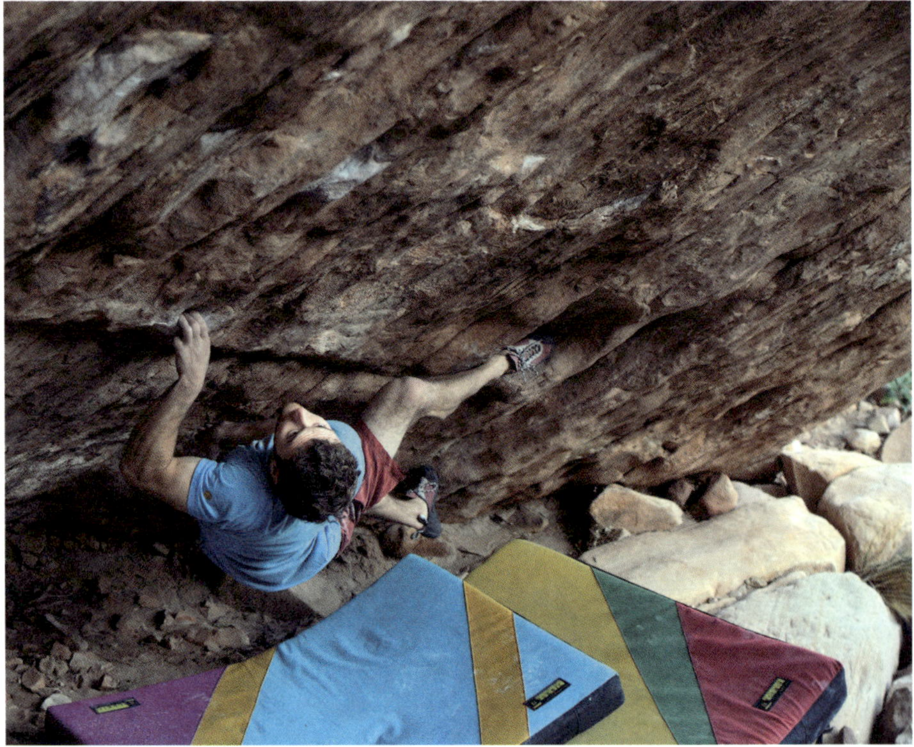

MATT PINCUS ON *THE JABBERWOCKY*, RED ROCKS, USA. © DAVID MASON

always and will always be in the context of a lifetime of my own climbing and pushing my performance. I have competed internationally, and bouldered and sport climbed all over the world to a high standard; in all these avenues, I have pushed my body hard. I hope that sharing my knowledge on nutrition will help you navigate this somewhat confusing area of climbing performance that has the power to unlock your further potential.

Before studying the subject myself, I made many mistakes with my own nutrition. In particular, I would like to touch on my personal experience of **relative energy deficiency in sport (REDs)**. This book is not about me, but it feels relevant to highlight that I have navigated the journey through REDs because it affects my perspective on sports nutrition and therefore, inevitably, the feel and content of this book. From diagnosis to recovery and beyond, I learned – and am still learning – so much about the nuances of the human body, nutrition, food, identity, body image and much more. While lighter is not always better, strength-to-weight ratio does still have a role to play in climbing performance, and reconciling these two somewhat conflicting concepts is no small task. My personal REDs experience fundamentally changed my outlook on nutrition for climbing and I hope that this book is able to communicate some of the key messages that have, over time, become central to how I think about food and eating. With a sporting culture that has deeply ingrained ideas about body weight and image, climbing still has a lot of room for growth and I hope that this book can make a contribution to that.

INTRODUCTION

Nutrition is a fundamental part of climbing training, performance and recovery. Optimal nutrition practices help support climbing on the day as well as long-term development in the sport. Good nutrition is also important for health and emotional well-being, with social connection and food enjoyment being crucial parts of the full picture. There is a lot to understand and navigate within this topic, not to mention the numerous fad diets and food marketing that promises the world. So, where do we start?

Recent research suggests that climbers are missing the mark with their nutrition. Studies have shown that an overwhelming number of climbers are not eating enough to meet their energy needs, may be suffering from low energy availability, are undereating carbohydrate in particular and are potentially low in some micronutrients such as iron.[1] Is this suboptimal nutrition practice driven by misinformation, lack of information, intentional restriction or unintentional under-nutrition?

In reality, it's likely a bit of everything.

It's fair to say that climbing culture has coveted the lean and light physique for as long as many of us can remember, and, while it is impossible to get away from the weight-sensitive nature of the sport completely, there is a shift happening. Gradually, the narrative is getting more nuanced, more informed and more sensible. Climbers are becoming increasingly savvy; realising that endless restriction and the search for lightness are not conducive to long-term development in climbing performance. Slowly, as a community, we are getting stronger and we are learning to eat to climb.

Let's set the scene for a continued narrative around positive nutrition for climbing. This means a focus on **adding**, *not taking away*; boosting the system rather than following a reductionist approach. It isn't possible to do a nutrition 'quick fix' in one meal, one snack or from one day of eating. It's consistency over time that makes the difference. It's just like training for climbing: you don't get strong fingers after just one fingerboard session, but if you turn up to your fingerboard consistently for six months, the gains will come. Similarly, being consistent with positive, supportive nutrition most of the time will reap benefits in the long term. This allows for flexibility around food which is vital for practical, social, cultural, emotional and psychological reasons.

This is because food – and eating – is a biopsychosocial entity; it is not as simple as just fuel. Food can be used positively in different ways in different contexts. For example, a climber might use Haribo sweets before or during a long redpoint or multi-pitch; we may think of sweets as 'unhealthy', but in this context they are quick-acting, smart nutrition. A big plate of vegetables is very nutritious with lots of vitamins and minerals, but it is probably not the ideal choice just before a climb as it will make you feel full and there is a large digestive load from all the associated fibre. Chocolate biscuits are an appropriate choice for enjoyment and social connection – after all, who doesn't love a cup of tea and a biscuit with friends?

Another important part of understanding nutritional science for any sport is acknowledging that it is ever evolving. New research is conducted all the time to question, develop

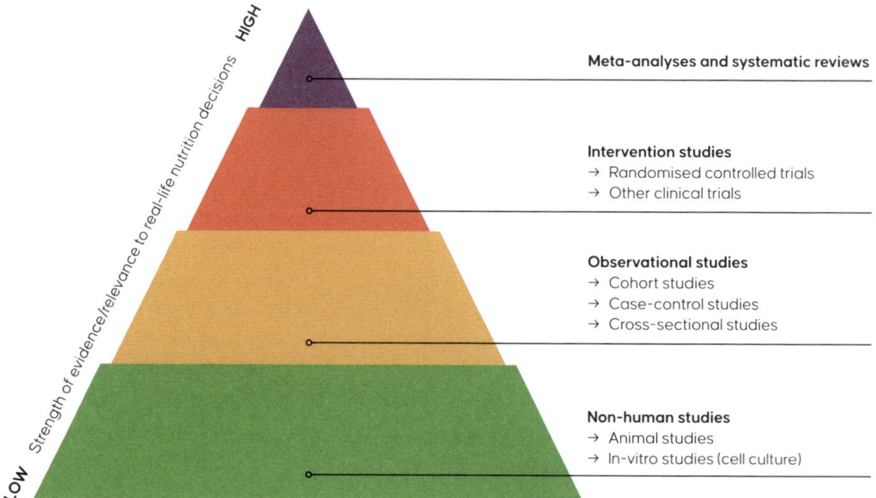

Figure 1: The hierarchy of evidence by Alice Callahan. Licensed under CC BY 4.0.

and expand on what is considered current knowledge and understanding. There are literally hundreds of thousands of research studies looking at sports nutrition and exercise metabolism, and it is from these – and the emerging research into climbing nutrition specifically – that we can find the answers to how best to fuel and recover.

In this context, and before reading what this book has to offer, it is important to discuss the concept of evidence-based nutrition and why it is so important. Evidence-based nutrition means nutritional strategies that are underpinned with a good level of high-quality evidence to support their efficacy. One study cannot determine a solid answer, but a *body* of evidence can be more revealing. When looking at research, it helps to understand the hierarchy of evidence; some research is more compelling than other research. Essentially, the type of study or review and how well it is done will determine how much weight it holds.

At the bottom of the pyramid in figure 1 (above), there are animal and in-vitro (meaning test tube or dish) studies. While these are a great and less expensive way to investigate biological mechanisms, the results cannot be extrapolated to humans or real-life situations. Often research begins here in preliminary stages before moving to another type of study.

Next there are observational studies. In these, information about groups of people and their dietary intake or patterns is collected and associations can be drawn. Often, a group of people are observed over a certain time period, either prospectively or retrospectively, to gather data. While observational studies can find strong associations, the reason they sit where they do in the pyramid is that they do not find conclusive cause and effect. This is because there may be confounding factors at play, for example, hypothetically if vegans are found to have a longer lifespan this could be due to their food choices, but they are also a group of people who are likely to make other health-promoting life choices such as not smoking.

The next level up is intervention studies, the classic of which is the randomised

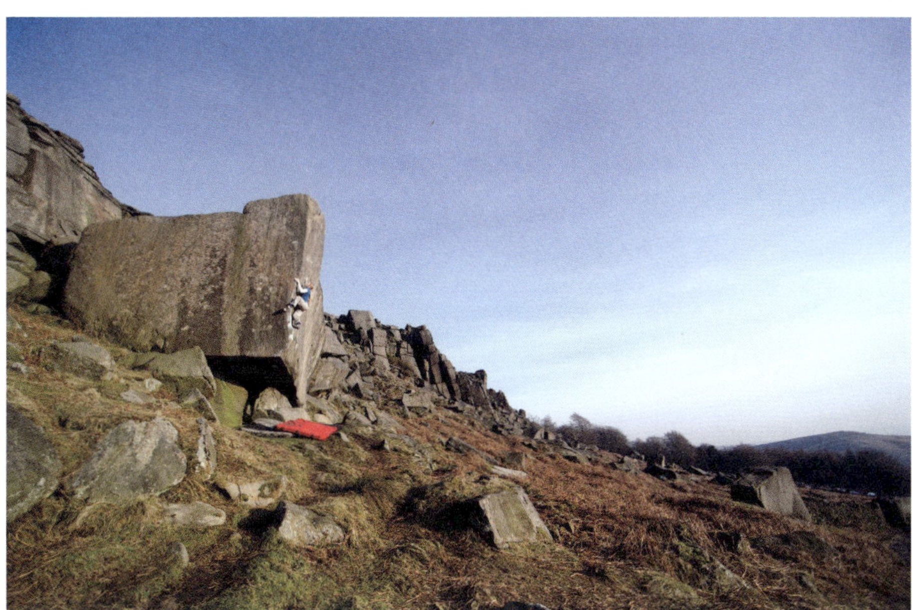

THE AUTHOR ON *CARELESS TORQUE*, STANAGE PLANTATION, UK. © **NICK BROWN**

controlled trial (RCT). These involve (as the title suggests) an intervention, which is essentially a change or treatment imposed by the researcher and a control group. This type of research, when done well, can elicit a cause-and-effect result.

Finally, there are meta-analyses and systematic reviews. These are studies of studies. They look at all the research in a given area, evaluate the quality of all the studies and draw overall conclusions. These are really useful as there are often many studies on a topic, all with varying quality and conflicting results.

There will be a strong emphasis on evidence-based knowledge in this book to build trust in the recommendations and provide signposting (via references) for more information if desired. Of course, as with any subject, there are changes over time as new things are tested and discovered, so it is important to keep an open mind.

While evidence-based science is really important, context and lived experience are also paramount. That's why this book includes ten stories from climbers of a variety of backgrounds, disciplines and experiences. These stories are ghostwritten by me based on interviews and the aim is to show more depth, nuance and context for various nutritional approaches and journeys. Not all the nutritional approaches taken by these climbers are completely evidence based or ideal; in fact, some are less than ideal! But, as readers, we can learn from their shared experience. Importantly, these stories are generous contributions to opening up the narrative that we have around food and eating in climbing.

Annoyingly, the answer to a lot of nutrition questions is, 'Well, it depends … '. The purpose of this book is to help you gain a deeper understanding of nutrition in the context of climbing and all its many considerations. To give you the power and the knowledge to answer the questions you have, make informed choices and be flexible in what you eat to fit the needs of the moment, in the context of long-term benefit.

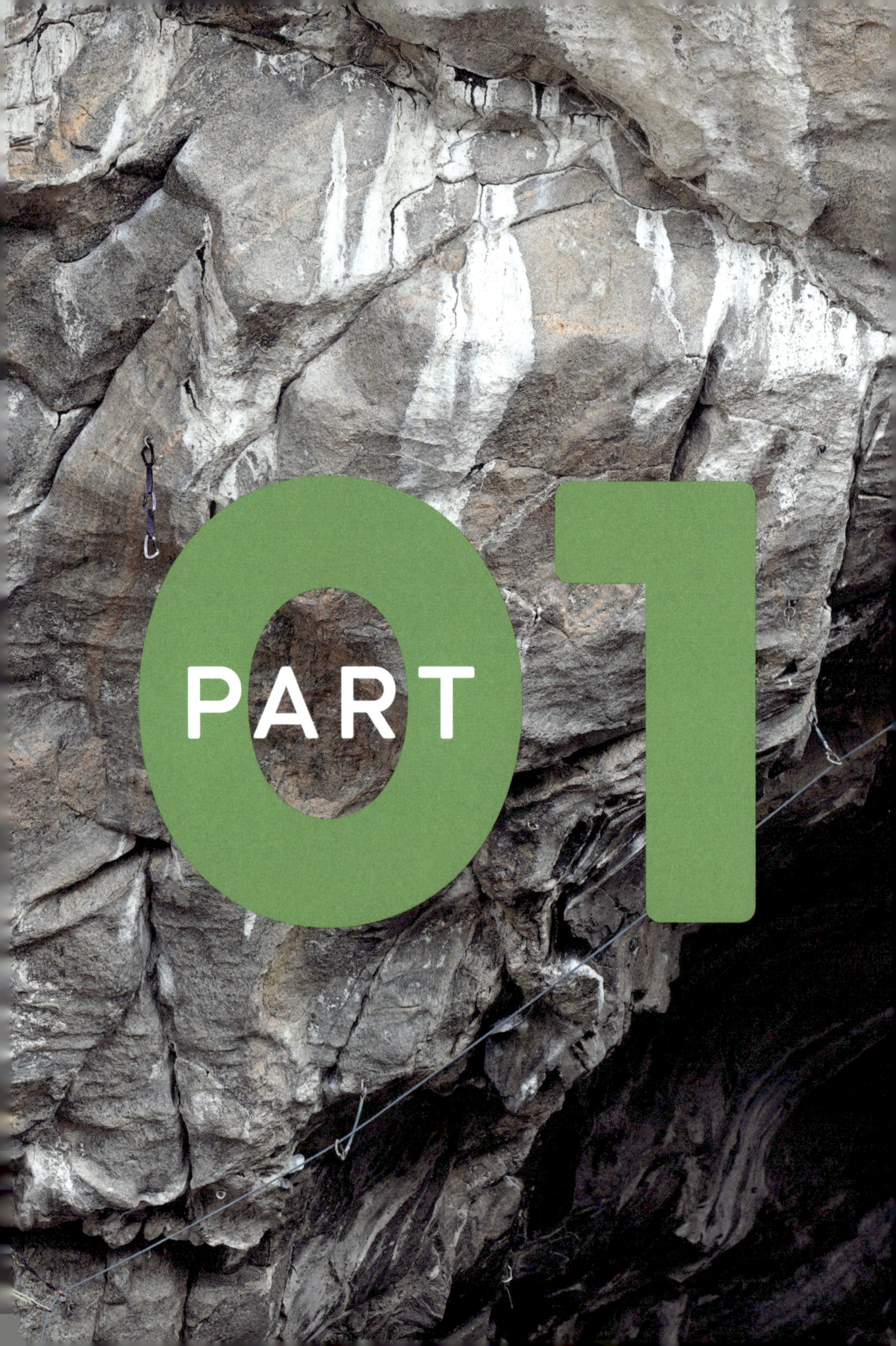
PART
01

PRINCIPLES

KATHERINE CHOONG ON *NORDIC FLOWER* (L1+L2), FLATANGER, NORWAY © **KEITH SHARPLES**

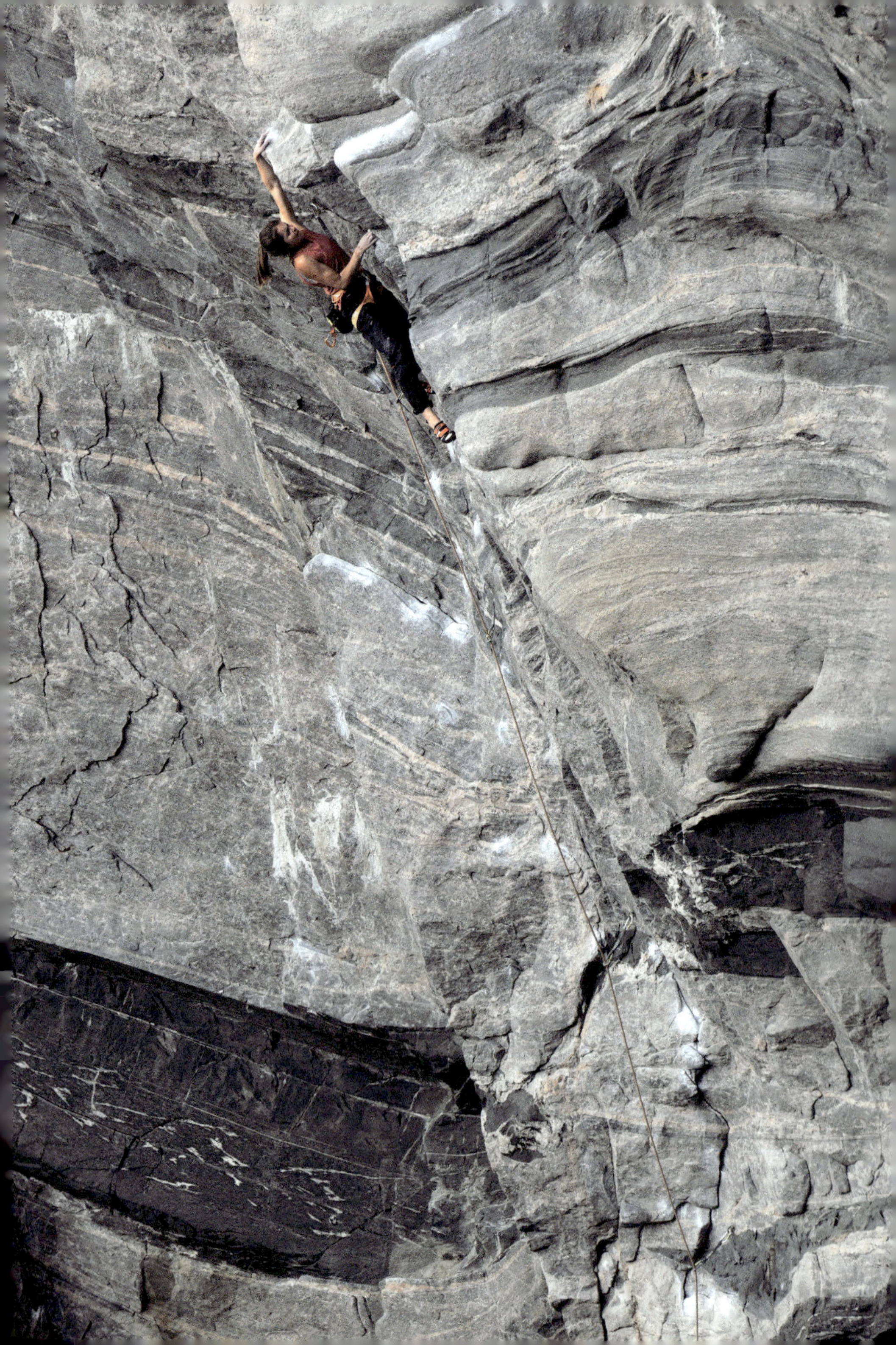

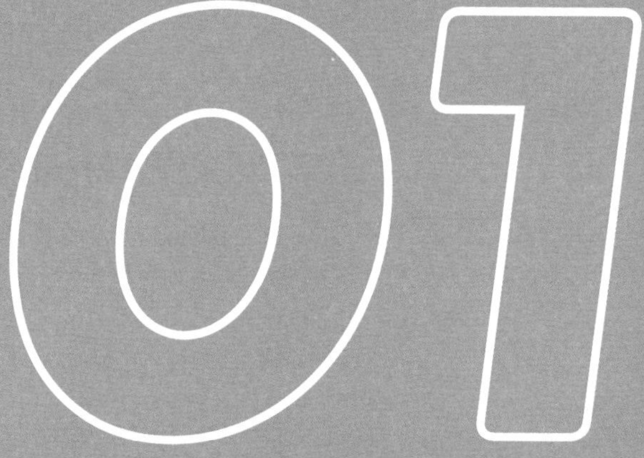

ENERGY
EAT TO PERFORM

EVENTYRBLANDING, FLATANGER, NORWAY © KEITH SHARPLES

Why is energy such an important concept in nutrition?

Energy is the foundation of good nutrition and provides the basic opportunity for us to use our bodies for things like climbing. Optimising nutrition should begin first and foremost with ensuring that there is enough energy in the system. For example, there is no point in speculating about ideal macronutrient ratios or meal composition if there is not enough energy going in.

To be able to maximise our performance in climbing and the adaptations gained from any training, energy availability for climbing and training must also be maximised. This is a long-term view; the ability to respond physiologically and become a better athlete is dependent on the quality, intensity and volume at which we can expose our body to a stimulus – climbing, or training for climbing, in this case. This will be greater, both long and short term, if energy is not a limiting factor in our sessions or in recovery from sessions. Recovery, both within and between sessions, is a crucial part of this picture. Better and faster recovery means higher quality, more volume and more intensity is possible in a given time frame, and thus greater adaptation and progression over time. Not only will our physiological adaptation be maximised with this approach, but when we have more available energy to practise the sport, we also get more time to hone the technical elements.

The basic premise of this perspective on energy, and nutrition in general, is to think about what can be added rather than taken away. **Try to steer towards a mentality of boosting your system, and away from the reductionist approach of minimum effective dose.** In many sports, and particularly in climbing, this may require a paradigm shift from what has been the sport's cultural norm for some time.

Energy systems in climbing

So, how is energy used when we climb? There are three main energy pathways in our cells that are used when exercising. They all have different ways of making ATP (adenosine triphosphate), a unit of energy, which our muscles can then use to create force. Which pathway is most dominant will depend on the intensity and duration of the effort in that moment: climbing can be lower intensity and continuous, or shorter, higher-intensity bursts of effort, or a combination of both of those things. It is not an on/off switch between these different systems but more of an interchangeable dominance depending on demand.

- ***Phosphocreatine system (PCr)***
  The PCr system is the fastest way to get energy as it uses readily available creatine phosphate in a cell to create ATP. It is fast but limited in availability and slow to replenish. The PCr system is used in short, hard bursts of effort, especially in the first ten seconds. Think about maximal-effort moves, or a deadlift or a sprint.
- ***Anaerobic glycolysis***
  In anaerobic glycolysis, the cell uses glucose (from carbohydrate) to create ATP when no oxygen is present and the intensity demand is high. This system will take over dominance from the PCr system after the initial burst and it can sustain energy provision for up to two minutes. Think about hard boulder problems or a series of challenging moves on a route.
- ***Aerobic glycolysis***
  Aerobic glycolysis uses both carbohydrate and fat to create ATP in the presence of oxygen. This is the most sustainable and efficient way to create energy but requires lower intensities of effort. Think about

walking to the crag, easier sections of climbing or recovering between bouts of higher-intensity work.

The objective intensity at which we switch energy system dominance is also dependent on our strength and fitness; one person may complete a certain climb with aerobic system dominance, while another might be using more of their anaerobic pathways on the same climb. This is dependent on our aerobic threshold (the maximum intensity at which we could indefinitely continue using aerobic glycolysis to create ATP), particularly in the forearms as these are often the limiting muscle groups for climbing performance. This threshold, when describing the use of the finger flexors in climbing, has been coined *critical force*.[1]

Energy intake

The energy used by the body to climb – and for everything else that goes on behind the scenes to exist and function – has to come from somewhere: food. *Energy intake* describes the energy value of the food that we eat. *Energy availability* describes the amount of energy intake we need to allow our body to function optimally – before accounting for the energy needs of exercise. This is discussed in more detail in chapter 11. Making sure there is enough energy availability is crucial for our health and performance. It is the starting point in terms of understanding what we need from the food we eat and how we can use nutrition to feel and perform better.

Energy intake from food is measured in kilocalories (kcals) and, although it would be great to offer a simple answer for how much we need to eat, it is something that is constantly in flux.[i] There are methods that can be used to estimate our needs, but that is all they are, estimations. If they are used, it must be as a starting point rather than as an absolute figure to stick to. The energy needed for any given day or period of time will be highly dependent on multiple factors such as our activity level and relative fitness, body temperature, environment (for example, altitude) and previous food intake, as well as body size, composition, age and biological sex.

As a very general concept, if we eat less than we expend, weight loss may occur (fat and muscle loss), and if we eat more than required then we might gain weight (fat, or muscle if training stimulus is present). This 'calories in versus calories out' concept is widely used to describe the balance of energy between consumption and expenditure within the body and, while it does have foundation based on the rule of thermodynamics, it oversimplifies what is going on in the body and can be misleading if followed too rigidly in practice.

By this rule, as mentioned above, any deviation from perceived energy balance – the matching of estimated input and output – would result in weight loss or gain. Due to the flux of both sides of this equation, and the elaborate physiology of the body, it can be more complex than this. It is helpful to think of energy intake requirements as a range rather than an absolute figure. For example, increasing energy intake may lead to increased climbing energy and output, and up-regulation of certain bodily functions (thus increasing one side of the equation unknowingly) rather than weight gain, and, conversely, a reduction in intake may lead to down-regulation of certain bodily functions and reduced energy in climbing, rather than immediate weight loss.

i A calorie is the amount of energy needed to raise the temperature of 1 gram of water by 1 °C. A kilocalorie is 1,000 calories. In practice, and in this book, these terms are used interchangeably, with the informal term 'calorie' representing kilocalories.

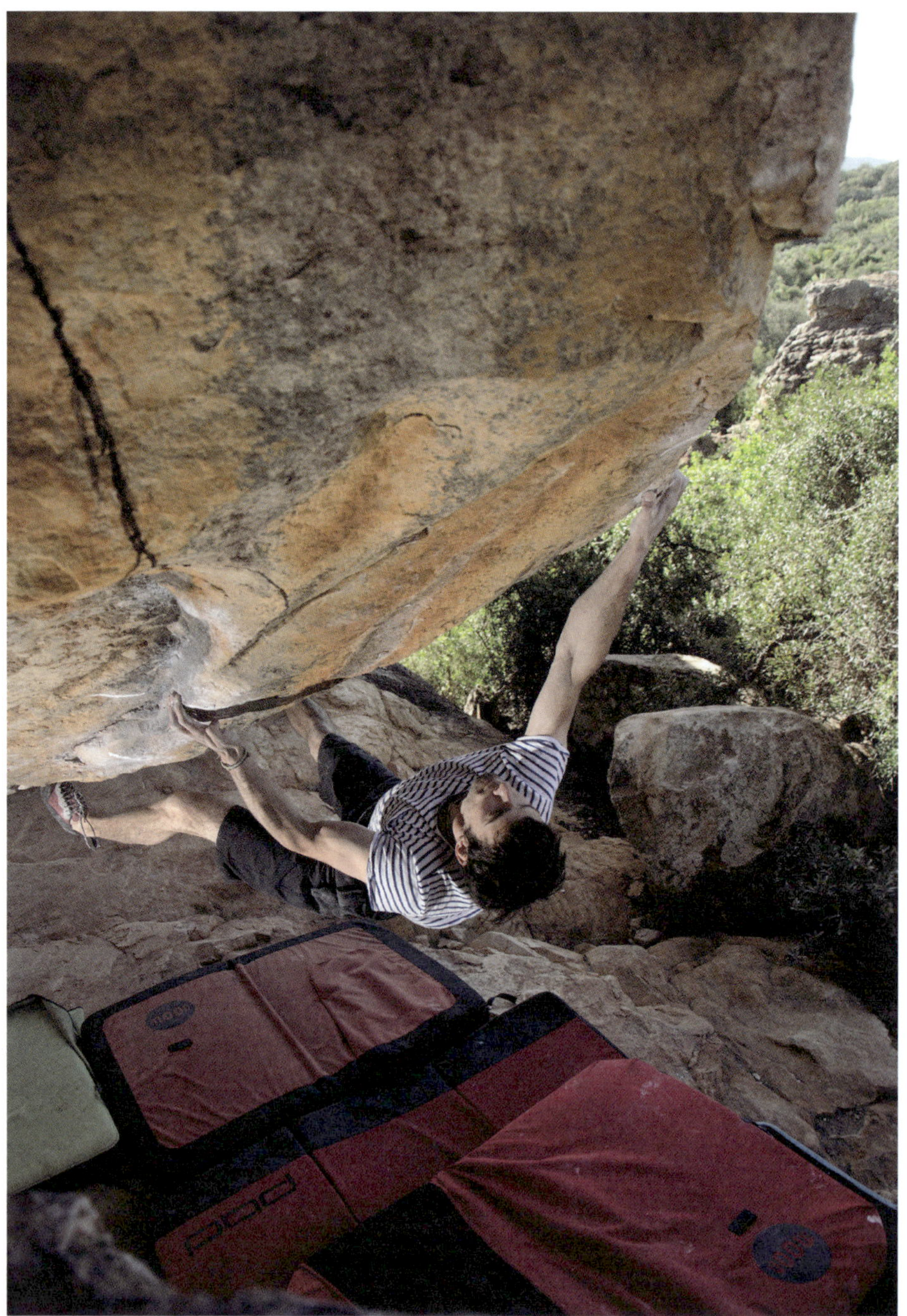

DAVID MASON ON *BLACK SHADOW*, ROCKLANDS, SOUTH AFRICA. © **NICK BROWN**

The body is highly adaptable and dynamic, especially in an athletic population, making it key not to distil these concepts down too much. This is compounded by the reality that measuring both intake and output of energy is very difficult and often inaccurate. Nuance and flexibility, alongside knowledge, are vital in gaining a functional and optimal approach to energy intake.

Measuring energy needs

In an ideal world, methods with higher accuracy such as indirect calorimetry – a non-invasive method that measures gas exchange – would be used to measure base-level energy needs, but, in a real-world situation, this is not always possible. As a starting point, resting energy expenditure (REE) can be calculated more practically by using one of a number of equations, depending on the availability of measurements and metrics. One way these equations differ from each other is that some consider body composition – relative amounts of fat and fat-free mass – while others do not. In an athletic population, such as climbers, where muscle mass (part of fat-free mass) is often higher than in the general population, an equation that takes into account body composition (if known) will likely be more accurate. Muscle mass is more metabolically active than fat mass and, as such, having more of it will mean a higher energy expenditure even at rest. In the case of climbers with higher muscle mass, equations that do not include body composition will often come out with a lower estimate than those that do due to this difference, leaving the climber with a concept of their energy needs that may be too low. Figure 2 presents the three equations found to have the most reliability in athletes and climbers, along with an example.[2]

Figure 2: Example equations for measuring REE.[ii]

The following examples use a 30-year-old male climber; 180 centimetres tall, weighing 80 kilograms with a fat-free mass of 68 kilograms (15 per cent body fat).

ten Haaf (2014) – weight-based (doesn't account for lean mass):
REE (kcals/day) = (11.936 × weight in kg) + (587.728 × height in m) – (8.129 × age in years) + (191.027 × sex (M=1; F=0)) + 29.729
Example REE = 11.936 x 80 + 587.728 × 1.8 - 8.129 × 30 + 191.027 × 1 + 29.279
= 1,989 kcals/day

De Lorenzo (1999) – weight based (doesn't account for lean mass):
REE (kcals/day) = -857 + (9.0 × weight in kg) + (11.7 × height in cm)
Example REE = -857 + (9 × 80) + (11.7 × 180)
= 1,969 kcals/day

ten Haaf (2014) – fat-free-mass based (accounts for lean mass):
REE (kcals/day) = (22.771 × FFM in kg) + 484.264
Example REE = (22.771 x 68) + 484.264
= 2,033 kcals/day

ii While many older, well-known equations such as the Harris–Benedict and Mifflin–St Jeor are still frequently used, a 2023 systematic review and meta analysis by O'Neill et al. into the accuracy of prediction equations in athletes recommends the use of the 2014 ten Haaf equation, and a 2023 study by Chmielewska et al. suggests that the De Lorenzo and ten Haaf equations are the most reliable for sport climbers.

If body fat percentage information is available, the results of REE equations can also be checked against energy availability thresholds. These are the thresholds under which a person is likely to have dysfunction – both health and performance – due to insufficient energy availability. The thresholds are currently understood to be no lower than 30 kilocalories per kilogram of fat-free mass for women, and no lower than 9–25 kilocalories per kilogram of fat-free mass for men.[3]

For the example individual in figure 2, this means ensuring that their daily intake – **not** including calories for any activity or exercise as these must be added on top – must ideally not be below 1,700 kilocalories.

Figure 3: Total energy expenditure.

EXERCISE ACTIVITY THERMOGENESIS

- → The energy cost of exercise, such as climbing or training.
- → Varies depending on the intensity and volume of exercise.

NON-EXERCISE ACTIVITY THERMOGENESIS (NEAT)

- → The energy cost of non-exercise activity, such as standing, walking or working.
- → Varies depending on the intensity and volume of occupational activity and general lifestyle.

THERMIC EFFECT OF FEEDING

- → The energy cost of digesting food.
- → Varies depending on the amount and composition of food.

RESTING ENERGY EXPENDITURE (REE)

- → The energy cost of background basic bodily functions at rest, such as breathing, pumping blood around the body, maintaining a stable body temperature and hormone production.
- → Varies depending on age, height, body mass, body composition and biological sex.

It is worth mentioning that these equations are quite dated and lack reliability, but we do not currently have new options.[4] They offer starting points, estimates for our baseline energy needs; the energy required by our body to perform basic bodily functions such as breathing, pumping blood around the body, maintaining a stable body temperature and hormone production. Any activity, however small or large, must be added on top of this, adding yet another layer of estimation (see figure 3, adapted from Hills et al., 2014).[5]

There are some estimations in the literature for the energy cost of climbing, but these values can vary a lot depending on the relative difficulty of the climb, our ability relative to that difficulty, our familiarity with the climb and how steep the climb is.[6] Bear in mind that these numbers are all rough estimates and are therefore open to a reasonable level of inaccuracy, especially in sports such as climbing where energy needs vary so wildly and our understanding of them is not concrete.

Given that there isn't a gold-standard way to determine the energy requirements of climbing in all its varieties and forms, a very simple (but also very rough) way to estimate the energy needs of a day is to use what is called a physical activity level (PAL) multiplier. This essentially multiplies the REE value. For example, a restful day with no exercise at all might have a multiplier of 1.2 (remember, the REE alone represents zero activity, just basal requirements at full rest), a light climbing day might use a multiplier of 1.3 or 1.4, and so on. These multipliers must include **all** activity in the day, not just climbing. Consider any other activities such as dog walking, running or cycling to work as well.

Using this strategy of estimation, our

example climber might use something like this to get some starting ideas around his energy intake levels:

Rest day (full rest) = PAL of 1.1–1.3

Light day (a light climbing session) = PAL of 1.3–1.5

Moderate day (one or more high-intensity or longer-duration sessions) = PAL of 1.5–1.7

Heavy day (high-demand day with multiple high-intensity and/or longer-duration sessions) = PAL of 1.7+

And using his REE from the ten Haaf equation (which accounts for lean mass), the resulting figures would look something like this:

Rest day = 2,236–2,643 kcals

Light day = 2,643–3,050 kcals

Moderate day = 3,050–3,456 kcals

Heavy day = 3,456+ kcals

These are really rough ranges, but they can provide a starting point from which our example climber can then experiment. Bear in mind that the body is dynamic and adaptable, so these numbers will vary over time and in different situations even for one person. It's a constantly changing conversation.

While it can be useful to understand what makes up total energy needs, it is not wholly necessary to calculate and stick to exact numbers. This kind of approach, while informative, can lead to rigidity in eating patterns that do not serve us as individuals. The most important thing is understanding that adequate energy intake – that lies in a range not a fixed number – is key to our health and performance. Understanding some numbers as a starting point from which to experiment is a good way to go. The human body is very good at letting us know when energy is needed, and learning to listen to the signals it sends is a skill worth cultivating (intuitive eating is discussed more in chapter 12).

What about genetics?

There is also the strong force of genetics to consider, and with this comes the well-established concept of homeostatic weight regulation mechanisms.[7] One of the key components of this concept is that of a 'set point', which was considered as early as the 1950s in obesity research.[8] This theory dictates that we each have a genetic body fat range that the brain aims to maintain and regulatory feedback systems that work to keep us within this range. So, essentially, there are physiological mechanisms at play that keep us in a range of body fatness that is genetically determined.

This is not everything and it will still interact with our environment – food availability and choices, lifestyle and activity levels – but it is a powerful part of the picture. That is why we see a hereditary element to body size and obesity and a strong drive in the direction of weight regain after weight loss. It is worth mentioning, in the context of the obesity epidemic, that the upper range of this set point appears to have weaker biological moderation than the lower ranges. In other words, it is easier to push this set point upwards and maintain weight gain than it is to lower it and/or maintain weight loss.

Understanding appetite

One of the reasons that it isn't necessary – despite temptation – to outsource all this decision-making to our conscious brain is the presence of various internal feedback systems. One such neurobiological system is that of appetite hormones.

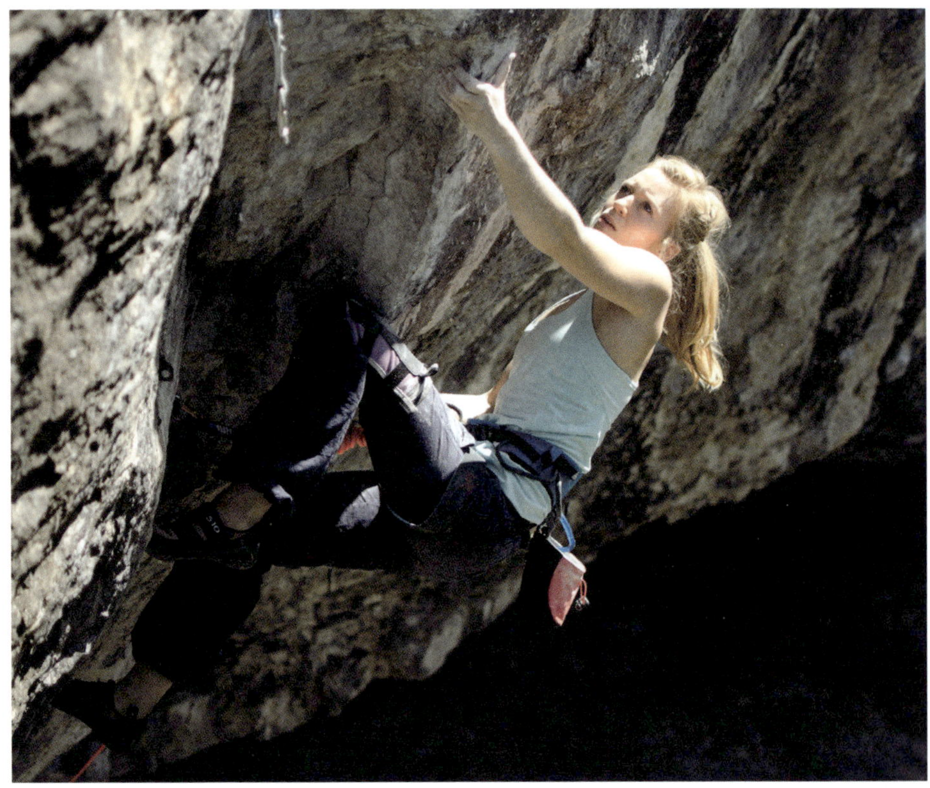

THE AUTHOR ON *MECCA: THE MIDLIFE CRISIS*, RAVEN TOR, UK. © NICK BROWN

Without going too deep into this, there are many hormones at play which can affect and control our appetite; some act on our brain directly and some circulate peripherally.[9] Key players here, among others, include ghrelin, cholecystokinin (CCK), peptide YY (PYY) and leptin. These homeostatic hormones stimulate the body to register hunger (ghrelin) or satiety (CCK, PYY and leptin), respectively. Ghrelin, CCK and PYY are produced in the gastrointestinal tract, whereas leptin is produced in fat cells. In a well-functioning system, these hormones reflect nutritional status and body fat stores: ghrelin will be higher in periods of food scarcity; CCK and PYY respond to nutrients in the gut (especially protein and fat), and leptin is positively correlated with the presence of fat stores.

Insulin is also an appetite regulator. Insulin in the blood rises sharply after a meal and crosses the blood–brain barrier to signal that the need for food is reduced. These hormones are all in constant flux, determined by internal biological and nutritional status, sending signals to the brain about what our body needs.

Of course, there are more layers of complexity to consider. Food palatability and sensory information registered by the brain are also at play and often have an impact on energy intake before any endocrine processes have made their mark, making food choices and interoceptive awareness highly relevant to energy intake.[10] Exercise can also suppress appetite, further complicating the signals that we receive.[11] Not to mention that our psychological brain – conscious and unconscious – is not unbiased, affected as everyone is by cultural influences that dictate what a 'meal' or 'snack' *should* look like, how much a person of a certain size *should* eat and what a body, especially an athletic body, *should* look like. Appetite, it turns out, is not simply physiological but biopsychosocial.

When the complexity of all these systems – only very lightly delved into above – is considered, it seems presumptuous to think that a simple equation could give us a static, reliable number for how much to eat and when we should eat. While it might feel gratifying to calculate a number and then just stick to it, this is not the flexible, long-term approach that benefits the most successful athletes. The harder-won battle is cultivating a relationship with our body and food intake that has a high level of interoceptive awareness combined with nutritional knowledge enabling a dynamic, flexible and responsive approach to food. Ideally, nutrition and particularly energy intake should be viewed from a position of curiosity and willingness to experiment.

Pay attention and notice how your body feels and performs, increase intake a bit, and then observe again. A trial-and-error approach in this direction will encourage a positive and collaborative relationship with food that is constantly evolving and adjusting. Best of all, it leaves you open to discover what your body is capable of with a maximised input.

In short, learn the basics, by all means make some rough estimates in numbers, but don't forget to trust and listen to your body.

KEY TAKEAWAYS

→ Energy intake is a pillar of good nutrition; make optimising energy intake a priority.

→ Boost your body with the maximal effective dose for long-term progression; steer away from a reductionist approach.

→ There are three main energy systems in climbing: the PCr system, anaerobic glycolysis and aerobic glycolysis.

→ Energy expenditure (measured in kilocalories) is made up of resting energy expenditure, thermic effect of feeding, non-exercise activity and exercise activity.

→ There are some methods for calculating calorie needs, but these give just rough estimates as starting points from which to experiment.

→ Genetics and body fat 'set point' play a powerful role in weight management.

→ Appetite regulation is a complex biopsychosocial system. Using calculations and estimates for energy needs can be informative, but remember to listen to and trust your body.

WHAT CAN I DO?

→ Have a think about whether you eat enough calories overall on most days.

→ Where can you **add** food in? How can you further support your body to optimise output and recovery?

→ If it feels helpful, work out some numbers so you have an idea of a rough range and track a day of food intake to see how close you are to that range.

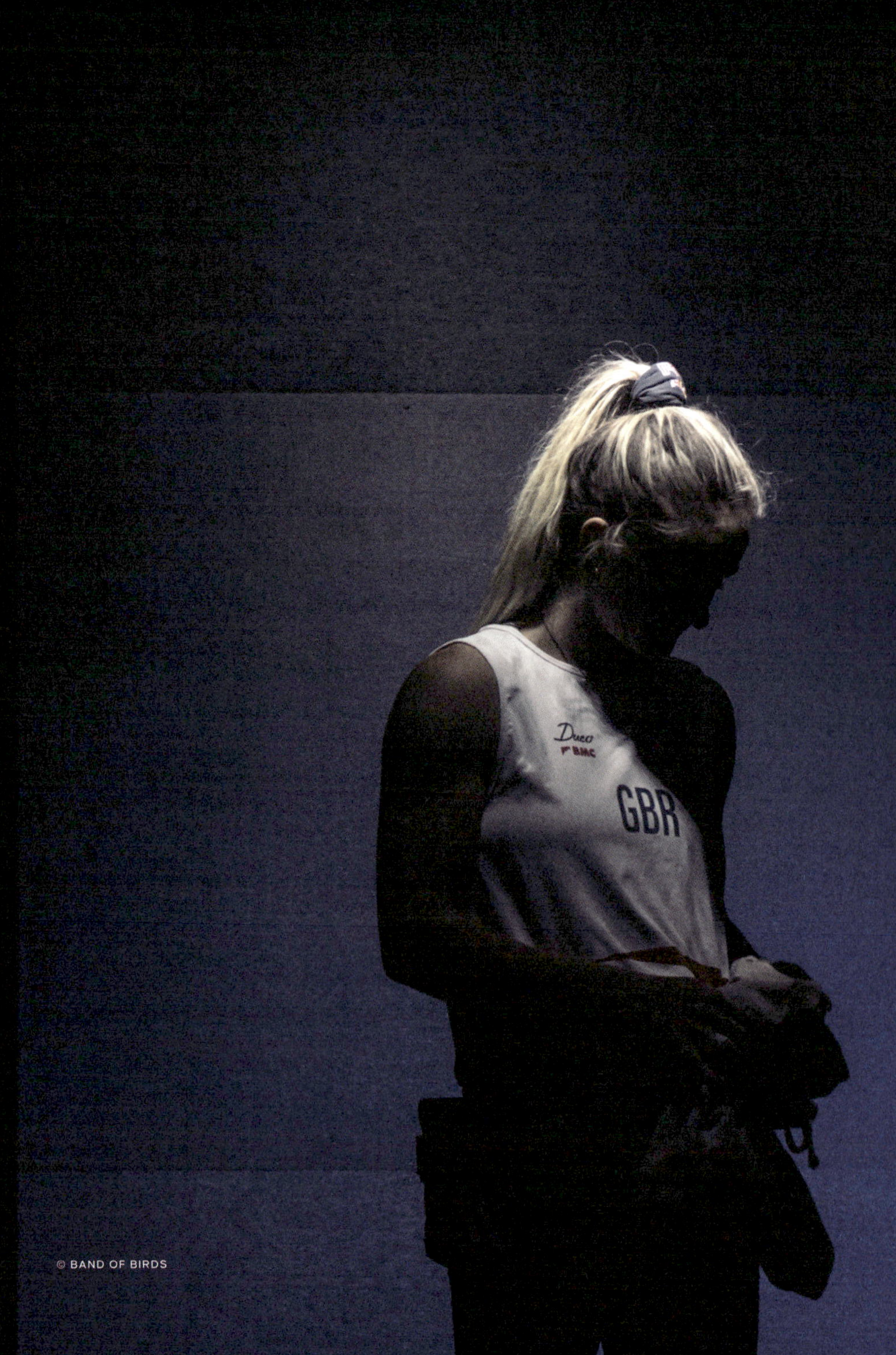
GBR

SHAUNA COXSEY *BECOMING AN ATHLETE*

Shauna needs little introduction. With 33 world cup medals to her name, 11 of them gold, and two overall world titles, she has been a force within the global competition climbing scene. Shauna generously shares her journey with nutrition and performance in a strikingly honest and open manner.

When I was 18, I decided I wanted to change my approach to being a professional climber – I wanted to be a professional athlete. Let me explain.

The pivotal moment came for me in 2012 when I broke my leg. I didn't land weirdly or anything, it just broke when I jumped down off a boulder. It was a stress fracture and a DEXA scan showed that I had low bone density. I was 48 kilograms, I knew I was pushing myself to be light and I also knew it had started to impact my health. So, there I was, with my broken leg, sitting on my sofa alone watching the London Olympics on the TV. I realised then that I wanted to be like the athletes I was watching, and not light and frail.

Growing up in our sport, I always looked up to the elite climbers before me who won medals and climbed hard. I wanted to be like them in some ways but, since my leg break, not in others. Don't get me wrong, these people were huge inspirations to me, but many of them looked different to the athletes that I saw in other sports. They didn't look like the robust, healthy, muscular men and women I was watching take medals in athletics and swimming. I didn't look like those athletes either. At that moment, my trajectory changed. I wanted to take the vibe of those Olympic athletes I was watching on the TV and bring it to my climbing. I wanted to morph from the injured climber that I was into a true athlete.

My body had sent me a strong message: low bone density is no joke. I realised that my nutrition in particular was going to play a significant role if I wanted to be a successful athlete. So, I got a coach, I got support for my mental game and I got nutritional support. I started to build a team around me and this has been fundamental for me over the years. My nutrition needed to improve; I needed to shift away from unhelpful habits and behaviours to a supportive and nourishing relationship with food. It's hard to get away from the reality of climbing being a weight-dependent sport, it's etched into the core of what we do – we literally lift our bodies and carry them up walls. Of course moves feel easier if you take off some weight. This is a side to our sport that I think is really scary in terms of health and well-being.

From then on, I worked with dietitian Rebecca Dent to sort out my nutrition. The key thing for me was education. Learning about nutrition really helped me to understand the *why* behind the things Rebecca would recommend. It was the most important change for me: knowledge really is power. So, I learned about the importance of things like proteins, carbohydrates and fats for performance, as well as why I needed to increase my intake of calcium, iron and other vitamins to support my bones and overall health. We focused on a food-first approach, making sure my meals and snacks were all balanced and met the demands of my training. At the same time, we worked hard to understand my body composition through taking skinfold measures and DEXA scans so that weight wasn't our only data point.

Of course, as with all challenging changes, the journey wasn't linear. There were bumps in the road; times when I found the process easier, times when it felt really very hard. There were some key tactics that were very individual to me and really helpful. For example, breakfast has always been a challenging meal for me; I don't feel that hungry and don't like to eat at that time of day. It has always been an easy meal to skip. So, we made it predictable, logistically easy and as palatable as possible. It was the same each day, often prepared by my husband Ned so I didn't have to portion it out. I just had to turn up and eat. I still have to do this now from time to time.

I gained a solid ten kilos but with that ten kilos came some of my best performances and it was at that higher weight that I won the majority of my medals. I learned that my best strength-to-weight ratio wasn't found at my lightest weight. In fact, if my weight started to drop again, it often came with diminished performance, tiredness and frequent illness. I knew the weight at which I was really healthy, I knew where I might perform my best but couldn't stay long, and I knew the weight at which I was too light.

The competition circuit can be intense. A lot of travelling, lots of different food cultures, hotel rooms, planes and trains. I often travelled with food to keep things as controlled and predictable as possible. The last thing any competitor wants is to go into a world cup feeling like they haven't fuelled well or, even worse, get sick. So, I took my go-to snacks, my breakfast prep and my recovery meals with me to many places around the world. Because breakfast has always been tough for me – and especially so at competitions due to added nerves I think – I had to make it particularly manageable. Not only was it super important to get it in, it had to have the right ingredients to help me perform well and be very portable. So, I used to take a hand blender and make a smoothie each morning in my hotel room with Huel, powdered peanut butter, oats, soy milk and banana; that way I knew I was giving myself the best possible preparation for the day ahead. It took the decisions away and allowed me to handle that particular meal in a mechanical fashion.

Next, before the actual climbing starts at world cups there is an isolation zone where everyone warms up and waits for their turn to climb. The time spent there can vary depending on which round it is and where a competitor is ranked. It always felt like I was the person with the most snacks! There are often some provided, but not always and not necessarily what I might want. My snack game was strong, and I made sure I never ran out. When the climbing started, I didn't actually eat anything during the round but would drink Red Bull in little sips between boulders to give me a boost. I also had water with a HIGH5 solution added which contained carbohydrates

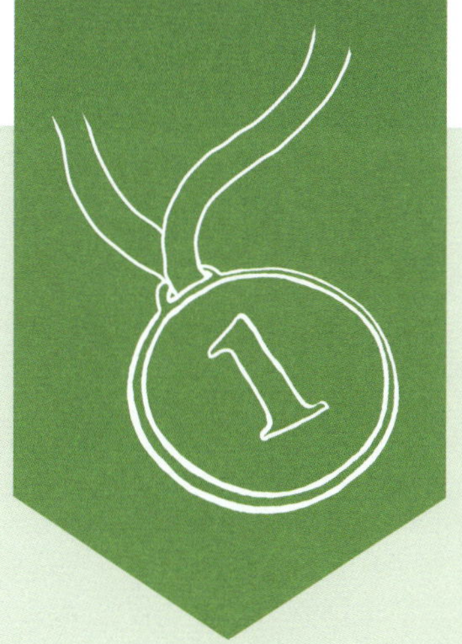

and electrolytes, as well as some backup CLIF BLOKS if I needed them. My hydration was always done really intuitively – I didn't do any measuring of sweat rates or anything, I just went on feel and that worked fine for me. Immediately after the competition round I always had a Nākd bar; it probably wasn't the absolute best nutritionally, but it was something I knew I could stomach as eating post round was rarely something I wanted to do and I ate it alongside taking some BCAAs. Later on, I would have a recovery meal that was a balance of proteins, carbohydrates, fats and vegetables.

Climbing and performing at a top level was and is my career, my livelihood and my passion. I'm lucky of course, but it came – and does come – with pressure. I've had a lot of injuries over the years and I do wonder – although of course I'll never know for sure – whether my early errors of not eating enough played a hand in how many I have had to deal with. As a professional athlete I have had to find a really fine balance between eating enough to stay healthy and progress in training while also keeping a body composition that is optimised for performance. This is not a simple task and it's been hard both physically and emotionally at times. I have many medals and I'm an Olympian but, in my eyes, my biggest achievement is that throughout it all I have kept my love for climbing to this day.

All the competing seems like a lifetime ago now, but my nutrition is still really important as I push my body towards my outdoor climbing goals. And the newest challenge? Being a parent and all that comes with that while keeping on top of my own needs! Pregnancy and breastfeeding are whole separate topics, but to touch lightly on those areas, as other mothers out there know, they are both intense on the body! Being pregnant and then recovering post-partum came with a whole set of physical, mental and nutritional challenges. Breastfeeding my daughter was a joy and a privilege, but it also carried a huge energy cost and could be draining; I really struggled to keep my weight up when breastfeeding and training. Now we are in the toddler phase, I need to be really organised. I have less time than ever and my attention is often split. Frankie is my priority, but I need to make sure that I also pack snacks for me next to the ones I never forget for her. Parenting seems to involve keeping lots of balls in the air at once and I try my best to make sure the nutrition ball doesn't get dropped. My body certainly lets me know if it does.

Being a mother has also intensified my desire for the priorities in our climbing culture to change and change dramatically. My daughter loves climbing and I want her to grow up in a sport that champions the strong not the light, the healthy not the emaciated. I've done my best to play a role in moving our sport in this direction through my role as president of the IFSC Athletes' Commission over the last six years, but there is still a long way to go. We need to look after the athletes that are competing now, but I also feel strongly that we have a responsibility to the community as a whole and the climbers of the next generation. As with most persistent issues, there isn't a straightforward solution, but I hope that we can start to get our priorities in the right places as time moves forward. Climbing is now an Olympic sport and with that comes more exposure, more money and, ultimately, more pressure on athletes. I'd be lying if I said I wasn't worried.

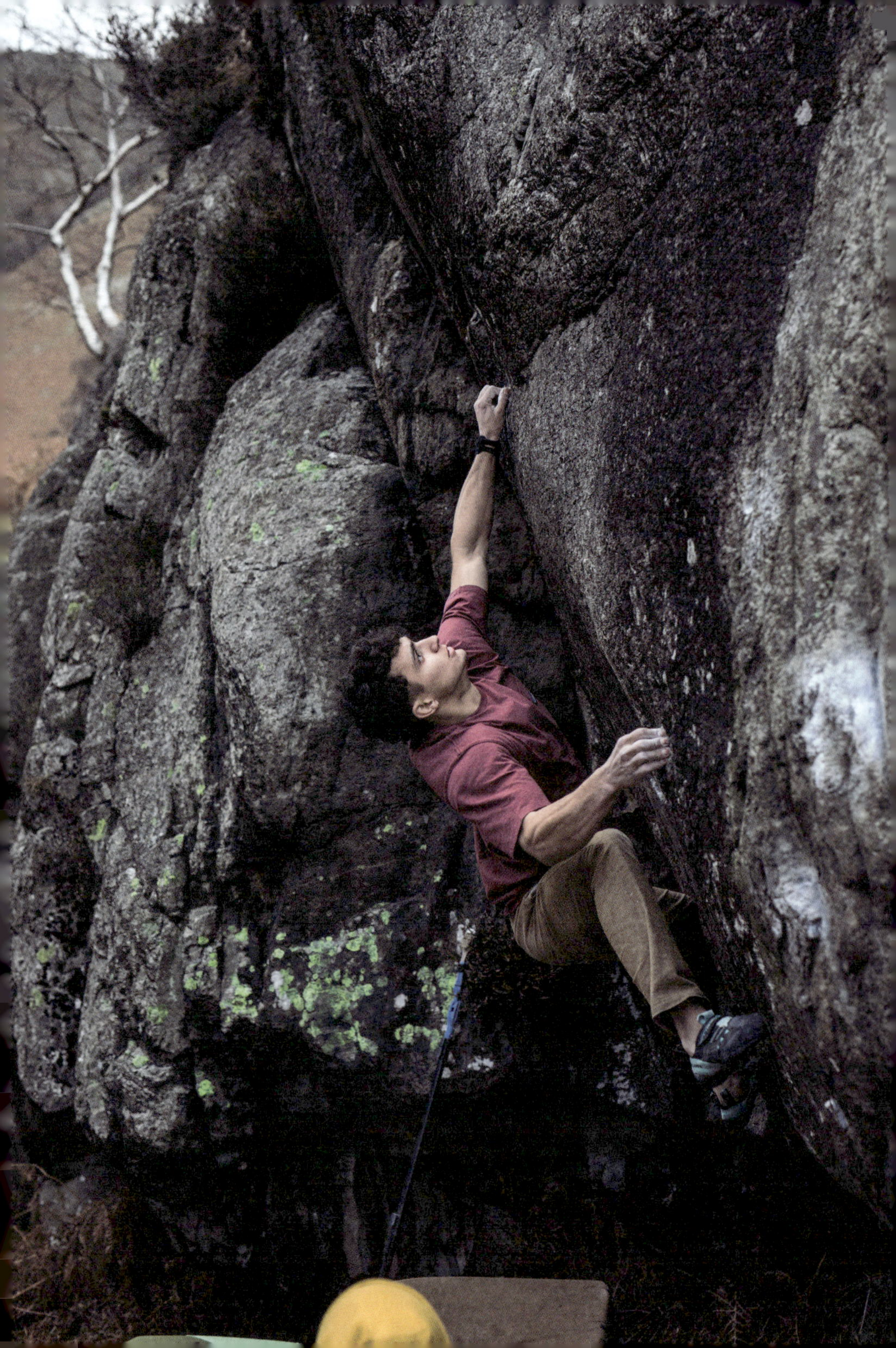

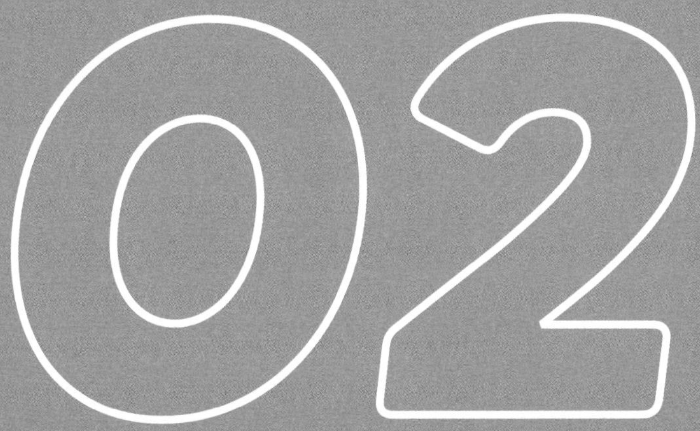

MACRO-NUTRIENTS CARBO-HYDRATES

FUEL TO BURN

AIDAN ROBERTS ON *TRUFFLES ON BICYCLES*, LANGSTRATH, UK © **SAM PRATT**

Macronutrients are categories of food that our body needs in large amounts in order to function well. These categories – carbohydrates, proteins and fats – all provide energy in the form of calories and they all have unique jobs to do within the body's complex systems.

What are carbohydrates?

Carbohydrates are molecules that can be broken down, transported and used by the body to produce energy. One gram of carbohydrates provides 4 kilocalories of energy. The body uses carbohydrates for many processes, including those in the brain and muscles. If carbohydrates are eaten and not needed straight away, they can be stored as glycogen in muscles or the liver so they are available for the next time they are needed. This means we all have a store, albeit finite (approximately 400 to 500 grams' worth, depending on the person), of available energy in our system, and it's important, as athletes and climbers, to keep this store topped up so we don't run out. As mentioned in chapter 1, there are different energy systems at play when we climb, and some – the anaerobic systems – require carbohydrates in order to function. Therefore, how much, what type and when carbohydrates are eaten can be manipulated to support optimal training and performance.

Types of carbohydrates

The chemical definition of a carbohydrate includes monosaccharides and polysaccharides, which are different length chains of sugars, but it can be more helpful to think of this macronutrient in terms of simple versus complex carbohydrates, or their relative glycaemic index and load. This just means thinking in terms of how the body breaks them down, how fast the energy is available and, therefore, in what scenarios they are beneficial. It's all food at the end of the day, but a little knowledge of types of food and application can go a long way to helping our performance in sport.

Simple versus complex carbohydrates

Simple carbohydrates – single units or shorter chains – like bread, jams, fruit and sugary snacks are essentially already in a very useable state. They can be digested fast and put to use very quickly in the body. Refined or 'added' sugars sit in this category, and, while they are great sources of quickly available energy, they often lack the nutrient density and other benefits (for example, fibre) of the naturally occurring simple or complex carbohydrates. Timing and context here is everything. Would eating only refined sugars be good for your health? No, but during a climbing session, something with refined sugar can give you the quick boost you need to perform without the added stress of digestion and fullness.

Complex carbohydrates – longer chains – like many vegetables, wholegrain rice, bread and pasta, and quinoa and legumes are slow release and will give a steady stream of energy throughout the day, but they also take longer to digest. Complex carbohydrates are often accompanied by a greater array of vitamins, minerals and fibre; fibre has additional beneficial effects on the gut and gut microbiome.

Glycaemic index and load

As always, food is nuanced and some foods will be a combination of simple and complex carbohydrates, and, of course, we usually eat mixed meals. This is where the more detailed concepts of glycaemic index and glycaemic load can be helpful in visualising how different carbohydrates are digested and absorbed by the body.

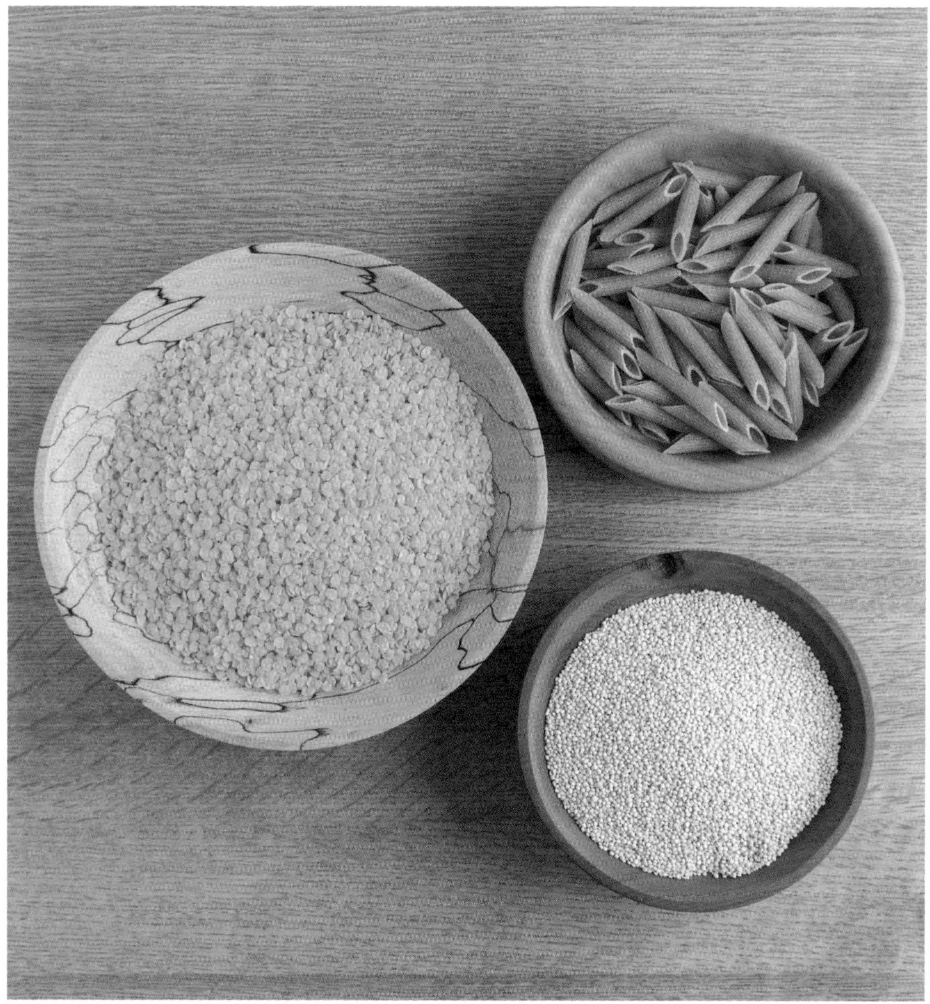

RED LENTILS, WHOLEGRAIN PASTA AND QUINOA ARE ALL GREAT SOURCES OF COMPLEX CARBOHYDRATES WITH THE LENTILS ALSO OFFERING A SIGNIFICANT PROTEIN CONTRIBUTION AT 9 GRAMS PER 100 GRAMS (COOKED).

The glycaemic index (GI) of a food is a measure of how quickly that particular food will cause blood sugar levels to rise. Glucose (pure sugar) is given a score of 100 and everything else is compared against this measure. The GI of a food will depend on the amount and type of carbohydrate it contains as well as what else it contains, for example, protein, fat and fibre. A GI of below 55 is considered low GI, while above 70 is considered high GI. The term glycaemic load (GL) simply adds in the dimension of the serving size to give a value for the 'load' of that particular meal rather than an absolute score for a certain food type. This can really change the picture, as a food with a high GI such as watermelon may only have a small load if the serving size – and therefore the amount of carbohydrate actually consumed – is low (see figure 4). Of course, when foods are combined,

FOOD	GLYCAEMIC INDEX (GI)	GLYCAEMIC LOAD (GL) PER 100-GRAM SERVING
Cornflakes	84	73
Rice cakes	82	67
Rye crispbread	65	53
Mars bar	68	42
Granola bar	61	39
Bagel	72	39
White bread	70	35
All-bran cereal	42	32
Wholegrain bread	69	32
Parsnips	97	20
Baked potato	85	18
Boiled couscous	65	15
Boiled sweet potato	54	13
Wholegrain rice	55	13
Banana	53	12
Pineapple	66	8
Grapes	43	8
Kiwi fruit	52	7
Carrots	71	7
Apple	39	6
Boiled lentils	29	6
Watermelon	72	5
Peanuts	12	3

Figure 4: Glycaemic index and load for some example foods (adapted from Cordain et al., 2003).[1]

the GL will change too and meals are very often a mixture of foods. For example, eating some white bread on its own will have a different GL to a white bread sandwich with butter, cheese and ham. Glycaemic index and load are not something that should be measured or tracked on an individual level, but rather concepts that are useful to understand.

Bear in mind that low GI/GL does not always equal 'healthy', and vice versa; it simply tells us how quickly a carbohydrate affects blood sugar levels. It's a completely normal physiological response for blood sugar levels to spike after eating foods containing carbohydrates, and, unless there is a specific medical reason to manage this, it does not need to be monitored closely. A basic understanding of how foods affect blood sugar is useful for maintaining stable energy levels and knowing when certain food types are useful. For example, eating

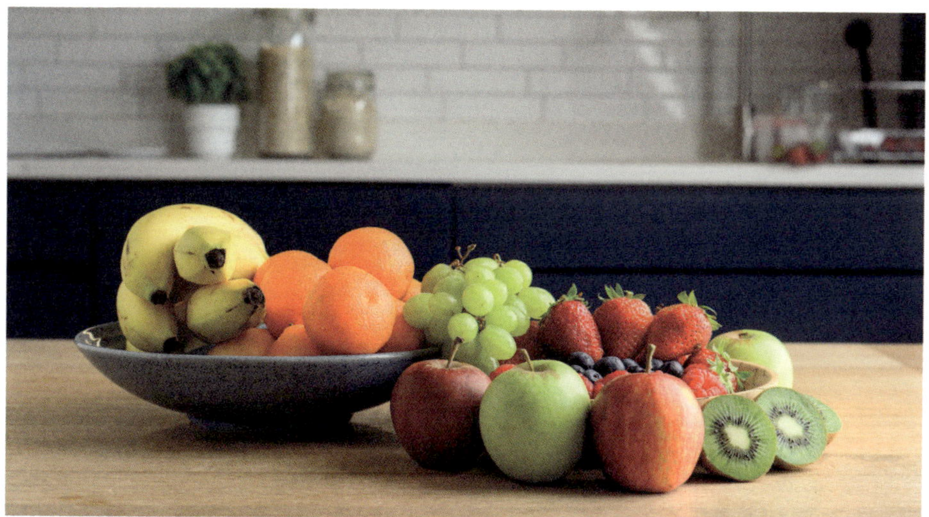

FRUITS ARE A GREAT SOURCE OF CARBOHYDRATE (SOME MORE THAN OTHERS) AND FIBRE.

higher GI foods before and during exercise makes a lot of nutritional sense so that the muscles have ample quickly available fuel to work. Usually, but not always, selecting the lower GI option will mean choosing a more complex carbohydrate with higher nutrient density and fibre that will give longer-lasting energy which may be more appropriate at mealtimes further from the exercise window.

Fibre

Fibre is a type of carbohydrate that is not completely broken down by the digestive system; it passes through the gut relatively unchanged. Fibre helps to keep food moving through the gut, can prevent constipation, affects (as mentioned above) how quickly sugar reaches the bloodstream, and can have a positive effect on our gut microbiome (see page 60). A diet high in fibre is associated with better health outcomes and lowered risk of certain diseases.[2] The British Nutrition Foundation recommends that adults consume 30 grams of fibre a day.[3]

There are two main types of fibre in the food we eat: soluble and insoluble. As its name suggests, soluble fibre can dissolve in water, while insoluble fibre cannot. Soluble fibres are often the softer, more moist parts of fruits and vegetables (i.e. not the skins), whereas insoluble fibres are the harder, coarser components such as the skins or shells of seeds and grains. Therefore, many foods, when eaten as a whole, contain both types of fibre. These types of fibre are managed differently in the gut and have unique properties that make them helpful. For example, resistant starch is a type of soluble fibre that is fermented in the gut by gut bacteria, a process that produces short-chain fatty acids which are beneficial to the body. Eating a range of dietary fibre can help with an array of things such as diversity of gut bacteria, immunity, relieving constipation and reducing bowel inflammation.[4]

It is worth bearing in mind that eating too much fibre, increasing fibre intake too quickly or eating fibre before exercising can cause discomfort in general, or in particular during exercise. This does vary among individuals, so a trial-and-error approach with gradual changes is recommended. Equally, make sure that fibre isn't replacing much-needed calories; this is easy to do by accident as fibre can be very filling but is low in energy.

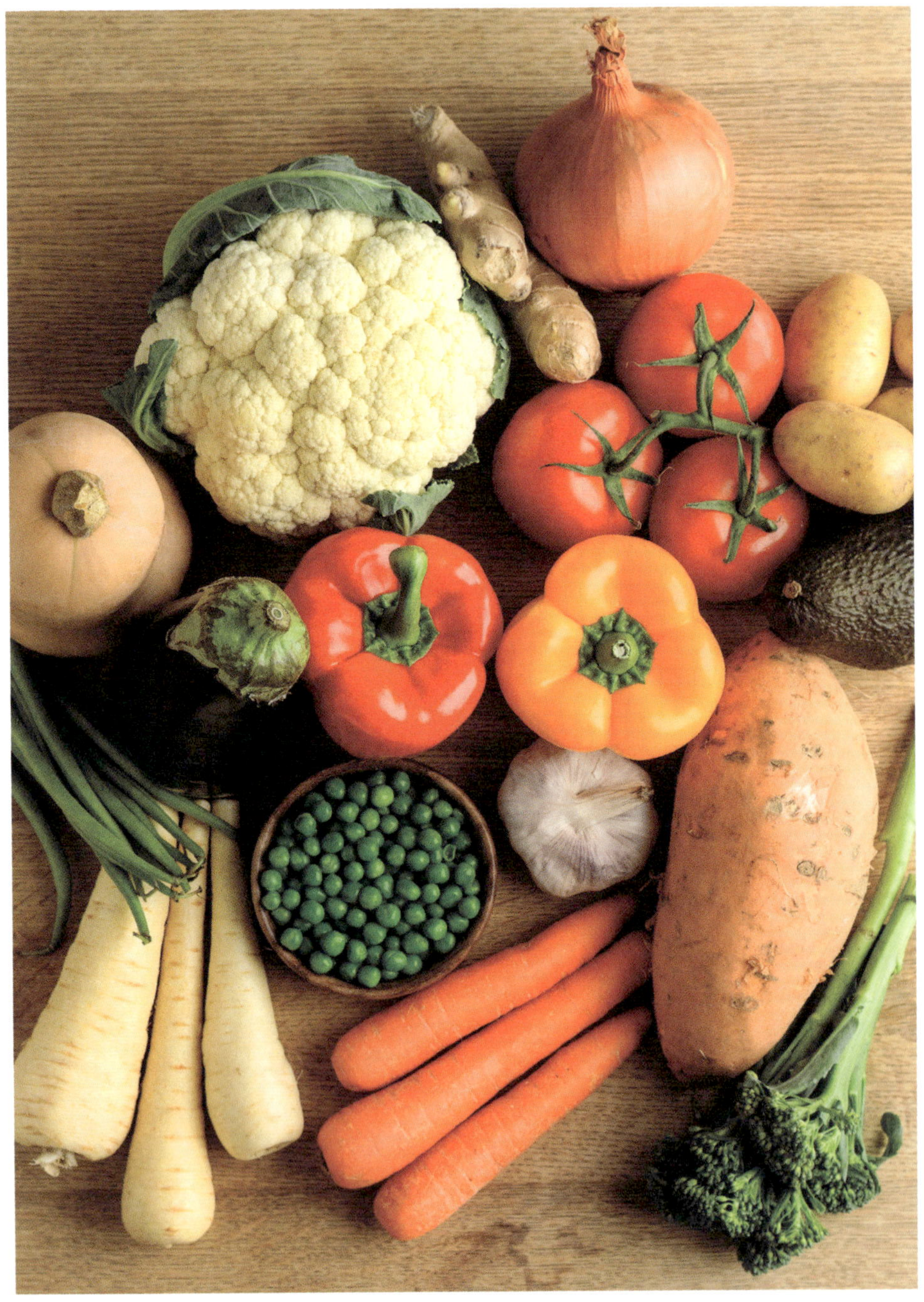

MANY VEGETABLES CONTAIN CARBOHYDRATES AS WELL AS AN ARRAY OF VITAMINS, MINERALS AND FIBRE. FOR EXAMPLE, A MEDIUM BAKED SWEET POTATO CAN PROVIDE APPROXIMATELY 30 GRAMS OF CARBOHYDRATE AND 5 GRAMS OF FIBRE, ALONG WITH VITAMINS A, C, B6 AND POTASSIUM.

Carbohydrate recommendations for climbers

Carbohydrate is the key energy source for high-intensity exercise such as climbing. As mentioned previously, when our muscles work anaerobically, they need to have carbohydrate available for the chemical processes that produce energy to deliver force. While all exercise uses a combination of energy systems, the anaerobic element is crucial for any big efforts; think hard moves, sustained sequences or anything that requires some serious oomph.

So, how much carbohydrate should climbers be eating in a given day? We have some ranges from the available climbing literature to suggest daily intakes of 3–7 grams per kilogram of body weight, with a reduced need of 3–5 grams per kilogram of body weight for boulderers.[5] These are large ranges because the type, intensity and duration of climbing in a day can affect carbohydrate needs significantly. As a *rough* guide, if you are having a very short session (less than one hour) go to the lower end with around 3–4 grams per kilogram of body weight; for a moderate-length session (one to three hours), aim for the middle of the range at roughly 5 grams per kilogram of body weight; and if you are having a long session of over three hours, aim for the top end of 7 grams per kilogram of body weight – or more. As always, be flexible and willing to experiment – you may need to adjust these suggestions depending on how you feel.

For example, a female boulderer who weighs 60 kilograms should be looking at a range of 180–300 grams of carbohydrate per day – the actual amount within this range will depend on session length and intensity; a male route climber who weighs 80 kilograms may consider a range of 240–560 grams over the day. These are just starting points for thinking about carbohydrate intake and can be adjusted up or down to meet the demands of activity on a particular day. It will be a process of trial and error for each individual.

What does this look like in food?

FOOD	AMOUNT	CARBOHYDRATE (g)
Oats (dry)	100 g	~64
Wholegrain rice (cooked)	100 g	~27
Quinoa (cooked)	100 g	~18
Wholegrain pasta (cooked)	100 g	~33
Banana	Medium size	~30
White potatoes (boiled)	100 g	~17
Wholegrain bread	1 slice	~15
Lentils (cooked)	100 g	~16
Fresh orange juice	300 ml	~33

Figure 5: Example carbohydrate foods.

Timing your carbohydrate intake

When thinking about the timing of your carbohydrate intake it can be helpful to visualise what the aim of eating it is. This splits nicely into the concepts of **fuelling** and **recovery**.

Fuelling: on the day

Eating before and during sessions helps to make sure that you have the available carbohydrate in your system to support your muscles and brain to do the work you are asking them to do – and to do it well. While this section discusses carbohydrate intake on the day of a session, what is eaten 24 to 36 hours before a session can contribute, especially if you are preparing for a day with high carbohydrate needs (see Fuelling: carbohydrate loading, opposite).

Before a climbing session, specific timing matters. On the day, if a meal occurs one to four hours before your session, aim for complex carbohydrates and a larger proportion of your daily intake (at least 1 gram per kilogram of body weight). This time frame means you have ample opportunity to digest food and store carbohydrate for later use. Less than one hour before a session, aim for a smaller portion of a simpler source of carbohydrate that can be quickly absorbed and used with minimal digestion effort.

During a session, if it lasts longer than 90 minutes, consider a top-up of simple carbohydrates (30–60 grams) to optimise your session quality and duration.[6] This could be as simple as a banana and some oatcakes. If you are out for a whole day, this gets more complex and you have to consider regular top-ups that include other macronutrients (see chapter 8).

Fuelling: carbohydrate loading

Generally, carbohydrate loading is the practice of eating a higher intake of carbohydrate (often 8–12 grams per kilogram of body weight) in the day or days leading up to a performance window with the aim of maximising the storage of glucose as glycogen in the muscles and liver. This is based on evidence that glycogen depletion is a key part of why performance declines during sustained bouts of exercise, especially high-intensity efforts.[7] The idea with 'loading' is that, when the time comes to try hard, we have the maximum amount of this precious fuel available and we are less likely to fail due to it running out.

But, is there evidence for this specifically in climbing? As a sport that is most often limited by the capacity of a smaller group of muscles (the forearms), it is logical to question whether taking on higher levels of carbohydrate would make a difference or whether it would just weigh us down. The answer is that we don't really know; more research is needed. Limit climbing – whether endurance or strength focused – is high intensity by nature, and, although often limited by the forearms, it does require whole body involvement, so it would make sense to ensure that glycogen levels do not limit performance. This may be particularly pertinent in disciplines that require full-body, gymnastic movements over a longer effort. Any weight gain – due to water retention that occurs with carbohydrate consumption – could be reasonably offset in the short term by using a low residue (low fibre) diet.[8]

As this is a bit of a grey area in climbing, it could be something you can experiment with: do you feel like you perform better when you eat more carbohydrates in the days leading up to a big session or redpoint? Even if loading at high levels of carbohydrate (8–12 grams per kilogram of body weight) feels too much, remember that optimal carbohydrate availability is part of being prepared and it isn't something that is achieved in one meal before you head out to the crag. Making carbohydrate a key part of your dietary intake in the 24 to 36 hours before a strenuous climbing day is likely to contribute to better energy levels and more gusto on the rock.

Recovery

After a session, it's all about refilling your tank; replacing used energy sources (glycogen stores) so that the energy is available for the next climbing session. As with fuelling before climbing, this can be a mixed meal containing a larger proportion (~1.2 grams per kilogram of body weight) of the day's carbohydrate intake, including complex carbohydrates to gain the benefits of greater nutrient density and fibre.[9] Practically speaking, if a session finishes and it isn't possible to eat a meal or you don't want to (exercise can reduce appetite), it is still essential to take on some recovery carbohydrates. This can be achieved through simpler means such as a recovery shake or a smaller snack initially, prior to a proper meal later on.

Is a low-carbohydrate high-fat (LCHF) diet useful for climbers?

Nowadays in sport, and climbing specifically, it can be hard to talk about carbohydrates without mention of low-carb or ketogenic approaches to nutrition. It's a tricky area with plenty of n=1 experiences and anecdotal praise for this somewhat-extreme dietary practice. While there are clinical situations where adopting a continuous low-carbohydrate approach may be helpful, such as for those with high body fat or diabetes, it is more nuanced, and the evidence less supportive, when we look at the athletic population.[10]

There are two main areas that make this approach attractive: fat adaptation and weight loss. Both of these could positively affect performance and therefore require consideration.

Fat adaptation

Fat adaptation is the concept of creating a nutritional environment within the body whereby fat is the preferable fuel source and can be used easily, sparing carbohydrate stores for bigger, higher-intensity efforts. This makes intuitive sense as humans have limited glycogen stores in the body but much larger fat stores – even in relatively lean athletes. So, given fat and carbohydrate are used interchangeably anyway, why not try to adapt to using this bigger store most of the time, saving the carbohydrate for when it is really needed?

The downside of this approach is that if carbohydrate availability is *chronically* lowered, research has shown a down-regulatory response in the body's ability to use carbohydrate called reduced glycolytic capacity.[11] It's a 'use it or lose it' situation where, for all the best intentions around 'saving' carbohydrate for higher-intensity efforts, when these efforts are needed, that pathway isn't as available. The body effectively becomes less flexible metabolically and those big oomph moments are where the deficit shows.[12] So, if high-intensity efforts are part of a climber's desired performance – and most climbing demands high-intensity efforts at some point – LCHF is likely to leave them wanting.

Weight loss

The second attraction to LCHF is weight loss. Many people report weight loss when they shift to a LCHF diet, especially initially. This can, in part, be due to lower carbohydrate stores in the body. As mentioned before, carbohydrate is stored as glycogen in the liver and muscles; this process also involves the storage of some water too: for every gram of glycogen stored, 3 grams of water are stored with it. So, if a person reduces their carbohydrate intake, their glycogen stores will deplete fast and along with the loss of those stores there will also be a loss of water weight. This is where the initial drop in body weight comes from when people transition to LCHF diets. So, it can create a lighter body mass, but, in a sport that requires high-intensity efforts, at what cost?

Fats and proteins are also known to be more satiating and more slowly digested than carbohydrates. The idea here is that eating a higher proportion of these foods – in lieu of carbohydrates – will help a person eat less overall, thereby consuming fewer calories and creating a deficit that induces fat loss. While this does make some sense and may work for some, it is also flawed. Fats carry 9 kilocalories per gram compared to the 4 kilocalories per gram of protein and carbohydrates, meaning that eating a high-fat diet requires less food to reach the same amount of calories eaten. Essentially, with weight loss, it comes down to creating an energy deficit for which there are many methods; see chapter 11.

What about LCHF performance?

Performance data to date in athletic populations is not supportive of LCHF. While every study has participants that present across a spectrum, the overwhelming sense in sports nutrition at the moment is that it's not worth it.[13] One of the key researchers in this area is Louise Burke, an Australian sports dietitian, academic and author who has put a lot of her time and career into looking at LCHF diets in athletes. Her most well-known series of studies were dubbed the Supernova studies and they involved in-depth study of international race walkers in a scenario where their food intake and training could be closely controlled.[14] She looked at high-carbohydrate, periodised-carbohydrate and low-carbohydrate intakes. The low-carbohydrate group performed significantly worse than the other two groups. This result has been found repeatedly.[15]

While race walking is not climbing, it is possible to translate physiological and nutritional findings across sports when we consider the needs of a sport and the determinants of performance within it. Climbing is a sport with high-intensity, anaerobic function at its centre. While climbers do use aerobic pathways, they are not used effectively in place of anaerobic pathways when the demand is high. Chronically low carbohydrate will limit climbing performance output and essentially remove the 'top gear' in terms of climbing and training intensity. Research specifically in climbing suggests the need for more awareness of the pitfalls of a LCHF diet as it becomes more popular and climbing athletes, when studied, consistently undereat carbohydrates.[16]

Periodising carbohydrate intake

Periodising carbohydrate intake describes a flexible approach where intake is manipulated according to the demands of a day or session for a specific outcome. This concept is nicely depicted in the 'Fuel for the Work Required' model developed by Impey et al. in 2018.[17] The idea is that carbohydrate intake can be higher or lower on certain days or sessions and this might include some carbohydrate-restricted – also known as 'train low' – sessions. The evidence for train low protocols is mixed and, while there is some data to suggest these sessions may elicit some metabolic benefits, there is a risk of under-fuelling (specifically carbohydrate) and reducing the quality of a training stimulus and the strength adaptation from it, especially in higher-intensity sessions.[18] If sessions are done in a fasted or low-carbohydrate state, it's important that these are low-intensity sessions where carbohydrate needs are low, and that carbohydrate needs at other times of day are met.

However, adapting carbohydrate intake to support heavier or lighter days accordingly (for example, within the ranges stated on page 23) can actually help with the aforementioned metabolic flexibility. This means the body retains the ability to utilise fat effectively at rest and during lower-intensity activity, while maximising the rate of carbohydrate use, and therefore performance, during high-intensity efforts. What this means practically is that there are some days when your climbing session will benefit from higher carbohydrate support, and other days – light effort or rest days – when eating at the lower end of the recommended range is totally fine. So, rather than having a set amount each day on repeat, try to be flexible and adaptable to the needs of your session.

KEY TAKEAWAYS

- → Carbohydrates are a key macronutrient for climbing due to the high-intensity nature of the sport.
- → Simple carbohydrates can be useful when fast-acting energy is needed; complex carbohydrates are slower to digest and give longer-lasting energy.
- → Glycaemic index (GI) and glycaemic load (GL) can be used to understand how a food affects blood sugar levels.
- → A rise in blood sugar after eating is a normal physiological response.
- → Fibre intake is key for gut health; the recommended intake for adults is 30 grams per day.
- → Consider carbohydrate intakes in the range of 3–7 grams per kilogram of body weight per day with a flexible approach to meet the demands of your activity level.
- → Consider carbohydrate intakes before, during and after climbing to ensure optimal fuelling and recovery.
- → Low-carbohydrate high-fat (LCHF) diets, while anecdotally popular, have not been shown to be beneficial to performance.
- → Periodising carbohydrate intake may be a key method to maximise both performance and metabolic flexibility.

WHAT CAN I DO?

- → Have a think about how much carbohydrate you eat habitually and around training or climbing sessions: do you think you are eating enough?
- → If it feels helpful, work out some numbers from the ranges in this chapter to estimate your carbohydrate needs for different days: how far off are you, or are you meeting those targets?
- → What types of carbohydrates do you eat most and are there any other sources of this macronutrient that you could **add** to help you keep variety and optimise intake?
- → Have a think about how much fibre you eat on an average day: are you getting your 30 grams?
- → Consider the timing of carbohydrates before, during and after your sessions: could you improve in any of these areas?
- → Which days of the week or sessions do you think you need to really focus on optimising your carbohydrate intake to support your performance and recovery?

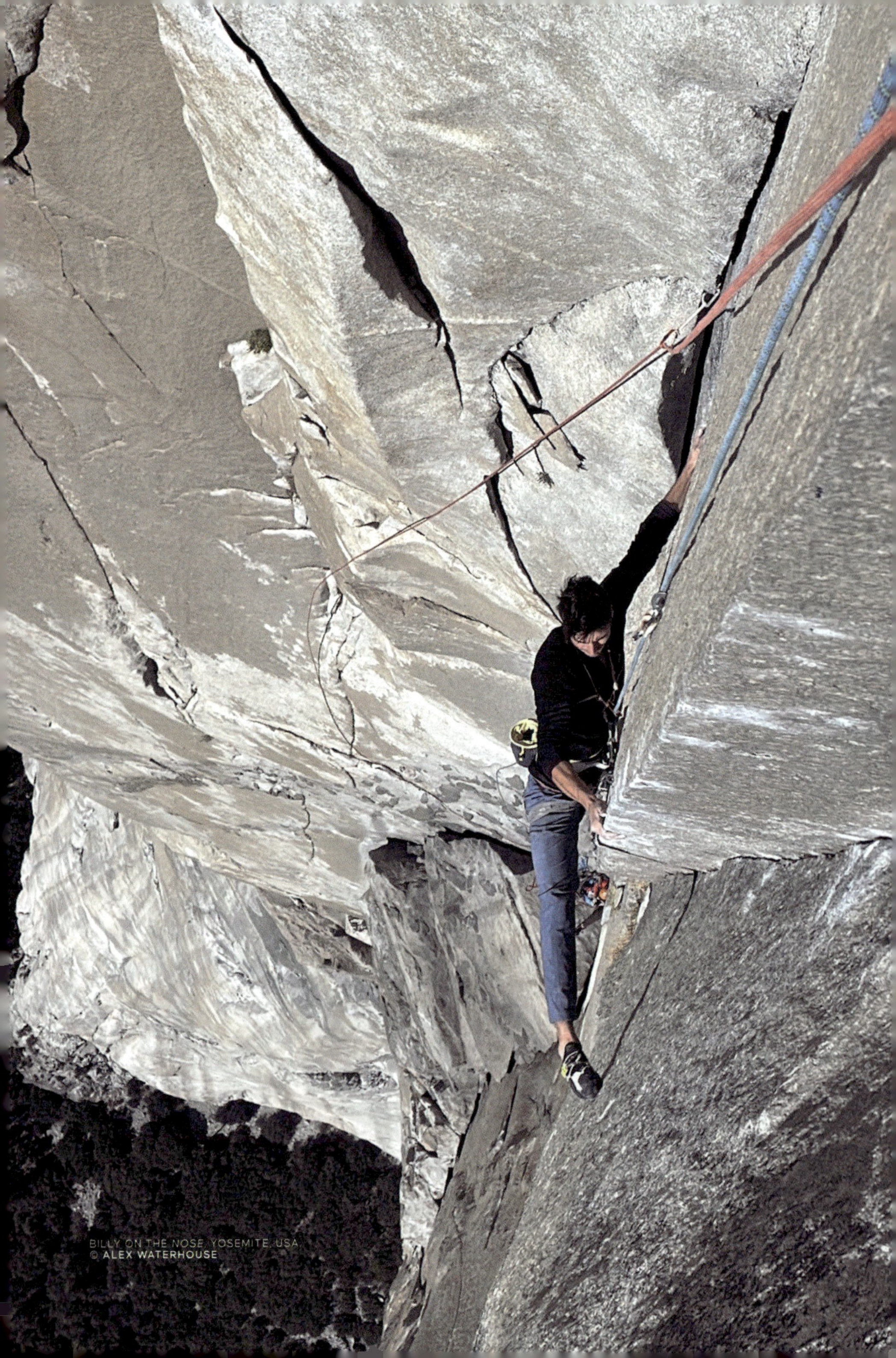

BILLY ON THE NOSE, YOSEMITE, USA
© ALEX WATERHOUSE

BILLY RIDAL
FREE-CLIMBING THE NOSE

Billy Ridal and Alex Waterhouse were competition climbers until they set their sights on free-climbing the *Nose* on El Capitan. With little experience of this type of climbing and a lot to learn, they embarked on the challenge with admirable confidence and ambition. Billy shares his insights into their food and nutrition during their time in Yosemite Valley, where performance is key but logistics are also crucial to success.

Alex and I had been predominantly competition climbers; that was our bread and butter, the place we thrived, felt comfortable and performed well. We had both been competing nationally and internationally since we were about ten, and coincidentally we both brought that part of our climbing lives to a close at the same time. We were done with competitions and were trying to figure out what we both – individually – wanted to do climbing-wise. It turned out we were pretty aligned there too. El Capitan loomed large in both our minds as the epitome of rock climbing; a bucket-list bit of rock if there ever was one. With very little experience between us (I had done a few two-pitch trad climbs in the past, Alex had maybe ventured to five pitches), we decided that we wanted to free-climb the *Nose* on El Capitan. Competition climbers are meant to be ambitious and confident, right?

So, we set about learning the skills: more trad climbing, anchor building, rope management, hauling and so on. We tried to get fit to do a lot of climbing in a day, while still keeping our top-end strength for the performances we knew we would need to pull out on the harder pitches. Given the lack of experience we had, it sounds ridiculous as a goal, but really, as competition climbers, we were well trained for high-pressure performance. And that is, partly, what climbing the *Nose* comes down to. Two extremely hard pitches ... albeit after tons of climbing and hauling on unfamiliar terrain with jaw-dropping levels of exposure. I was optimistic that while this goal was out of our wheelhouse, between us we had a diverse enough climbing skill set that we would be able to apply ourselves well in that environment. There was also YouTube. We learned a *lot* from YouTube.

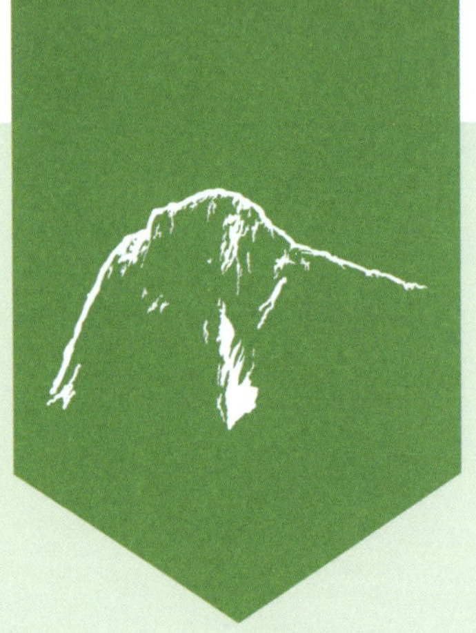

If I'm honest, we didn't really think about food and nutrition until we got to the Valley, but when we arrived I realised it was going to be a significant factor. Our preparation had been focused on developing the physical and technical skills of the task and, as a result, things like nutrition hadn't been centre stage. We had a month to work on the route, figure out logistics and get ourselves ready for an attempt, and it was during this time that we figured out the whole food scenario. Interestingly, a lot of the advice that we came across seemed to stem from aid climbing where it's all about calories and ease of eating, but we wanted to include a bit more nuance to make sure our bodies could work at their absolute best.

There was definitely an element of trial and error involved! On the first few days we took cream cheese bagels for lunch; these exploded in our haul bag. One time we took ramen noodles; I wouldn't recommend them either – they are extremely faffy and use a lot of water. Slowly, we worked out our food choices and it boiled down to (pun intended) instant coffee with instant oatmeal packets in the morning, mostly snacks during the day, and then an evening meal of some kind of rice or grain packet with some tinned fish or chicken or a can of chilli. The only exception was the first day of our send push when we took sandwiches with fresh fillings for that initial day's lunch; we thought it was worth delaying any micronutrient deficiencies for as long as possible! Our daytime snacks consisted of bars of varying sorts, trail mix, Cosmic Brownies (these were a must for Alex) and Oreos for when we needed a morale boost. We tried to mix up the meals to keep ourselves interested and we tried to make sure we got a good macro split, with a focus on getting enough protein and carbohydrates as well as, of course, enough overall calorie intake. We put electrolytes in our water to help stay hydrated. We didn't go for freeze-dried meals because despite the lightweight benefits, they were super-expensive to buy in the Valley shops. Next time, we'll plan ahead and bring some.

Our set-up was three food bags: breakfast bag, snack bag and dinner bag. The snack bag was always in an easy-to-reach place so we could eat whenever we needed in the day. Of course, there is a balance between taking enough food and also the effort of carrying and hauling it. Many climbers take a reductionist approach here and get by on as little as possible. We did the opposite. The climbing on the *Nose*, particularly the two hardest pitches, was going to demand our best performances and we didn't want food scarcity to hold us back mentally or physically. Of course, that means more effort and potentially building fatigue from hauling, but we felt that doing more and eating more suited us better than doing less and eating less. So, we packed extra food and water, we made stashes and we never ran out. In fact, by the end of the month I had gained three kilos. Some muscle, I suspect, from the manual labour that is big walling, but probably not all. We did always eat a lot of large pizzas when we were off the wall ... but that's probably not relevant!

The happy ending is that we both successfully free-climbed the *Nose*. I guess that means we made some decent decisions along the way, both with our climbing and things like nutrition. We learned a lot about everything to do with big wall climbing in the process, including food management. If we were to do it again, I would definitely try to get some freeze-dried meals more economically!

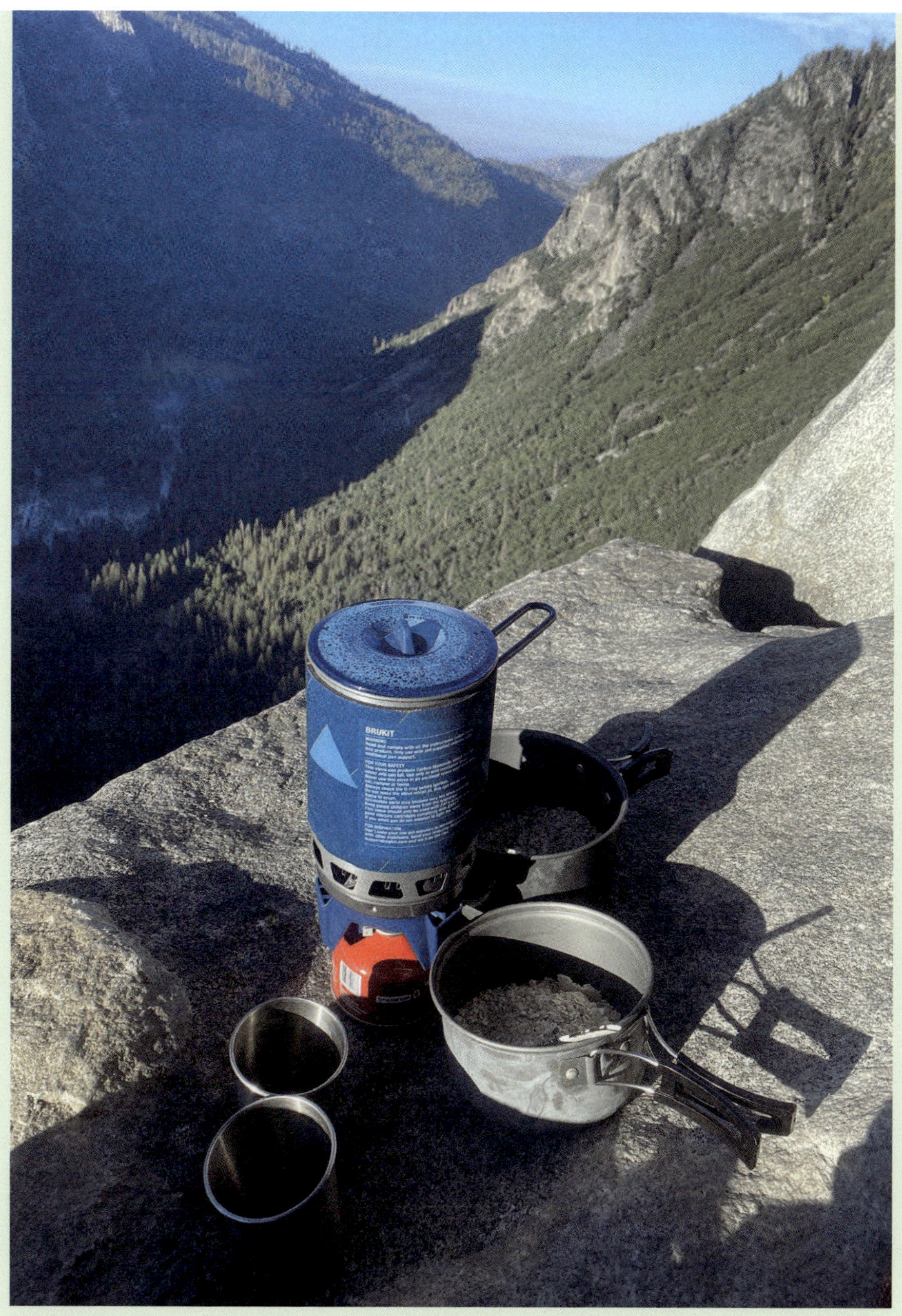
BRUKIT

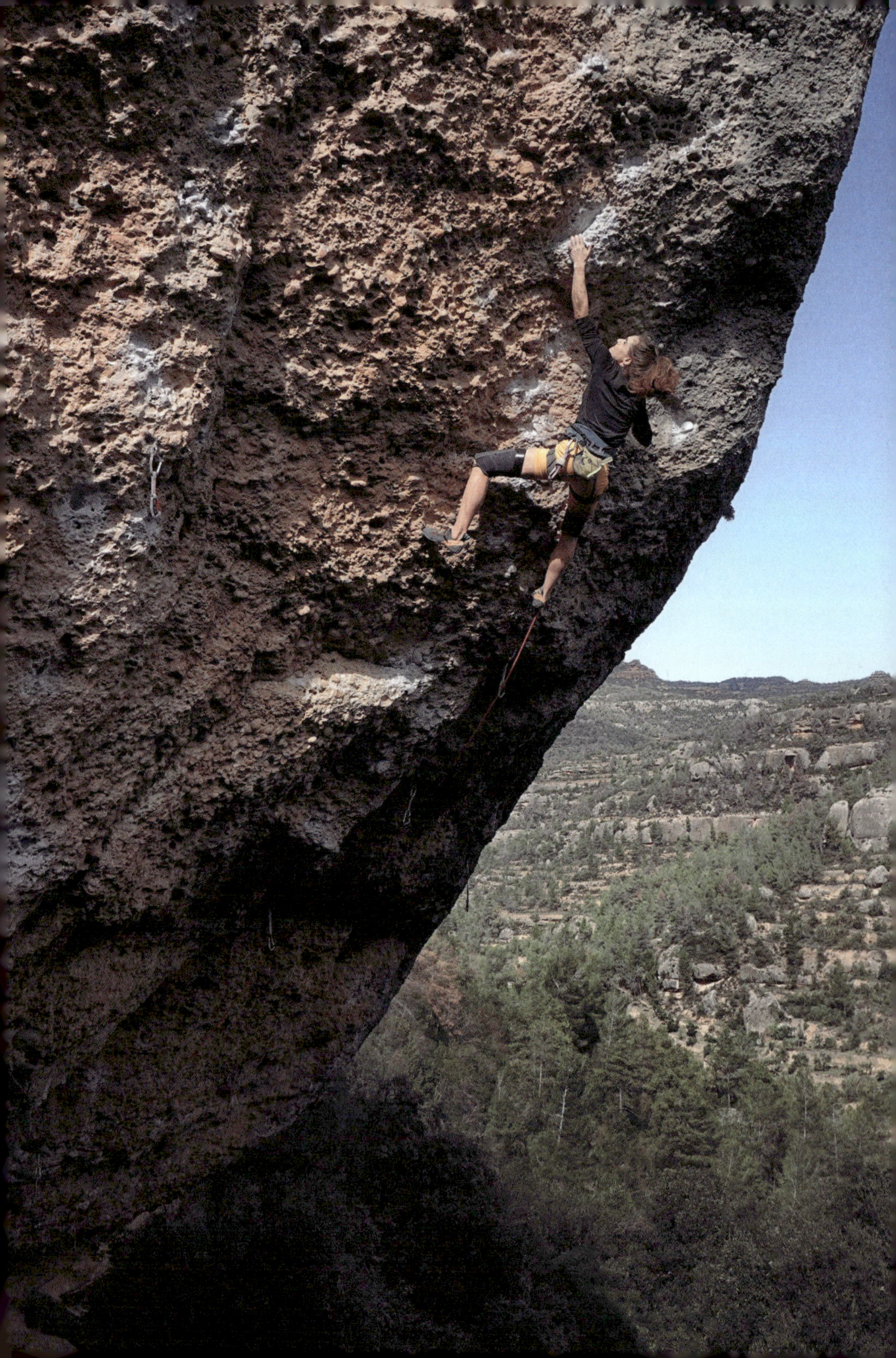

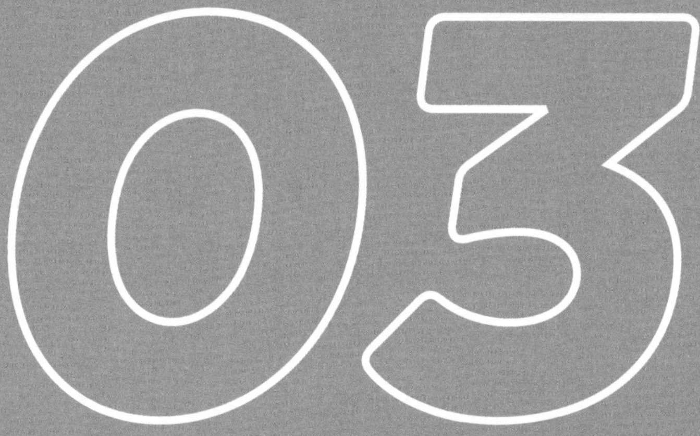

MACRO-NUTRIENTS PROTEINS

THE BUILDING BLOCKS FOR ADAPTATION

SATIVA PATATICA, MARGALEF, SPAIN. © KEITH SHARPLES

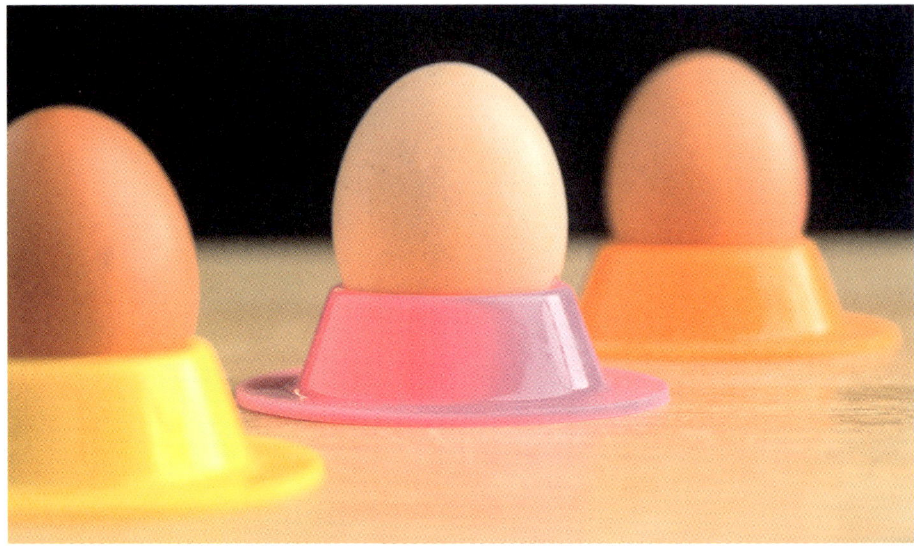

A LARGE EGG TYPICALLY CONTAINS 6–7 GRAMS OF PROTEIN.

What are proteins?

Proteins are the building blocks that our body uses for growth, repair and adaptation of muscles after training or climbing. Proteins also have many other functions in the body, including the creation of enzymes, antibodies and red blood cells. As such, they play a role in health as well as athletic performance. As climbers wishing to optimise our nutrition, proteins are a key player as adequate complete protein doses throughout the day and following training will help our muscle development and recovery over time.

When thinking about muscle adaptation and recovery, there are two key processes at play: *muscle protein synthesis* and *muscle protein breakdown*. One is the creation of new muscle protein, and the other is the degradation of existing muscle protein (some of which is an integral part of adaptation). The net result is described as *muscle protein turnover*, and this determines levels of lean mass and adaptation to a training stimulus.

So, what does this mean for nutrition? Protein availability – particularly essential amino acid availability – is an influential player in this process. Ensuring there is adequate available protein in the system at the right times can be the key to maximising muscle protein synthesis, reducing unnecessary muscle protein breakdown and therefore optimising muscle protein turnover. It's worth mentioning that while protein intake primarily influences synthesis of new muscle protein, it is also key to make sure there is adequate overall energy in the system, especially if muscle gain is a priority. This minimises the use of dietary protein and/or muscle protein breakdown to make up any calorie deficit.

Types of proteins

Essential versus non-essential

Proteins are made up of amino acid chains, and different protein-based foods have different amino acid profiles. This means that the combination of amino acids varies from food to food. This matters because there are some amino acids that are 'essential' and some that are 'non-essential'. Essential amino acids are those that cannot be made in our body and so need to be provided by our diet.

ESSENTIAL	NON-ESSENTIAL
Histidine	Alanine
Isoleucine	Arginine
Leucine	Asparagine
Lysine	Aspartic acid
Methionine	Cysteine
Phenylalanine	Glutamic acid
Threonine	Glutamine
Tryptophan	Glycine
Valine	Proline
	Serine
	Tyrosine

Figure 6: Amino acids – essential and non-essential.

Foods that contain all nine essential amino acids in adequate amounts for processes such as growth, repair and muscle protein synthesis are called complete proteins. Complete protein sources come in the form of foods such as meat, fish, poultry, dairy (including whey protein), eggs, quinoa and soy products like tofu.

Many – but not all – plant-based proteins such as vegetables, grains, legumes, breads and nuts do not contain all the essential amino acids and therefore are considered incomplete. Incomplete protein sources can, however, simply be combined to create an overall intake where adequate essential amino acids are present. This is particularly pertinent if you are following a vegan or vegetarian diet.

Leucine

When thinking about muscle adaptation and recovery, leucine is a particularly key amino acid. Leucine works as a signalling amino acid for muscle protein synthesis, and the concept of a 'leucine threshold' for optimising post-exercise muscle protein synthesis is fairly well accepted in the literature, especially in older adults.[1]

What this means is that, ideally, protein intake after exercise should contain at least 2–3 grams of leucine to maximise the adaptation response in the muscle. Some protein-based foods contain more leucine than others, of course! As leucine is one of the essential amino acids, complete proteins such as meat, dairy and fish all have high levels of leucine, but many plant-based foods, such as tofu and lentils, do also contain it in smaller amounts.[2]

Branched-chain amino acids (BCAAs)

Branched-chain amino acid (BCAA) supplementation has been popular in sports nutrition for some time. The three BCAAs are leucine, valine and isoleucine, all of which are essential amino acids. These amino acids are key for muscle adaptation and recovery, but they can be easily sourced through food choices rather than an expensive supplement. Many reviews have determined no direct benefit to performance, alleviating muscle damage or increasing muscle protein synthesis by supplementing with BCAAs over simply optimising protein intake overall.[3] This is because when BCAAs are taken as a supplement alone, the other essential amino acids become a limiting factor in the process. Yes, these particular ones are key, but it is beneficial for athletes and climbers to consume *all* of the essential amino acids. Getting all of them from whole food sources means more nutrient density all round; think macronutrients, micronutrients and fibre. And money saved.

Protein recommendations for climbers

So, how much protein should climbers be eating? As already mentioned, protein is key for many processes in the body, but when looking at climbers and athletes in particular it comes into sharper focus due to its supporting role in recovery and adaptation. Of course, going climbing and training for climbing are the most important factors in progressing, but optimising nutrition helps to make the most of any effort we put in.

The current climbing literature suggests protein intake ranges of 1.4–2 grams per kilogram of body weight for boulderers, and 1.2–1.8 grams per kilogram of body weight for route climbers, both of which sit comfortably within the more general ranges suggested for athletes of 1.2–2 grams per kilogram of body weight.[4] The reason that bouldering has a slightly higher range is because the demands of bouldering are more strength and power based; this often means boulderers will have higher lean mass, as well as doing more strength and power-focused training.

If we go back to our example climbers from page 23, a female boulderer who weighs 60 kilograms should be looking at a range of 84–120 grams of protein per day, while a male route climber who weighs 80 kilograms may consider a range of 96–144 grams over the day. These are *starting points* for thinking about protein intake, and, while they do not need to be exact, consistency over time in hitting these kinds of targets can really benefit both recovery and lean mass development. As always, it's a process of trial and error for each individual in working out which protein foods work well and are enjoyable to include at different times in the day.

There are some scenarios where higher intakes of up to and beyond 2.4 grams per kilogram of body weight may be particularly beneficial. These include periods of time when our training or climbing load is especially high, when muscle gain is a goal, when recovering from injury or when undergoing a planned calorie deficit for weight loss.[5] For a high training load, muscle gain and injury rehabilitation, a higher intake really ensures that protein is not a limiting factor in any of these processes. In weight loss scenarios, it can help with maintaining lean mass and satiety.

What does this look like in food?

FOOD	AMOUNT	PROTEIN (g)
Whey protein supplement	30 g scoop	~25
Chicken breast	100 g	~32
Fillet steak	100 g	~29
Salmon steak	100 g	~23
0% fat Greek yoghurt	100 g	~11
Low-fat cottage cheese	100 g	~10-12
Eggs	1 egg	~6
Lentils (cooked)	100 g	~9
Quinoa (cooked)	100 g	~4.5
Wholegrain rice (cooked)	100 g	~3-5
Chickpeas	100 g	~7
Baked beans	100 g	~5
Wholegrain toast	2 thick slices	~10
Tinned mackerel in olive oil (drained)	100 g	~21

Figure 7: Example protein foods.

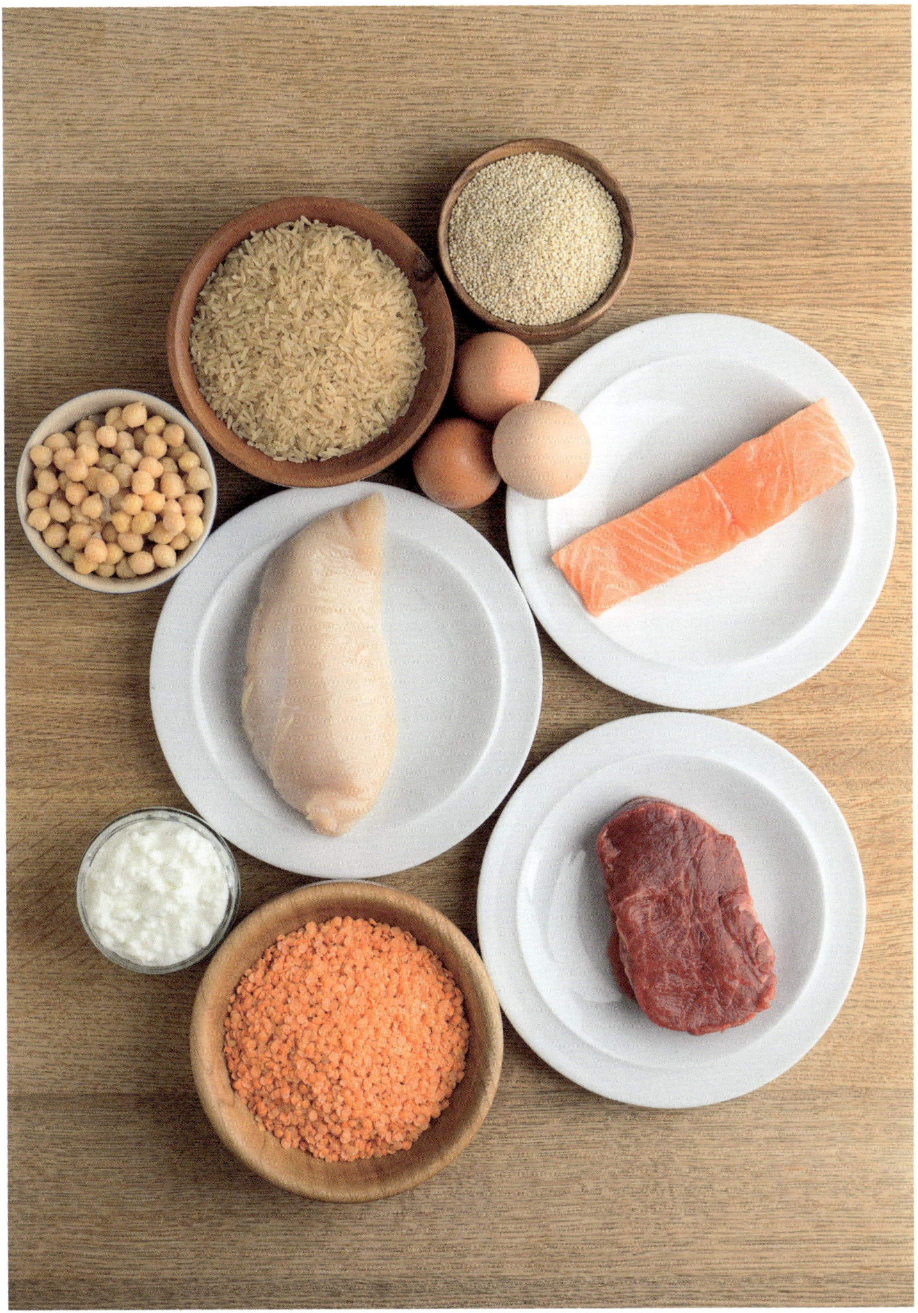

A 100-GRAM SALMON STEAK OFFERS APPROXIMATELY 23 GRAMS OF PROTEIN AND 11 GRAMS OF FAT, AS WELL AS BEING A GREAT SOURCE OF OMEGA-3S, WHILE A 100-GRAM FILLET STEAK PROVIDES 2-3 MILLIGRAMS OF IRON AND PLENTY OF B-VITAMINS ALONGSIDE ITS APPROXIMATELY 29 GRAMS OF PROTEIN.

Timing your protein intake

As with carbohydrate intake, there is some nuance with the timing of protein intake. After exercise there is a muscle protein synthesis response whereby muscles adapt to the training stimulus. As discussed earlier, this is countered by any muscle protein breakdown that occurs, resulting in an overall muscle protein turnover balance. Nutritional interventions aim to help increase muscle protein synthesis by ensuring that this process is not limited by inadequate amounts of essential amino acids.

Research into this process shows that there is an optimum dose–response of 0.25 grams of protein per kilogram of body weight, or an absolute dose of 20–40 grams of protein; these doses should be evenly distributed throughout the day (every three to four hours).[6] This maximises the muscle protein synthesis response to exercise which, over time, will enhance muscular adaptation.

In addition to this, there is some research to suggest that a pre-bed intake of protein (30–40 grams) can further promote overnight muscle protein synthesis; casein protein is a good option for this due to its slower digestion and release.[7]

Protein for older athletes

When it comes to older athletes, protein is a hot topic. There is a plethora of research into skeletal muscle function and maintenance in the *non-athletic* ageing population with the aim being to combat fragility, improve health outcomes and optimise quality of life.[8]

Where this intersects with the older *athletic* population, there has been support for the practice of increasing the protein dose recommended for older athletes to at least 40 grams every three to four hours. This is due to older athletes being less sensitive to lower doses of protein, a phenomenon known as anabolic resistance.[9] However, while older, more sedentary people may benefit from this, there is also some evidence and discussion suggesting that older athletes, due to their higher activity levels, may not need more than their younger counterparts and that it is inactivity, in fact, that drives the anabolic resistance seen in older people.[10]

So, it may be that older athletes need not worry about eating exceptionally high protein intakes; rather, ensuring that they meet current recommendations around optimal protein intake in line with their younger counterparts will be supportive in maintaining and developing lean mass.

If you are reaching your 40s and 50s, don't panic – your protein needs won't increase overnight, but equally try to make sure protein features regularly in your meals. Providing kidney function is still healthy, increasing protein intake to the recommendation of 40 grams per serving may not be necessary but could be protective in terms of ensuring adequate intake is maintained.

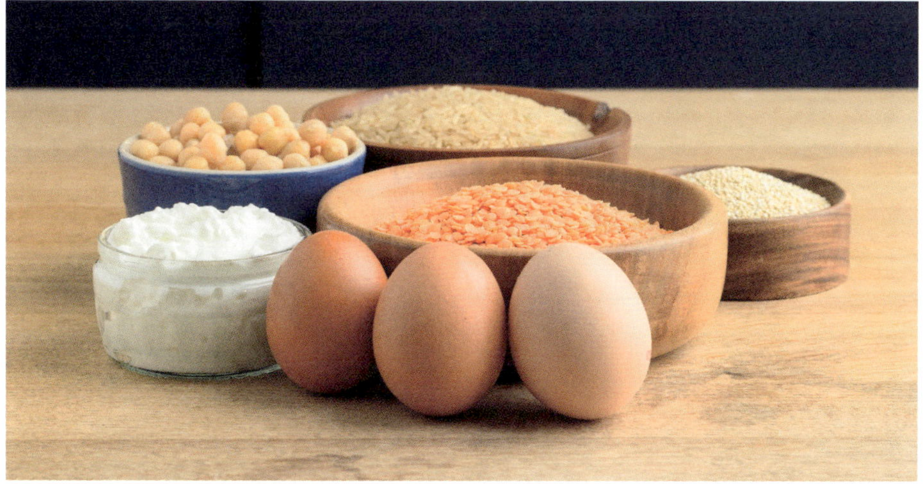

THERE ARE MANY VEGETARIAN AND VEGAN-FRIENDLY PROTEIN SOURCES, SUCH AS CHICKPEAS, LENTILS, QUINOA, EGGS AND DAIRY.

KEY TAKEAWAYS

- → Proteins are made up of amino acid chains and are the building blocks that the body uses for the growth, repair and adaptation of muscles as well as many other functions.
- → Amino acids are classed as essential and non-essential depending on whether they can be made in the body or need to be provided by the diet.
- → Muscle protein turnover = muscle protein synthesis - muscle protein breakdown.
- → Leucine is a key amino acid for optimising muscle protein synthesis due to its role in signalling.
- → Ideally, climbers should aim for protein intakes of 1.2–2 grams per kilogram of body weight per day spread out in doses of 20–30 grams every three to four hours.
- → Higher intakes may be useful in some scenarios: very intense training loads, injury, weight loss or intentional muscle gain.
- → Older athletes may benefit from higher doses (~40 grams) of protein depending on their activity levels.

WHAT CAN I DO?

- → Have a think about how much protein you eat each day: are you meeting the recommended ranges overall and per portion?
- → What are your go-to protein sources and are they complete or incomplete? What other sources could you **add** to your intake to help you meet your targets?
- → How is your protein intake spread throughout the day, and could you improve this to maximise muscle protein synthesis?
- → Do you have any special considerations for your protein intake, for example, are you vegan or vegetarian, an older athlete, or do you have a particularly heavy training load?
- → Are there particular meals where you struggle to include protein? What could you **add** to boost that meal?

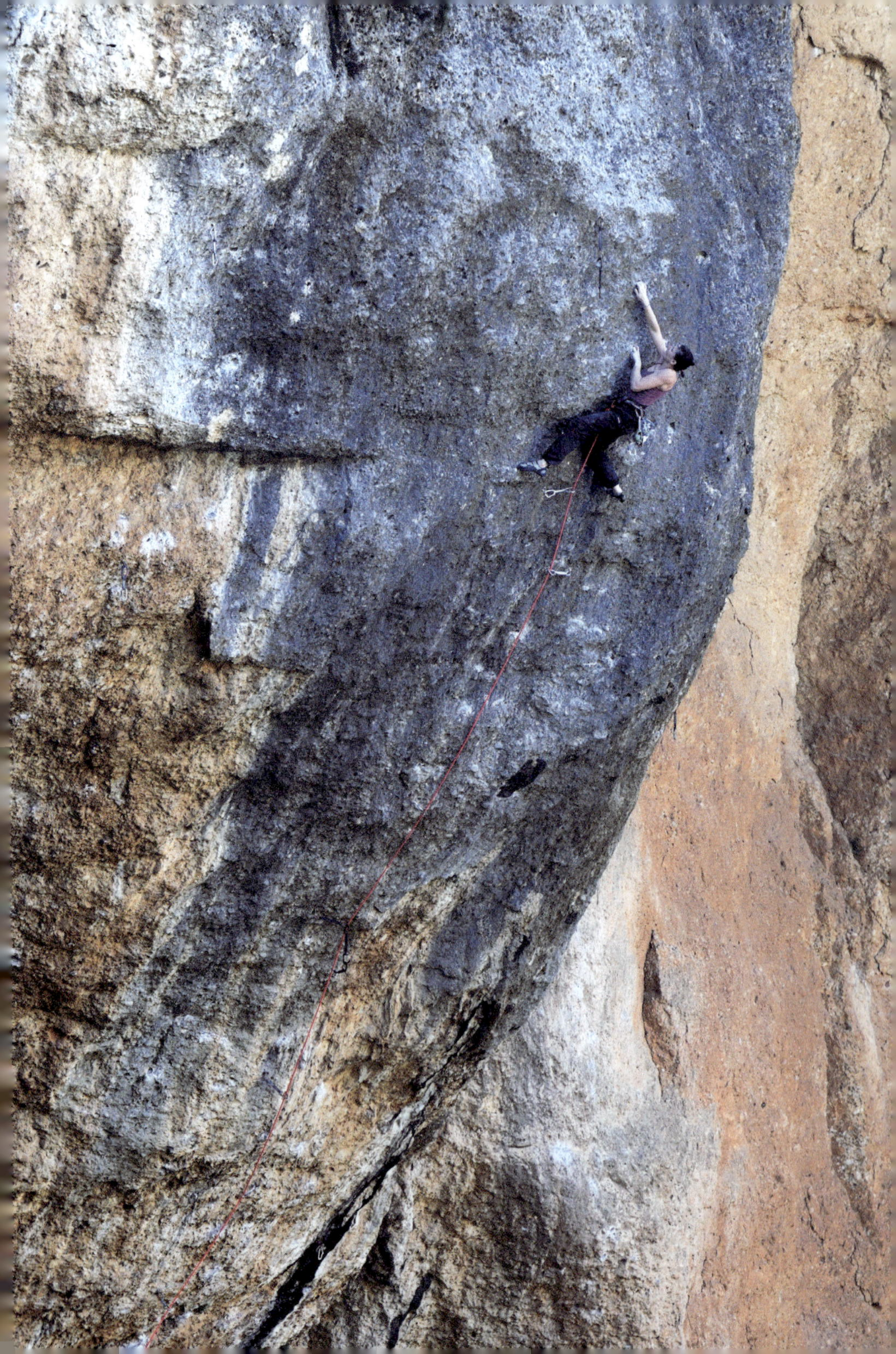

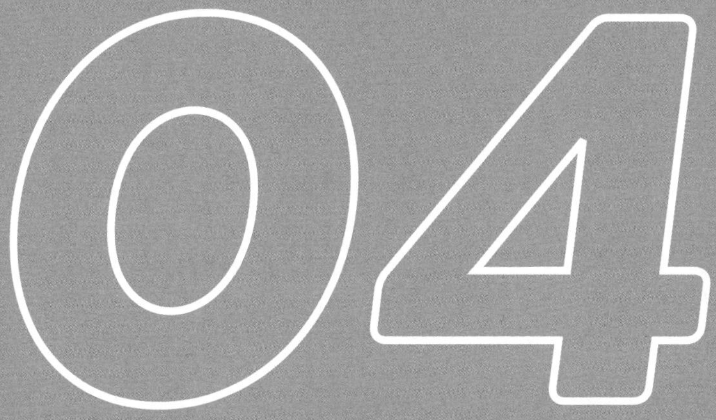

MACRO-NUTRIENTS FATS

KEY PLAYERS IN HEALTH AND IMMUNITY

LA VIA DEL QUIM, MARGALEF, SPAIN. © KEITH SHARPLES

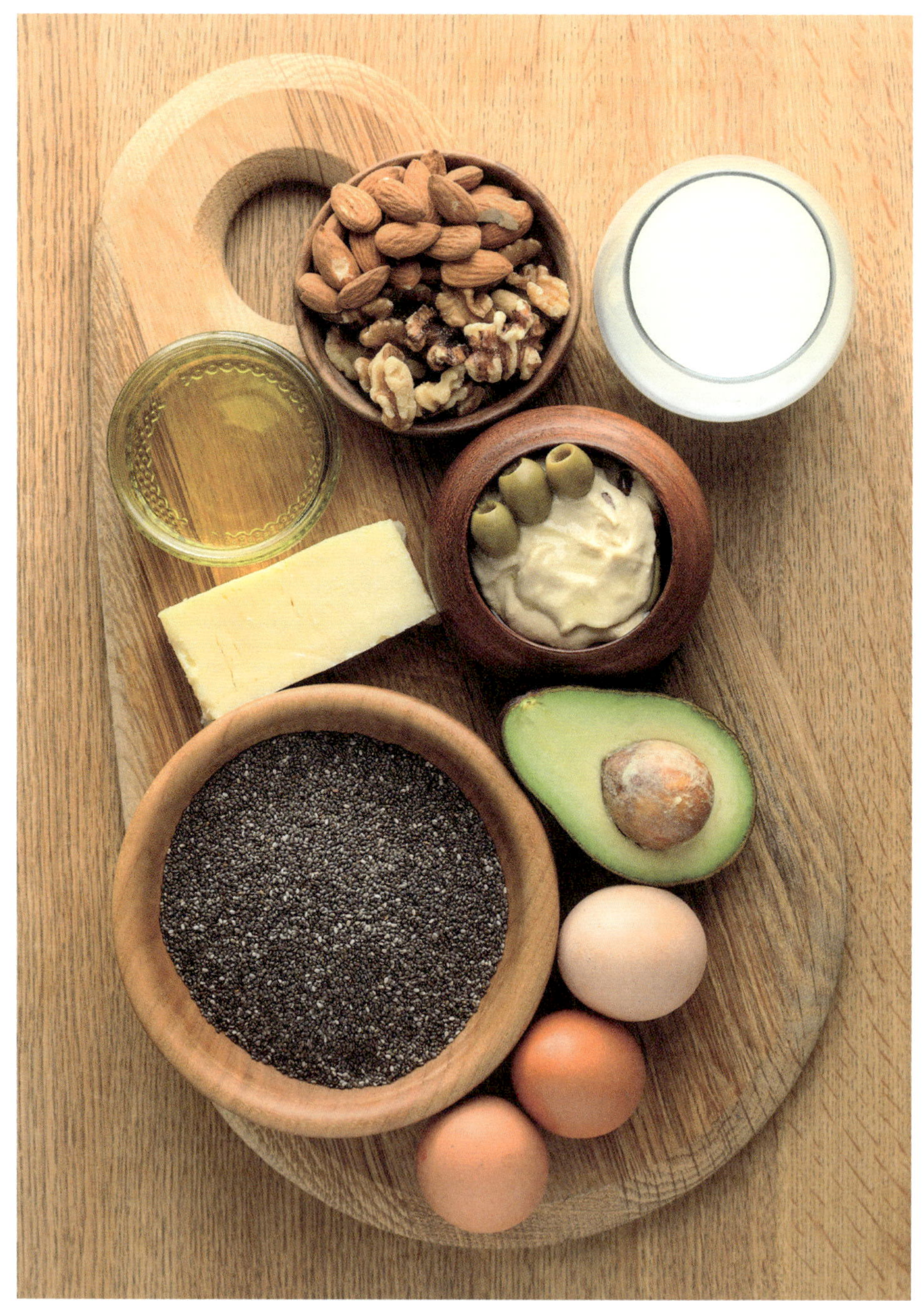

A MEDIUM AVOCADO (ABOUT 200 GRAMS) CONTAINS ROUGHLY 320 KILOCALORIES AND 29 GRAMS OF (MOSTLY) MONOUNSATURATED FAT AS WELL AS 13 GRAMS OF FIBRE.

What are fats?

Fats get a bad name as they often bring up images of excess body fat stores. This can fuel an unnecessary reductionist approach to eating fat-containing foods. In fact, dietary fats are really important for many things, including building strength, our hormones, the absorption of fat-soluble vitamins (A, D, E and K) and immunity. Fats also serve as an energy source for lower-intensity work.

Fats contain 9 kilocalories per gram, making them the most calorie-dense macronutrient (carbohydrates and proteins are both approximately 4 kilocalories per gram). Of course, this means that eating lots of fat-based foods can cause an inadvertent increase in energy intake that could cause body fat levels to increase. On the flip side, fats are also one of the most satiating macronutrients, along with protein.

As with everything, it's a balance, and it's important, especially as an athlete, not to let fat intake drop too low as this could compromise your health, recovery and adaptation. Don't be afraid of eating fats; they are important, especially when doing a lot of climbing or training.

Types of fats

There are different types of dietary fats – monounsaturated, polyunsaturated, saturated and trans fatty acids – and most foods will have a fatty acid profile that is a mixture of these. Foods are often defined by the type of fats that they contain the most of, which helps with their categorisation.

Unsaturated fats

Unsaturated fats are split into monounsaturated and polyunsaturated – these terms are all to do with how many double bonds are present in a carbon chain – and these fats are considered very beneficial to our health. Examples of foods containing unsaturated fats include salmon, mackerel, sardines, nuts and seeds, olive and rapeseed oils, and avocados.

Omega-3 polyunsaturated fats in particular may benefit athletes in areas such as muscle protein synthesis and muscle recovery.[1] However, data surrounding supplementation of omega-3 fatty acids (fish oils) for overall sports performance is mixed.[2] Good sources of omega-3 include fatty fish such as salmon, mackerel and sardines, as well as walnuts, chia seeds and flaxseed. If you don't like fish then this can be supplemented via fish oil capsules or algae-based capsules (if vegan/vegetarian), but if these foods feature regularly in your diet then supplementation is unlikely to be necessary.[3]

Saturated fats

The subject of saturated fats and health is still hotly debated. For many years there has been a lot of negativity around the health impact of eating saturated fats, especially in relation to cardiovascular disease. The messaging from governing bodies historically has been clear: limit saturated fat intake. However, more recent research and discussion is pulling this advice – and any limits which have been set – into review, suggesting no link between dietary saturated fat intake and increased risk of cardiovascular disease.[4] In fact, some foods that have in the past been demonised, such as whole dairy, are now considered beneficial to our health and cardiovascular risk.[5]

In contrast to this, a meta-analysis of randomised controlled trials by Hooper et al. in 2020 demonstrated a significant reduction in cardiovascular events when saturated fats were reduced for at least two years.[6] This study also showed that replacing saturated fats with polyunsaturated fats was most protective. So, perhaps the jury is still out.

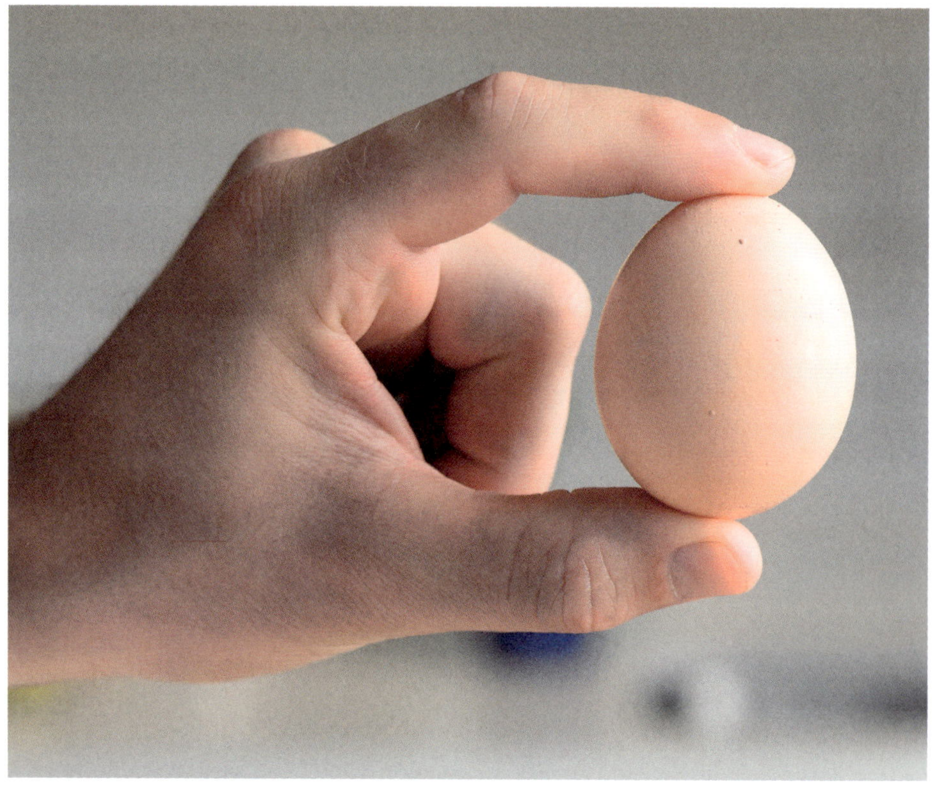

A LARGE EGG TYPICALLY CONTAINS 11 GRAMS OF FAT AS WELL AS B VITAMINS, VITAMIN D, CHOLINE, SELENIUM AND IODINE.

At this point, a sensible approach is to consider the diet as a whole, aiming for a balanced approach that contains a variety of fats from predominantly whole food sources. This more nuanced focus on variety and moderation of saturated fat intake, rather than strict saturated fat limitation, will likely result in an intake that has some saturated fat but also plenty of mono- and polyunsaturated fats as well.

Trans unsaturated fats

Trans unsaturated fats are mainly found in industrially processed foods and are associated with negative health outcomes including increased risk of coronary heart disease and all-cause mortality.[7] The use of trans fats has increased dramatically due to their relative cheapness to produce, their shelf life and their usability. They are solid at room temperature, making them suitable for many processed foods such as fried and baked foods, biscuits, pies and fast food items.

These types of fats are considered harmful and the World Health Organization suggests they should make up no more than 1 per cent of our dietary intake.[8]

Cholesterol

Cholesterol is a type of fat found in the blood. It is made predominantly of two types, HDL (high-density lipoprotein) and LDL (low-density lipoprotein). The body needs cholesterol for things like building cells, but high levels in the blood can also increase the risk of heart disease and stroke. While cholesterol is found in food, the body is very good at managing levels and the liver responds to an increase in dietary intake by reducing its cholesterol synthesis, reducing absorption and increasing secretion. This is why evidence from studies generally does not show a significant association between cholesterol in the diet and cardiovascular disease.[9] Dietary restriction of cholesterol is now considered only necessary in specific high-risk groups.[10]

Eggs in particular have had a lot of bad press over the years as they are a source of cholesterol and limits were previously advised on their intake. This advice has since been removed due to mounting research that suggests egg consumption has little effect on blood cholesterol and cardiovascular risk.[11] There are even potential protective benefits with higher intakes – more than one egg a day.[12] Eggs are also highly nutritious and particularly useful for athletes as they contain high levels of protein, B vitamins, vitamin D, choline, selenium and iodine.

Fat recommendations for climbers

There is no specific data for recommended fat intake in climbers. A review from Michael et al. in 2019 suggests fat intake in the region of 20–35 per cent of energy intake which sits in line with broader recommendations.[13]

While it is crucial that your fat intake does not drop chronically low, it can be manipulated in either direction for specific causes. For example, increased training demand or specific situations such as high altitude may require higher energy intakes and this can, in part, be compensated for by increasing fat intake to take advantage of the macronutrient's higher energy value. Or, conversely, if your energy needs are lower, for example during the off-season or intentional weight loss, your fat intake can be reduced. It is worth mentioning that female athletes who have menstrual dysfunction and other symptoms of REDs have been shown in some research to have dietary patterns that are low in fat (as well as low in carbohydrate and high in fibre) which may contribute to this dysfunction.[14]

What does this look like in food?

FOOD	AMOUNT	FAT (g)
Avocado	100 g	~15
Almonds	10 g	~5
Hummus	100 g	~10
Olive oil	1 tbsp	~14
Walnuts	10 g	~7
Chia seeds	10 g	~3
Smoked salmon	100 g	~4
Tinned mackerel in olive oil (drained)	100 g	~21
Olives	10 olives	~6
Whole milk	200 ml	~8
Cheddar cheese	100 g	~30
Eggs	1 egg	~11

Figure 8: Example fats.

Timing your fat intake

Fats should make a regular appearance in meals and snacks, but the timing of this macronutrient is less important than with carbohydrate or protein. For example, you could use fatty fish as a protein source, add olive oil to a salad or veggies, eat nuts/seeds, use nuts/nut butters or opt for full-fat dairy in some meals.

KEY TAKEAWAYS

- → Dietary fats are really important for many things including building strength, hormones, absorption of fat-soluble vitamins (A, D, E and K) and immunity.
- → Fat intake can sit in the broader ranges of 20–35 per cent of energy intake with regular appearances in meals and snacks.
- → There are different types of dietary fat (monounsaturated, polyunsaturated, saturated and trans fatty acids) and most foods will have a fatty acid profile that is a mixture of these.
- → Mono- and polyunsaturated fats such as fatty fish, nuts, seeds and olive oil are beneficial to health.
- → The subject of saturated fats and the link to cardiovascular health is still hotly debated. A sensible approach is to consider the diet as a whole, aiming for a balanced approach that contains a variety of fats from predominantly whole food sources.
- → Trans unsaturated fats found in processed foods are considered harmful to health and their consumption should be limited.
- → While high cholesterol in the blood increases risk of cardiovascular disease, dietary cholesterol intake is not a key driver.
- → Eggs are highly nutritious, need not be limited and are beneficial for athletes like climbers.

WHAT CAN I DO?

- → Is your fat intake in the 20–35 per cent of intake range? Could it be higher or lower?
- → Consider which foods make up most of your fat intake: is it a variety of types of fat or mostly one type?
- → Can you adjust your intake to increase mono- and polyunsaturated fats from whole food sources?
- → Consider all your meals in the last day: did some fat intake feature in each meal? If not, where could you **add** some mono- or polyunsaturated fats?

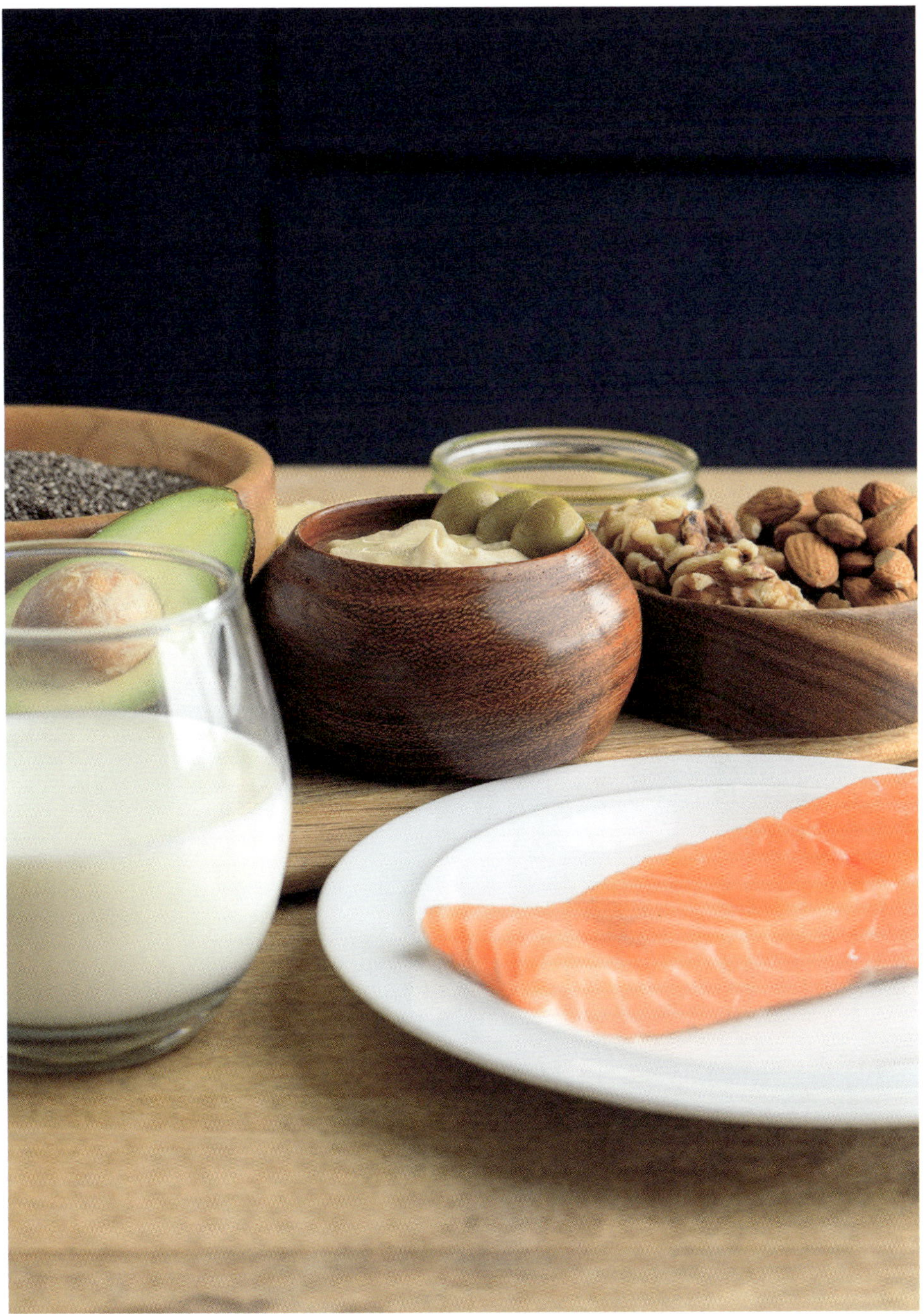

A 200-MILLILITRE GLASS OF WHOLE MILK CONTAINS 7.4 GRAMS OF FAT, OF WHICH 4.8 GRAMS IS SATURATED FAT. IT ALSO CONTAINS 9.4 GRAMS OF CARBOHYDRATE AND 7 GRAMS OF PROTEIN.

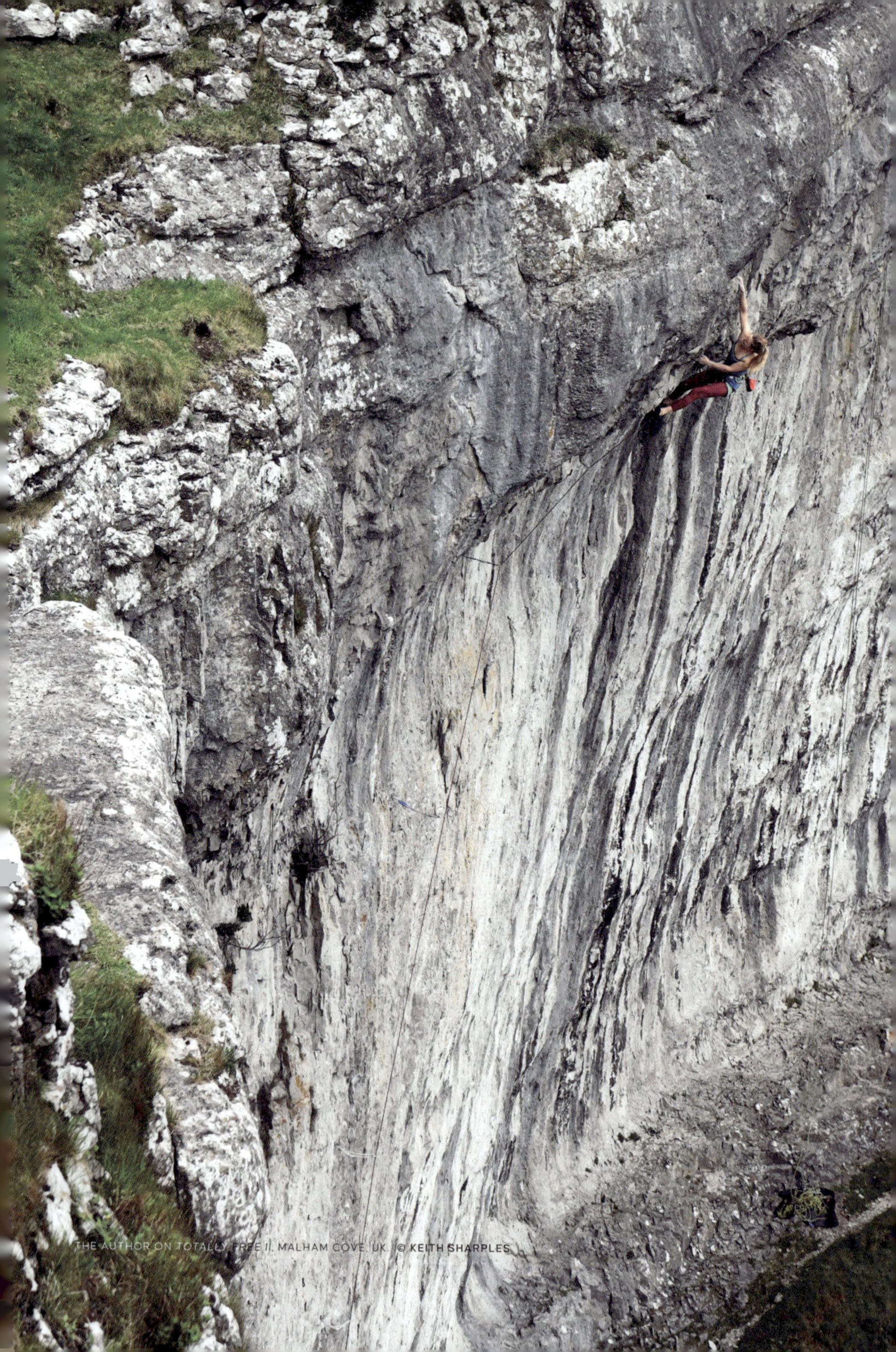

THE AUTHOR ON *TOTALLY FREE II*, MALHAM COVE, UK. | © KEITH SHARPLES

MINA LESLIE-WUJASTYK
STRAWBERRY PENCIL PICK-ME-UPS

This one is from me. It's a funny tale of how an unusual approach to crag nutrition helped me to finish off a particularly long sport route, *Totally Free II* (F8b). Sometimes, to fire on all cylinders, the best option is not the 'healthiest' food. All food has some value, even if it's just taste, but in this case I got taste and a send.

I fell off manteling the top of Malham Cove. Yep, right up there at the very top of the crag, level with where the tourists look at the view from the beautiful limestone pavement. I was pumped out of my brain at 69 metres up a 70-metre sport route having grunted my way through the previous few moves. I'd been on the route for over an hour and was seriously hitting a wall. The rope drag at this point was epic and I couldn't clip. I was on big holds trying to shake out and recover; the good aerobic capacity I thought I had cultivated had decided to leave the party. My legs were shaking, the dreaded sewing-machine dance. Only a couple of moves remained before I could mantel the crag and top-out the iconic route of *Totally Free II* that climbs the entire height of the Cove in one pitch. My body said no, not this time. I pushed on past the clip, elbows by my ears, one last-ditch effort before I was falling through the air.

Exhausted and depleted, I started to analyse what went wrong up there. How could I get a different result in that situation if I mustered the effort to try again? It felt like something was missing from my strategy. The science of training, nutrition, psychology and tactics is now commonplace in climbing. Increasingly we see evidence of a movement to analyse, to set goals, to construct plans and strategies. To perform at your top level you can't turn up unprepared. Gone are the days when climbing performance was simple; there's a plethora of terms to grasp now: do you work on your aerobic capacity or your anaerobic power? Is your limiting factor your isometric finger strength or your mental game? What's this ketogenic

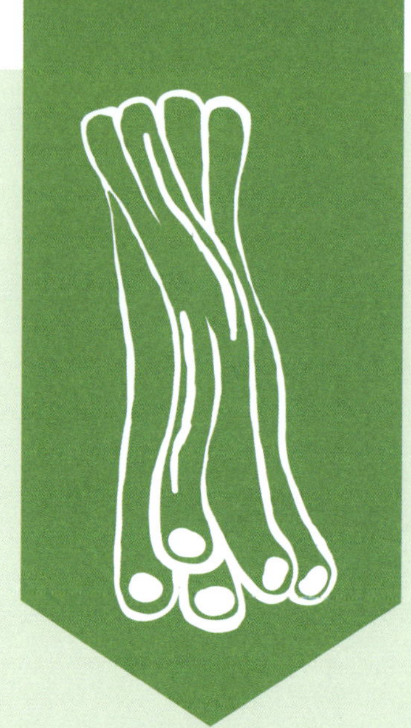

diet about and can you really pull hard without a good dose of carbohydrates in your belly? Spoiler alert on that last one: probably not.

Preparation comes in many forms, from physical strength and endurance to mental fortitude, from a well-timed 'peak' to a balance between training and rest. These things are all grafted out in the weeks, months and years before a climb, but what could I do to get an extra one per cent on the day?

I did a few things different the next time I went to try the route. I wore more thermals to stop my muscles getting cold, I used electrolytes in my water and I used a different rope system to minimise rope drag. *Totally Free II* is **long**; it's actually composed of three single independent pitches climbed as one. First, there is *The Groove* (F8a+), a total classic; then *Free and Easy* (F7c); and finally the *Breach of the Peace* roof (F7c). After pulling over the top, the climber unties, drops the rope, does a last mini scramble and then walks down off the back. On my failed attempt I had used one skinny (9.1-millimetre) single rope all the way. On my next attempt, I set off with two. I climbed *The Groove* with both ropes, clipping one in and trailing the other. At the top of *The Groove* there is a good rest and here I clipped the trailing line into three points and made sure I was on belay on that second rope before untying and dropping my first rope. This massively helped with drag on the top section.

But my most interesting, surprising and, I think, vital last-minute preparation came in the form of strawberry flavour, pencil-shaped sweets. At this point in my climbing life, my nutrition looked pretty wholesome most of the time; I felt I had fuelled really well before the attempt where I fell. Initially, I wasn't sure how I could improve on that front. I needed extra energy up there on that last section of climbing and I needed it fast. I was ready to try a new tactic.

The sweets aisle in the supermarket is not my normal habitat, I'm much more of a chocolate girl. It was bright and sickeningly colourful; the options were endless. Fizzy, fruity, chewy; I was out of my comfort zone. I picked at random: strawberry pencil sweets. I glanced at the ingredients list: all the bad-sounding things and *lots* of sugar. Perfectly luminous and flamboyant, I took them to the checkout.

Fast forward a day and I was back at the crag, standing at the foot of *Totally Free II*. Looking up it seemed a long way to the top, but this time, alongside a better rope plan and warmer clothes, I had extra ammunition. I checked my knots, chalked my hands and signalled to my belayer that I was ready to climb. It was time. To the casual observer nothing much had changed nutrition-wise, but I had a plan and it didn't involve additional fuel on the ground; that hadn't been enough last time. Oh no, this time I was taking a magic bullet up the route with me ... I had strawberry pencil sweets tucked into my sports bra. Whenever there was a rest, I reached down and took out a sweet or two. The sugar stops became like a series of punctuation marks, moments of weird juxtaposition between eating sweets and engaging with my physicality and the rock.

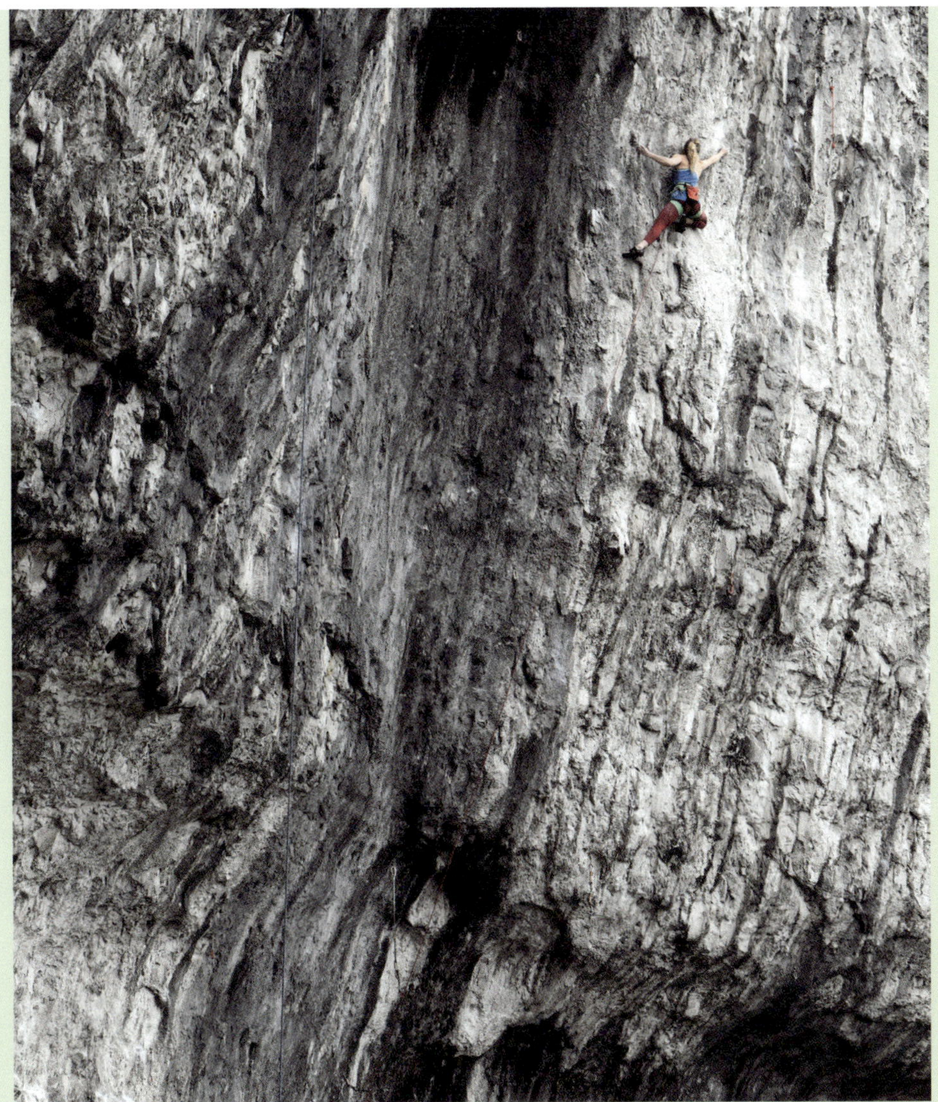

THE AUTHOR ON *TOTALLY FREE II*, MALHAM COVE, UK. © **KEITH SHARPLES**

To cut a long story short, I snacked my way up the 70-metre route. I didn't hit a wall. I didn't get the shakes. I pulled over the top of the crag, untied, dropped my rope and walked back down with a smile and the lingering taste of strawberries.

Of course, this anecdote, this observational study with me as a single participant, does not warrant cause and effect. My beloved strawberry pencil pick-me-ups may have had nothing to do with the outcome. Maybe it was the improved rope system, the warmer clothes, the electrolytes or just a better day. But I like to think they played a role, and I've certainly used them since.

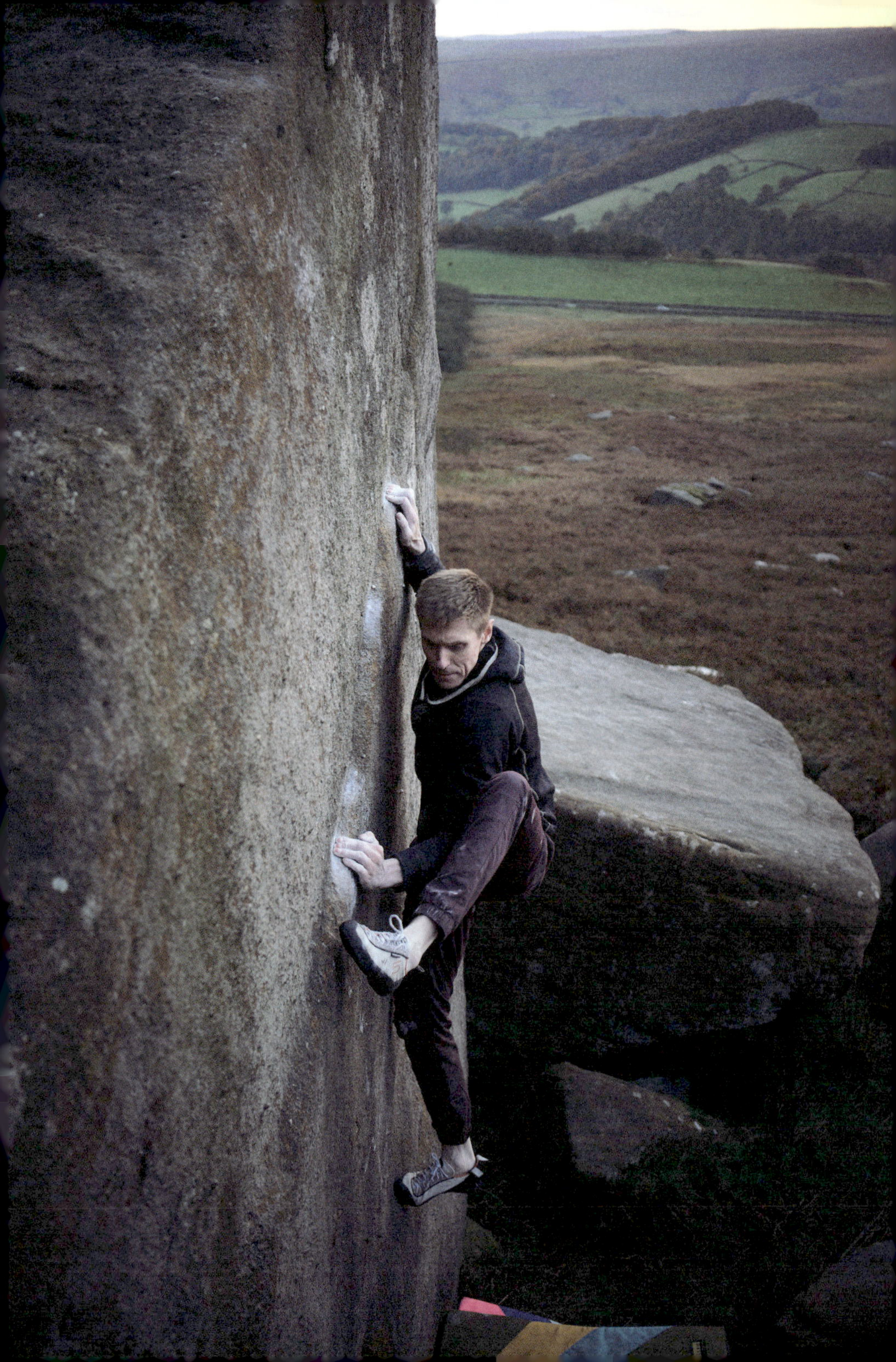

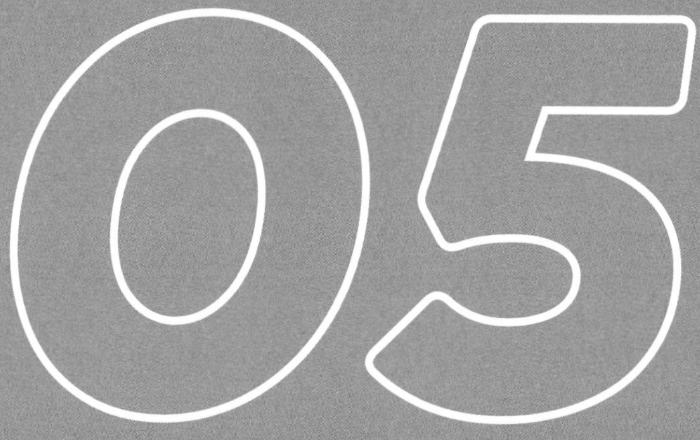

MICRO-NUTRIENTS
VITAMINS AND MINERALS

CHAR WILLIAMS ON *THE STORM*, STANAGE PLANTATION, UK. © JOHN COEFIELD

What are micronutrients?

Micronutrients are the vitamins and minerals in food. While they are needed in much smaller amounts than macronutrients, they are still very important for various functions in the body. There are many different vitamins and minerals, all with different roles, and they are found in varying amounts in an array of foods.

A good strategy when it comes to micronutrients is to aim for variety in food intake as this helps to cover all bases. For most people, this food-first approach of adding plenty of different whole foods to meals and snacks will be enough and supplementation will not be necessary. This can be achieved by including foods such as the following in your diet: carrots, beetroot, broccoli, tomatoes, radishes, kale, cauliflower, potatoes (white and sweet), blueberries, strawberries, citrus fruits, avocado, olives, nuts and seeds, as well as grains, oats, quinoa, red meat, dairy, and pulses and legumes such as beans and lentils. Think 'eating the rainbow' and you can't go too far wrong.

Having said this, there are particular micronutrients, outlined below, that play vital roles in sports performance, health and longevity, and that, as climbers, it is worth understanding in more depth. There are also some climbers who will need to focus a bit more on particular micronutrients, and potentially consider some supplementation use, for example vegans and vegetarians, women with heavy periods, or someone with a measured deficiency.

While a multivitamin may be a useful tool to cover all bases at certain times – for example, a trip where food variety is limited or a planned calorie deficit where food intake is reduced – it is best to aim for a food-first approach where possible with supplementation added in when there is a known deficiency.

Key vitamins and minerals for climbers

Vitamin D

Vitamin D is an interesting micronutrient as, unlike others, it is not primarily absorbed from food. It is synthesised in the skin from exposure to sunlight, with only 10–20 per cent derived from dietary sources. Foods that do contain vitamin D include salmon, eggs, red meat and fortified foods. It plays a role in immune health, exercise performance, injury recovery, bone health, muscular strength and neuromuscular function.[1] Deficiency can contribute to risk of bone issues including stress fractures, muscle weakness and injuries, and upper respiratory infections.[2]

In the general population, vitamin D deficiency is quite common due to the increasing amount of time we spend indoors, working hours and cultural habits.[3] More recent research also suggests a high risk for deficiency in elite athletes and specifically climbers.[4] If, for an individual, climbing is predominantly an outdoor pursuit, this may positively affect their vitamin D status through increased exposure to sunlight (depending on season and latitudes), but for an indoor climber who works a desk job, this will not be the case.

In the UK, the general population is advised to take a daily vitamin D supplement of 400 IU during the winter months, however it has been suggested that this is too low.[5] A dose of 1,000–2,000 IU in athletes may be more appropriate, however there is much controversy over specific dosing levels.[6] The best solution for athletes and climbers is to measure their vitamin D levels and supplement accordingly.[7] Again, there is controversy over adequate versus optimal levels and, while vitamin D toxicity is rare, high doses for no reason can be harmful.

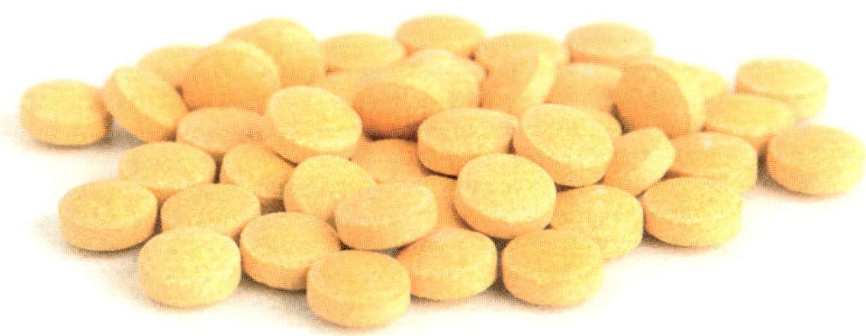

BLOOD TESTS ARE A USEFUL WAY TO IDENTIFY ANY DEFICIENCY AND INFORM SUPPLEMENTATION, IF NEEDED.

Iron

Iron plays a role in oxygen transport around the body – it makes haemoglobin in red blood cells – and energy production, as well as having an effect on exercise capacity and cognitive function.[8]

Athletes in general are at higher risk of iron deficiency: 15–35 per cent of female athletes and 5–11 per cent of male athletes.[9] In climbers, a study by Gibson-Smith et al. in 2020 reported that approximately 17 per cent of males and 45 per cent of females had a suboptimal iron status, with 30 per cent of the female participants meeting the criteria for iron deficiency.[10] Along with being at higher risk for deficiency, it has also been suggested that the daily recommended intake ranges (8.7 milligrams for men and 14.8 milligrams for women in the UK) may not be sufficient for an athletic population.[11] To compound this, Gibson-Smith et al. also found that from the climbers in their study, both men and women (21 per cent of males and 80 per cent of females) were not meeting the recommended intakes.

Clearly, iron is a key micronutrient which athletes and climbers should be mindful of. Symptoms of iron deficiency include fatigue, tiredness, dizziness and pale skin. If you are worried you might have iron deficiency, your best course of action is to go to your doctor and request a blood test.

Sources of iron are red meat, beans, eggs, nuts, wholegrains, legumes, soy/tofu, lentils, dark leafy greens and iron-fortified products, such as many breakfast cereals. It is worth noting that plant-based foods contain only non-heme iron which is not as easily absorbed as the heme iron found in animal products. Iron absorption can also be negatively affected by tannins, calcium and phytates (found in soy, nuts and legumes), so it is worth avoiding the consumption of tea, coffee and dairy in conjunction with iron-rich meals and considering sprouted, soaked and fermented versions of some foods to reduce phytates. Combining plant-based iron sources with foods containing vitamin C (oranges, strawberries) can help to improve absorption.[12]

There are specific scenarios where you may need to pay more attention to your iron intake, such as if you follow a vegan or vegetarian diet, are a woman with heavy periods, you are at risk of low energy availability and also if you have a very high training or exercise regimen.[13]

There is an additional – and very interesting – dynamic at play when it comes to exercise and iron intake/absorption. Hepcidin is a protein that regulates iron levels in the body and it has interactions with exercise – specifically exercise-induced inflammation – that can affect the absorption of iron. When a person exercises, this stimulates the release of hepcidin and impairs iron absorption for

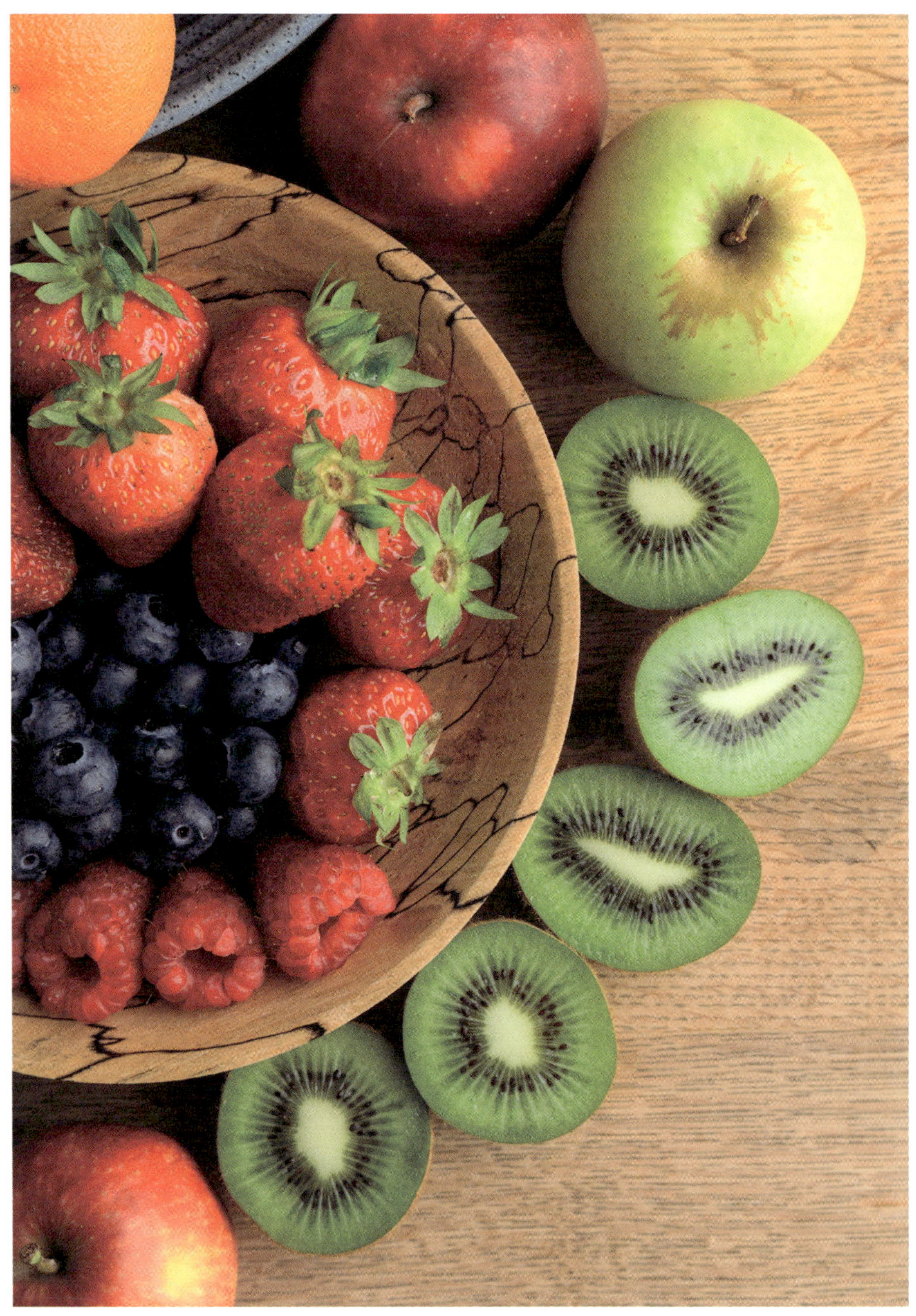

STRAWBERRIES, BLUEBERRIES AND RASPBERRIES ARE ALL HIGH IN VITAMIN C AND MANGANESE, WITH BLUEBERRIES HIGH IN VITAMIN K AS WELL.

the next three to six hours, which, if you are climbing or exercising a lot, could make optimal timing of eating iron very tricky. Hepcidin is also lower in the morning, so ideally iron-based foods should be eaten away from training with a preference for the morning.[14] To throw yet another spanner in the works, as mentioned above, the absorption of iron is negatively affected by tannins and calcium which are often found in breakfast meals!

It's easy to see why this is a difficult area, with climbers often displaying deficiencies. As with vitamin D, the best way to know whether you need a supplement is to get your iron levels tested.

Calcium

Calcium is a mineral that plays a key role in bone metabolism, muscle contraction (including heartbeat!) and nerve conduction. Research by Monedero et al. showed inadequate intake of calcium (and other micronutrients) in climbers, which suggests it should be something we keep an eye on.[15] In particular, not getting enough calcium can have negative effects on bone health which is often seen in cases of disordered eating and the avoidance of calcium-rich foods such as dairy. Alongside this, low energy availability (also prevalent in climbers) is a key player in bone health due to its negative effect on the production of hormones (such as oestrogen) that promote positive bone turnover. So, having enough food going in overall, as well as particular nutrients, is crucial.

The British Dietetic Association advises that calcium intake for adults should be in the range of 700 milligrams per day, with higher amounts needed for adolescents and those who are breastfeeding.[16] This can be managed through dietary intake with a focus on regular intake of calcium-rich foods such as dairy.[17] Other, non-dairy, sources include sardines, green leafy vegetables, tofu, nuts and calcium-fortified products; although, like with iron, there are issues with absorption when calcium is eaten with certain foods. For calcium, the absorption blockers are oxalic acid and phytates which are found in green vegetables and some grains.

Vitamin B12

B12 is an essential vitamin involved in DNA synthesis, keeping the nervous system healthy and making red blood cells. The role B12 plays in the latter is of particular note to athletes as there are potential performance benefits to red blood cell formation being optimised due to its relationship to aerobic capacity.[18] Having said this, there is little evidence to suggest that supplementing outside of a deficiency would have a positive performance effect; simply put, a B12 boost is only helpful if you are already running low. You should consider 'deficiency' as below 400 picograms per millilitre as this is where beneficial changes in blood cell formation may occur.[19] Low B12 status can cause symptoms such as weakness, fatigue, poor appetite and anaemia.

Vitamin B12 needs to come from food intake but is not present in plant foods (unless fortified), making deficiency a risk factor in vegan athletes.[20] A 2010 study by Gilsing et al. showed that 52 per cent of vegans were B12 deficient.[21] Foods that contain B12 include meat, dairy, eggs and fortified foods. The British Dietetic Association recommends 1.5 micrograms as the daily intake for adults which can be met by combinations of foods throughout the day.[22] Vegan climbers might benefit from regular checks on B12 levels to ensure their level of this vitamin is not compromised.

MICRONUTRIENT	*FOODS CONTAINING IT*	*EXAMPLE PORTIONS TO MEET REFERENCE NUTRIENT INTAKE (RNI)*
Vitamin D	Salmon, eggs, red meat, vitamin-D-fortified foods (breakfast cereals, non-dairy milks).	Supplementation of at least **400 IU** during the winter months. Sunlight should be adequate at other times in the UK.
Iron	Red meat, beans, eggs, nuts, wholegrains, legumes, soy/tofu, lentils, dark leafy greens and iron-fortified products.	**Men (8.7 mg) =** 40 g Weetabix (4.7 mg) + 78 g beef burger (1.9 mg) + one fried egg (1.3 mg) + 85 g broccoli (0.8 mg) **Women (14.8 mg) =** 30 g Bran Flakes (7.2 mg) + 80 g lentils (2.8 mg) + 90 g roast lamb (1.4 mg) + 80 g spinach (1.2 mg) + 40 g pine nuts (2.2 mg). (Milton Keynes University Hospital NHS Foundation Trust)[23]
Calcium	Milk, cheese, yoghurt, calcium-fortified soya, tofu, calcium-fortified cereals/non-dairy milks, sardines, pilchards, wholemeal bread, kale, some seeds.	**700 mg =** 200 ml glass of semi-skimmed milk (approximately 250 mg) + 200 g Greek yoghurt (250 mg) + 80 g boiled kale (120 mg) + 1 tbsp/12 g sesame seeds (80 mg) (British Nutrition Foundation)[24]
Vitamin B12	Meat, eggs, dairy products, fortified cereals, fortified plant milks, Marmite (yeast extract).	**1.5 mcg =** 100 g chicken (1–2.8 mcg), beef (2–3 mcg) or cod (2 mcg) **Plant-based options:** 200 ml fortified oat milk (0.76 mcg) + 30 g fortified Bran Flakes (0.7–0.8 mcg) Or 8 g Marmite (1.9 mcg) (University Hospitals Plymouth NHS Trust)[25]

Figure 9: Micronutrients in food.

KEY TAKEAWAYS

- Micronutrients are an important part of food intake with various crucial functions in the body.
- Most climbers can take a food-first approach, focusing on a varied whole food diet, to meet their micronutrient needs.
- The key micronutrients for climbers and athletes are vitamin D, iron, calcium and vitamin B12.
- Particular groups such as vegans, women with heavier periods and those in a state of low energy availability may be at higher risk for deficiency in some of these key micronutrients.
- The best way to determine if supplementation is necessary is through blood tests. This will determine if a deficiency is present and will inform supplementation protocols.

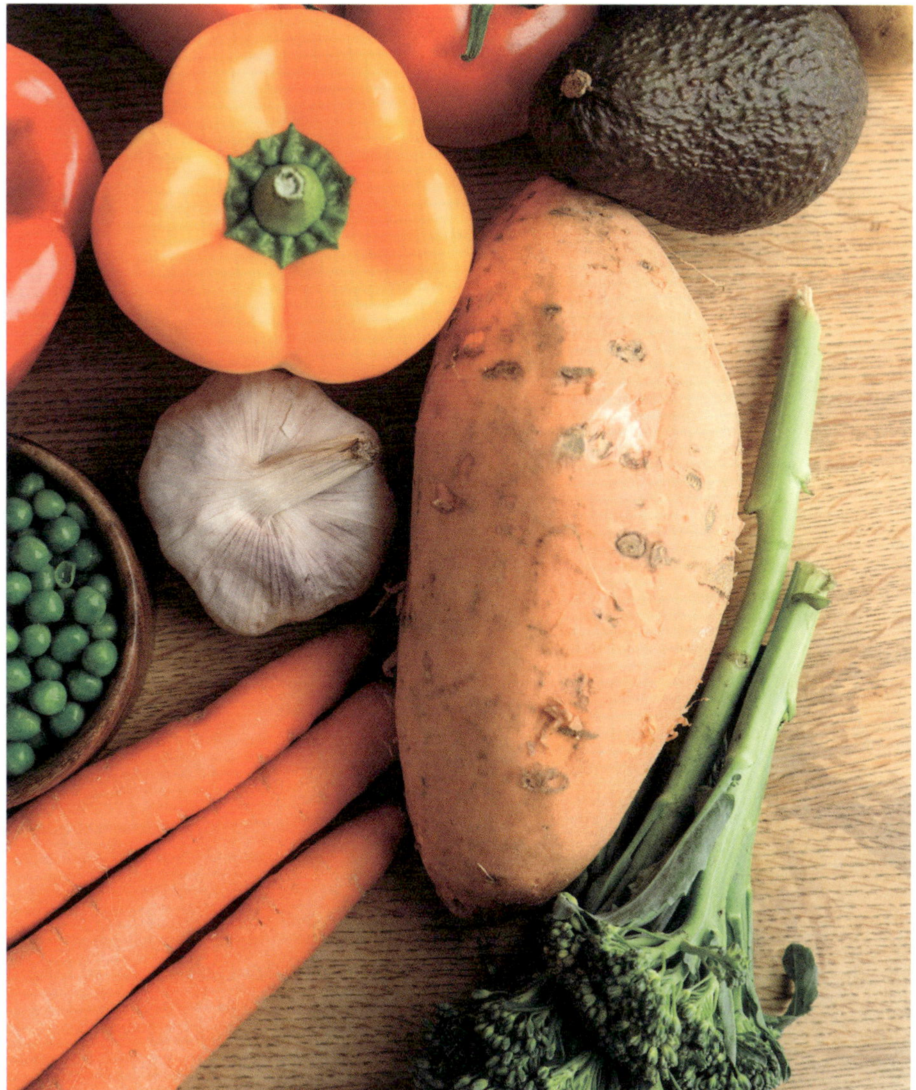

BROCCOLI IS A GOOD PLANT-BASED SOURCE OF IRON AND IT ALSO CONTAINS VITAMIN C WHICH HELPS WITH IRON ABSORPTION.

WHAT CAN I DO?

→ Consider whether you get a good variety of micronutrients through your food intake: are there any key micronutrients in this chapter that you think are missing from your diet?

→ Are you at higher risk from any deficiencies?

→ Do you have any symptoms that could warrant checking for deficiencies?

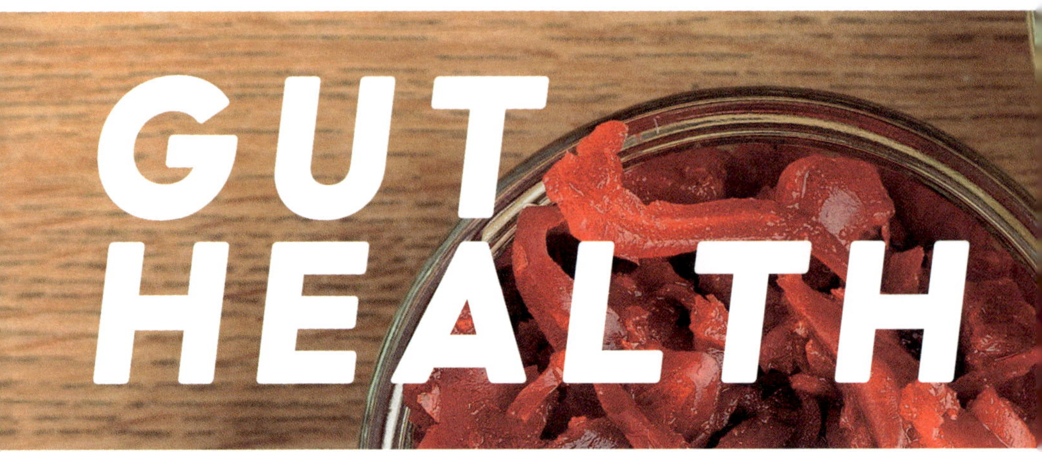

GUT HEALTH

Bacteria live in many areas of the human body, including the mouth, skin, lungs, vagina and intestines. It is estimated that 70 per cent reside in the gut, reaching a count of around 100 trillion.[1] The concept of gut health has been widely discussed, with a healthy gut microbiome touted as essential for those who want to feel their best. So, is gut health an overhyped trend or is it proving to be a key part of health, well-being and performance?

There is growing evidence that the gut microbiome in particular has a strong influence on health and immunity as well as mood via the gut–brain axis. It has also been suggested that a healthy microbiome may positively affect sports performance.[2] These bacteria are do-gooder bugs; among other things, they help to digest food and break down fibre to create useful things called short-chain fatty acids that play a significant role in health by regulating inflammation and promoting immunity.[3]

A 'healthy gut' is difficult to define, and, of course, knowing who the tenants in your tummy are is not information most of us have to hand. Generally speaking, a diverse set of microbes is a good thing. Easier to define from the outside is an unhappy gut. For example, the presence of regular symptoms like bloating, constipation, diarrhoea or excessive wind could indicate a gut that isn't balanced. Of course, most of us will get some of these symptoms some of the time without major issues, but chronic problems warrant some thought and investigation.

What can impact gut health?

Many factors influence the composition of the gut microbiome, some of which we can influence and some not.[4] For example, fixed things like type of birth delivery (vaginal or caesarean), age and genetics can impact the gut microbiome, as well as modifiable things like diet, sleep, stress and exercise. Eating too little can also have negative effects on the gut, as can alcohol.

Medication is also a player. Antibiotics, for example, are sometimes necessary and can be lifesaving, but they can negatively affect the gut as a side effect. Basically, they wipe out the good along with the bad. Exercise in general has been shown to exert a positive influence on gastrointestinal health status, which is good news for climbers.[5] However, proceed with caution as excessive exercise can be bad for the microbiome.[6]

Diet has a huge impact on the microbiome, with diversity being at the heart of it. Lots of variety of plant foods is ideal; think fruits, vegetables, grains, pulses, nuts, seeds and

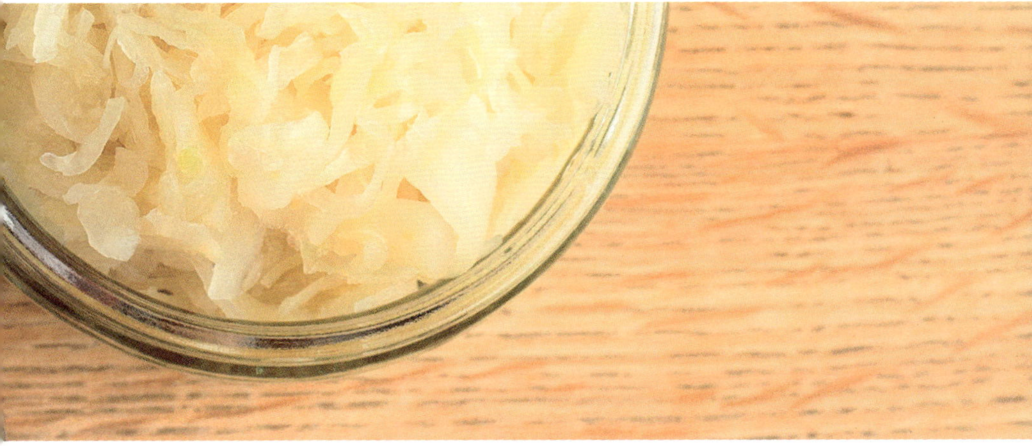

VARIETY IS KEY WHEN IT COMES TO GUT HEALTH. IF POSSIBLE, AIM FOR 30 DIFFERENT TYPES OF PLANT FOODS OVER THE COURSE OF A WEEK AS WELL AS FERMENTED FOODS.

spices – they all count! If possible, aim for 30 different types over the course of a week. In 2018, a study called the American Gut Project found that those people who ate more than 30 different types of fruit and vegetables over the course of a week had greater microbial diversity in their gut than those who ate ten or less.[7] So, ideally, mix it up and try different things rather than sticking to the same favourites all the time.

A word of caution though: make any changes slowly, adding a few new foods at a time. Increasing fibre intake quickly could cause some unwanted symptoms. And, of course, remember that not eating enough will negatively affect the gut so there is no point focusing on getting 30 different types of fruit and vegetables over a week if not enough calories are going in.

Example ideas:

→ Mix up the colours of your fruit and vegetables each week.
→ Add frozen fruits to your smoothies/yoghurt.
→ Season your food with spices and herbs.
→ Bulk out your meals with lentils or beans.
→ Vary your grains; use things like bulgur wheat or quinoa for variety.
→ Sprinkle seeds or nuts on your salads.

Probiotics and prebiotics

Probiotic foods are those that contain live bacteria that add to gut microbiome diversity. Classic examples are fermented foods such as sauerkraut, kombucha and kimchi, or dairy products such as yoghurt or kefir. Bear in mind that any pasteurisation process or the use of vinegar in fermentation kills the bacteria, so look for that on the label.

Over-the-counter probiotic supplements are getting very popular and, while there is evidence for their use in specific scenarios such as acute diarrhoea and some other intestinal diseases, there is still more work to be done to fully understand their role in health and disease as well as any safety considerations.[8] It has been suggested that supplementation with prebiotics and/or probiotics may be used therapeutically for athletes who have gastrointestinal issues, but it would be wise to consult a dietitian for more specificity on this.[9]

Prebiotics are the fibres that feed the probiotic organisms. While it is possible to buy prebiotics as a supplement, the best food for your microbes can be found in a varied whole food diet. Include lots of fresh plant foods, aiming for variety each day.

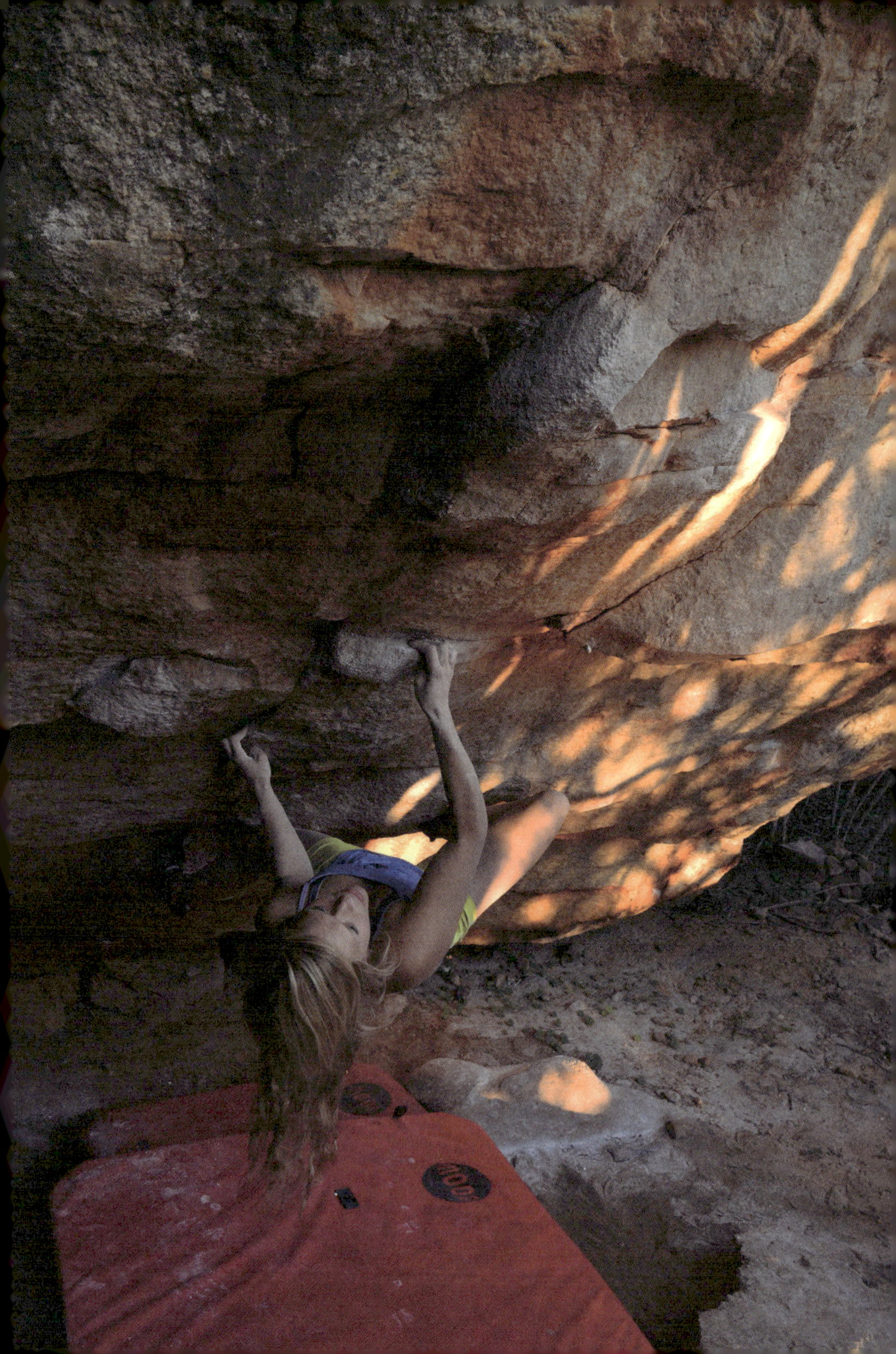

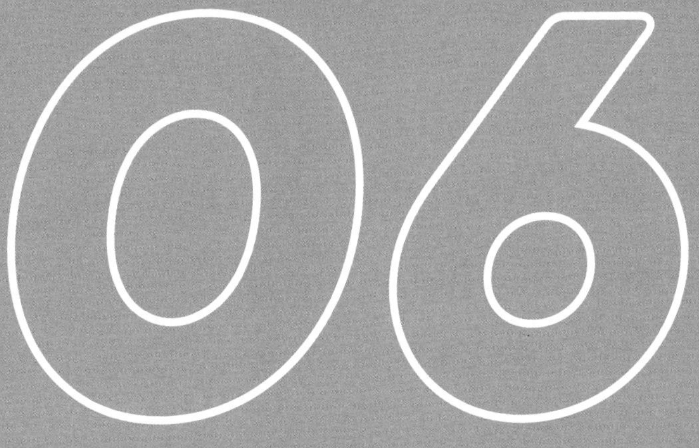

HYDRATION

THE AUTHOR ON *THE AMPHITHEATRE*, ROCKLANDS, SOUTH AFRICA. © **DAVID MASON**

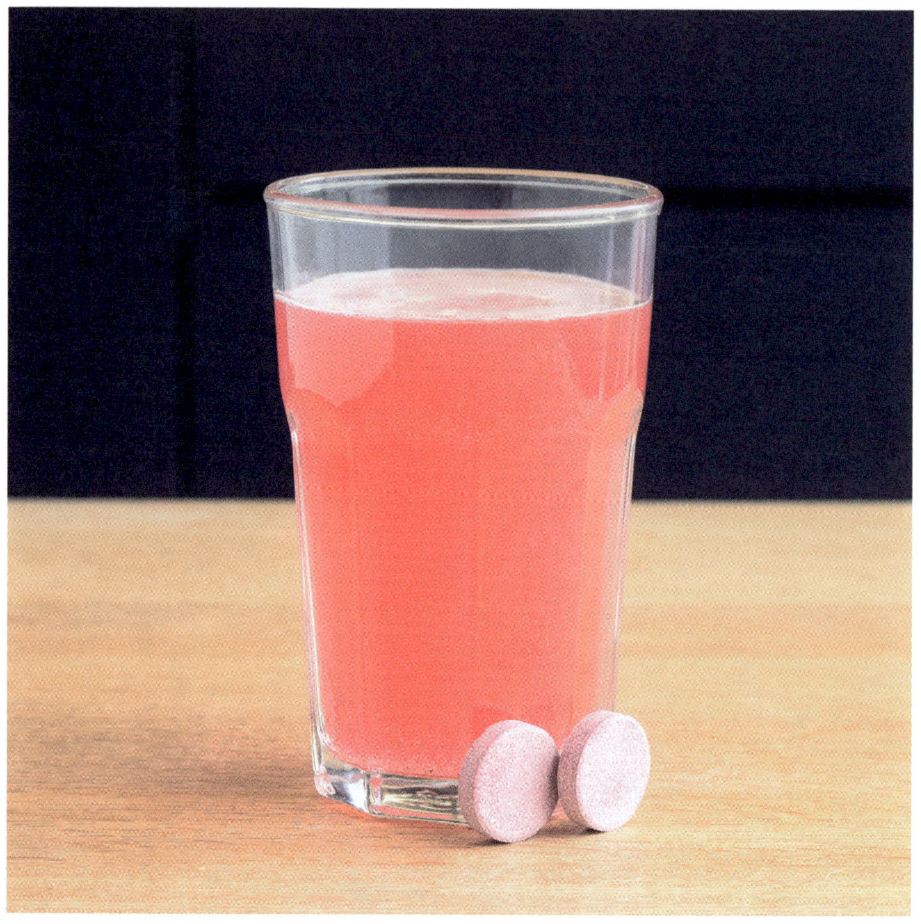

IF YOU'RE A HEAVY OR SALTY SWEATER, ADDING SOME ELECTROLYTES TO YOUR DRINK OR USING A SPORTS DRINK MIGHT BE BENEFICIAL.

Why is hydration important?

Fluids in the body contribute to many things including our blood makeup, kidney function, lymphatic system, digestive system, temperature regulation and lubrication of joints.[1] Our hydration levels can affect athletic performance, cognitive function and perceived effort, especially in endurance exercise and hot conditions. It may be helpful to know that, day to day, hydration is usually well managed by biological and behavioural mechanisms without much cognitive input. However, exercise presents an added challenge that can, in some cases, require additional thought.[2] As a baseline intake, before additional fluid for exercise is considered, most people need to drink in the range of 25–35 millilitres per kilogram of body weight per day.[3]

Fluid levels within the body can go in two directions: above or below an optimum range, i.e. overhydration or dehydration. Both of these scenarios, in mild forms, can be well managed by the body and exhibit little effect on performance, although both, in more moderate or severe forms, can negatively affect performance and health.

Dehydration

The loss of fluids above 2–3 per cent of body weight is considered a marker for where dehydration will begin to affect function and sports performance.[4] It is affected through a reduction in blood plasma and volume, impaired cardiovascular function, muscle blood flow and thermoregulatory capacity.[5] This is where one might expect to see the start of symptoms such as thirst, discomfort and disturbed movement economy, increasing to symptoms such as dizziness, fatigue and shortness of breath with more extreme dehydration.[6]

It has been suggested that climbers partaking in shorter routes or bouldering may be able to tolerate dehydration of 3–5 per cent, especially in cold conditions.[7] Having said this, as climbers, it's crucial not to dismiss crag approach efforts when considering our hydration for the day as these can be long and arduous in some cases and potentially have more of an effect on dehydration than the climbing itself.

Of course, there is a great deal of individual variation in response to dehydration and knowing what percentage of body weight is lost as fluid is a data point we will rarely have at the crag with us! Different people will also dehydrate at different rates depending on their individual sweat rates.

It's also worth considering electrolytes – sodium, potassium, magnesium and calcium, to name a few – when thinking about hydration. For low hydration needs, electrolytes in food will likely be sufficient, but if an activity or the conditions (heat) mean a lot of sweating, adding some electrolytes to your drink or using a sports drink might be beneficial.

Overhydration

Overhydration in exercise is more commonly associated with longer endurance sports and is not likely to be an issue in climbing itself, provided, as mentioned above, that the approach to the crag does not constitute considerable endurance exercise on its own. Despite being unlikely in most climbing scenarios, overhydration can be very serious. At the extreme, it dilutes the blood to the point where an osmotic gradient means that water moves into cells which can result in symptoms such as light-headedness, dizziness, nausea, puffiness and body weight gain from baseline, before progressing to a very serious medical condition.[8] At milder levels, drinking too much can be annoying as it means having to wee more often, and feelings of fullness or a sloshy tummy.

Practical hydration management

There isn't a straightforward answer to the question of how to monitor and manage hydration. There are lots of moving parts and many complexities to how fluid is controlled within the body. Hydration management is highly individual because we all have different sweat rates and also different sweat-sodium concentrations – how salty our sweat is – which can affect how quickly we become dehydrated in any one set of conditions. So, it is really an area that needs to be figured out on an individual basis. For some climbers, it will be an area of negligible interest, something that doesn't affect them much, whereas for others it will be a key piece of the puzzle for their well-being and performance.

General recommendations in climbing research are that climbers should aim to start climbing well hydrated and keep their urine colour pale by drinking 5–10 millilitres per kilogram of body weight approximately two hours before exercise, followed by 250 millilitres per hour with adjustments for conditions such as heat and humidity.[9] So, for our 80-kilogram male route climber (see page 23) this would mean drinking roughly 400–800 millilitres two hours before a session and 250 millilitres per hour during a session. And remember: this should be considered as *additional intake* in the context of the previously mentioned baseline daily requirement of 25–35 millilitres per kilogram of body weight.

Going into more depth on an individual basis, the main methods that can easily be used in practice for hydration management are **thirst**, **urine colour** and **sweat rate measurements**. As each one alone is not especially reliable, ideally a combination of these methods would be used to produce the most accurate assessment and therefore adequate management of fluid balance.[10] Daily changes in body mass, thirst and urine colour first thing in the morning may also be useful measures for tracking daily hydration.[11]

Thirst

Drinking to thirst essentially means relying on our body's innate communication for fluid needs. While thirst is not considered a very sensitive measure in longer-duration, higher-intensity exercise in the heat, researchers suggest that responding to thirst may be a sufficient method if exercise is lower intensity and lasts less than 60–90 minutes in cooler conditions.[12] This latter description would fit some climbers' sessions depending on the discipline, intensity of effort and time frame. Bear in mind that even if shorter duration (for example, a sport climbing redpoint), climbing is often high intensity; therefore, if performance is key, leaving hydration to thirst alone may not be ideal.

Also, while thirst sensation is purely biological, drinking behaviour can be affected by other factors such as fluid availability, perceptions about hydration and previous experiences around hydration management.[13] Essentially, having a bit of a plan in addition to responding to thirst is probably beneficial for most climbers. This could be as simple as using the general recommendations mentioned above as a starting point, or the more involved approach of measuring sweat rates to inform session hydration. It may sound obvious, but making sure you take plenty of fluids to the crag is an essential part of this.

Urine colour

Monitoring urine colour is another method for assessing hydration status and it is considered pretty sensitive for detecting dehydration.[14] It is relatively easy to do, making it an attractive option, but it may not be as accurate as some of the more involved methods partly because it is very subjective and quite basic as an approach. Essentially, aim for a pale straw

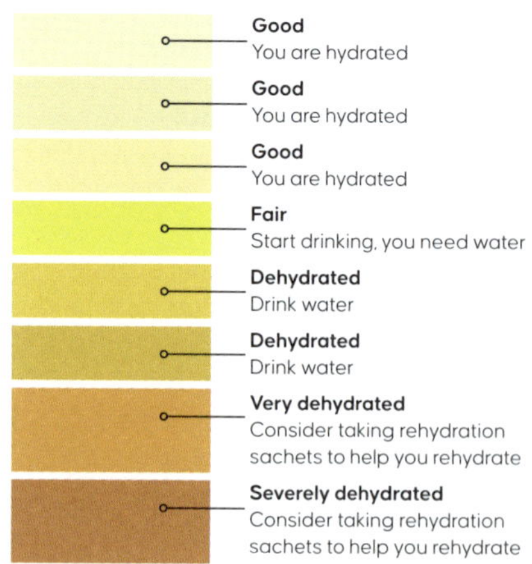

Figure 10: Urine colour chart (taken from Gunawan et al., 2018).[16]

colour; if your urine is darker than this, drink more. With methods such as thirst and urine colour, using them together is more effective than using just one or the other.[15]

Sweat rate measurements

Working out your sweat loss for a given time period or session involves measuring your body weight before and after the session while accounting for any fluid consumed during the session and any urine excreted. Calculating the difference in mass (see the sample equations below) will give you a value for fluid lost in the session which can be used to give you an indication of how much fluid should be taken on after the session for rehydration. Sweat rate can be determined by measuring over an hour or correcting for this time period (see the sample equations below).[17] This is useful for understanding roughly how much fluid you lose over a given time period so that you can plan your hydration strategy ahead of a session. For example, it might be useful to know how much fluid you need to take on a big wall stint by trying to replicate the conditions and measure in this way, thus avoiding carrying too much or not enough. Ideally these measurements should be done a few times, in conditions that represent a usual session, to give an average value.

Example:

As sweat rate measurement is a fairly specialist way of calculating fluid loss, we'll use the example of an indoor climber looking to understand her fluid needs for an upcoming bouldering competition as this allows us to simplify the calculations as it can all be carefully measured in the climbing gym. In this case, she will simulate a competition round and use this to calculate her fluid requirements for her forthcoming event. Let's say she weighs 60 kilograms pre-session, and she climbs intermittently in a bouldering round for approximately 45 minutes. During the round she drinks 250 millilitres of water and does not go for a wee. Her body weight after the round is 59.4 kilograms.

Sweat loss = 0.6 + 0.25 - 0
= 0.85 l (850 ml)

In this hypothetical situation she has lost 850 millilitres of fluid during the session. This is 1.4 per cent of her body weight and so she can be reassured that, in this scenario, she is managing her hydration well. As part of her post-session hydration recovery she can aim to replace this fluid loss.

Dividing her sweat loss value by the time in hours (0.75 hours in her case) also gives her a sweat rate value of 1.1 litres per hour. So, she knows that for each hour that she competes (in the conditions that she simulated),

Sweat loss (l) =

Body weight difference (kg) + Fluid intake (l) - Urine output (l)

Sweat rate (l/hr) =

$$\frac{\text{Body weight difference (kg) + Fluid intake (l) - Urine output (l)}}{\text{Time (hrs)}}$$

Adapted from Armstrong & Casa, 2009.[17]

she needs to rehydrate by approximately 1 litre of fluids. In an ideal world, this simulation would be done a few times before an event or big climb – mimicking temperatures and expected conditions, if possible – to increase its accuracy.

Hydration in the heat

Climbing in hot environments – or strenuous crag approaches in the heat – will have an impact on hydration needs. Interestingly, hydration in the heat has such an impact on athletes that several non-climbing sporting federations have implemented heat policies that allow the competition format to be changed in order to facilitate hydration needs.[18]

Climbing, depending on the discipline and location, may not be as vulnerable to hydration issues as other sports due to the intermittent nature of effort, the seeking of cooler environments and the shorter duration of continued effort. Having said this, many competitions take place in hot environments and many crags or crag approaches can also be hot.

When in hotter conditions, it may be worth increasing your fluid intake in line with thirst, urine colour and measured sweat losses (if possible). Fluid needs in the heat are very individual but consistent for each individual when conditions are mirrored, so, for example, competition climbers could simulate the heat environment they will compete in to help them plan their hydration needs.

To give rough guidelines, the IOC consensus statement on recommendations for sporting events in the heat suggests adding 1 litre per hour for each 5 °C increase in ambient temperature above 21.5 °C, as well as a key message that athletes should aim to take on sufficient fluids before their performance window so that they start hydrated.[19] But bear in mind that these recommendations are for endurance sports, not climbing specifically. It's worth noting that when exercising for long periods in the heat, it is normal to endure some dehydration, and hydration strategies should aim to minimise these rather than completely mitigate them.

Electrolytes are a particularly important factor in the heat due to higher sodium losses. Salty sweaters are encouraged to replace sodium losses before, during and after exercise, especially in the heat.[20] As mentioned before, this could be in the form of adding salt to food and drinks, or using sports drinks with added electrolytes.

Hydration at altitude

Altitude brings additional challenges to maintaining hydration. An increased breathing rate means that there is a higher level of water loss through respiration, urine loss is higher as the kidneys work hard to maintain a normal pH in the blood, and the dry air causes an increase in sweat rate.[21]

How much more fluid is needed will, as always, depend on the individual as well as the extent of elevation. Simply knowing that needs are higher at altitude is a good starting point so that you can be mindful of the benefits of drinking more. To individualise this, measure your sweat rate on any recce climbing trips, as well as monitoring your urine colour and responding to increased thirst. For more in-depth advice or ahead of trips that involve high altitudes, it may be worth seeking the advice of a dietitian.

So, what to drink?

This will really vary depending on individual sweat rates, salt losses, and the conditions and intensity of climbing.

If your hydration needs are relatively low

– for example, cold conditions, low-intensity climbing – then simple water may suffice. If your hydration needs are higher – hotter climates, higher-intensity climbing and/or you are a heavy or salty sweater – it may be beneficial to consider adding electrolytes and some carbohydrates to your drink.

KEY TAKEAWAYS

→ Fluids have many important roles in the body and hydration levels can influence various functions that affect performance as well as health.

→ Dehydration of more than 2–3 per cent of body weight is considered detrimental to sports performance, however short-duration climbing performance (think bouldering/short routes) may be able to tolerate up to 3–5 per cent.

→ Overhydration is more likely to be an issue in longer endurance sports, but it can be very serious and it is therefore prudent to be aware of the risks.

→ Practically, hydration levels can be monitored through thirst, urine colour and sweat rate measurements, or, ideally, a combination of all three.

→ Aim to start your session hydrated; guidelines for a day (excluding exercise) are 25–35 millilitres per kilogram of body weight.

→ Drink 5–10 millilitres per kilogram of body weight approximately two hours before exercise followed by 250 millilitres per hour with adjustments for conditions such as heat and humidity.

→ Consider crag approach efforts as well as climbing when thinking about hydration.

→ Hot environments and altitude both affect hydration, and more fluids (and attention to fluid intake) may be needed.

→ Consider adding electrolytes to drinks, especially if you are a salty sweater, have a high sweat rate or are climbing in hot conditions.

WHAT CAN I DO?

→ Think about your fluid intake on a daily basis: do you meet the baseline daily requirements of 25–35 millilitres per kilogram of body weight?

→ Make an effort to start your sessions hydrated.

→ Are you a heavy sweater and/or a salty sweater? If so, consider adding electrolytes to your drinks.

→ Use some of the techniques in this chapter to monitor your fluid intake and hydration levels and see how it affects you in your sessions and in your recovery afterwards.

→ If it feels helpful, calculate your sweat rate so you have a rough idea of your needs in a given environment.

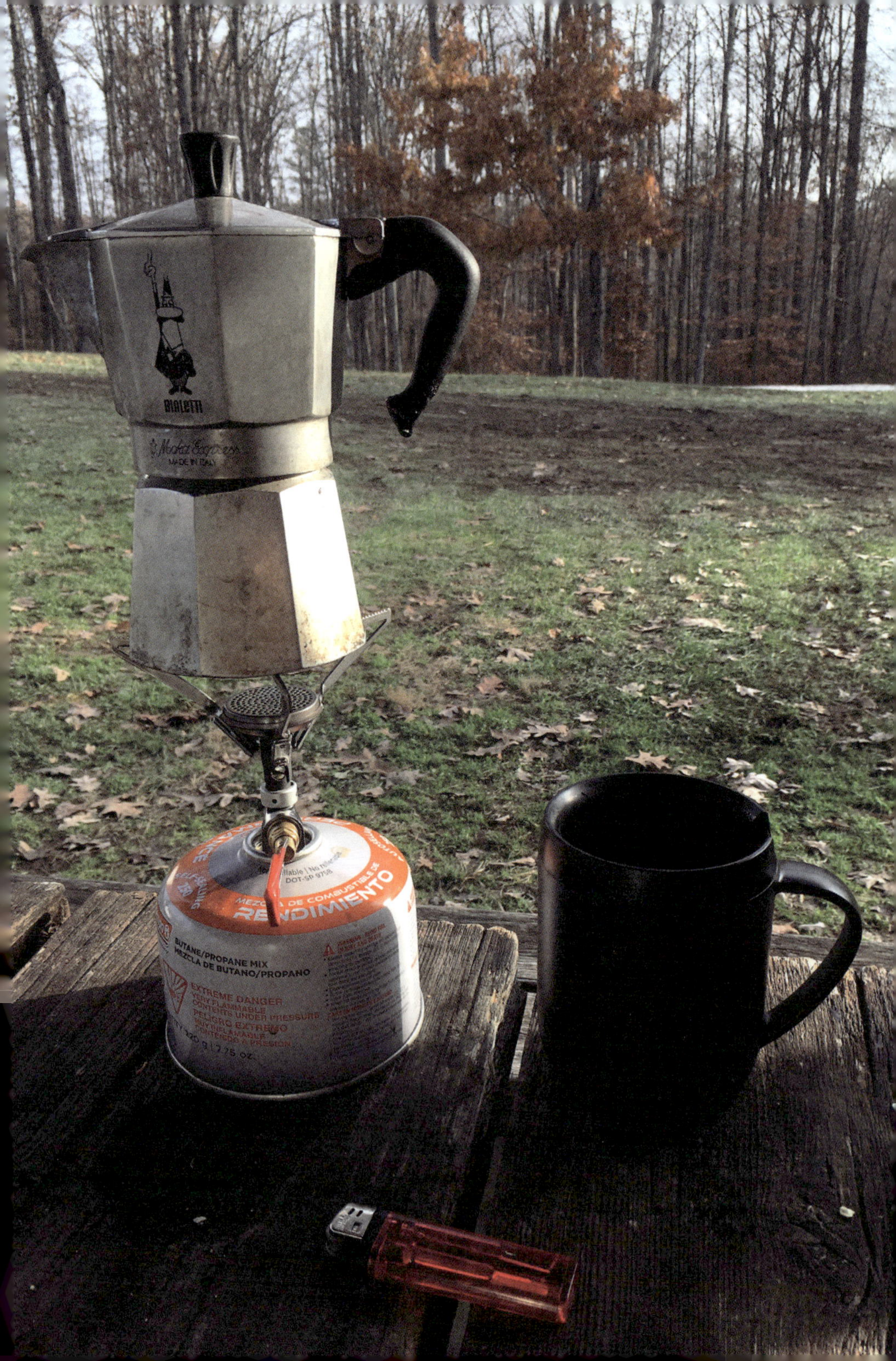

DOT-SP 9758
RENDIMIENTO
BUTANE/PROPANE MIX
MEZCLA DE BUTANO/PROPANO
EXTREME DANGER

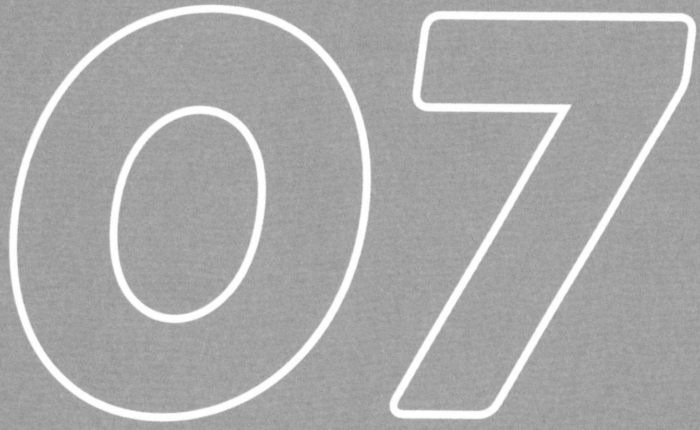

SPORTS SUPPLEMENTS

What are supplements?

A supplement is defined by the Oxford English Dictionary as, *'A thing added to something else to improve or complete it'*. In sports nutrition, it is exactly that. Supplements are additions that we may make with the intention of improving an aspect of our training, recovery or performance. While there is evidence to suggest that many supplements can give performance-enhancing effects, it is worth noting that this aspect of nutrition is really the cherry on the cake; the final thing to consider when all other boxes have been ticked. A food-first approach is the ideal, with supplements coming last as an added boost if appropriate.

Ask yourself these questions before adding a supplement:

- → Is my basic nutrition supportive already?
- → Do I have enough overall energy (calories) going in?
- → Am I eating appropriate amounts of carbohydrates, proteins and fats?
- → Do I consider the timing of my food intake around and during my sessions?
- → Do I eat a variety of colourful whole foods each day?
- → Am I hydrated and getting enough quality sleep?
- → Am I climbing or training regularly? (No amount of good nutrition or supplements will improve your climbing performance if you aren't giving your body the physical stimulus.)

If you can answer yes to the above and a supplement is being added:

- → Is the supplement **safe** to use?
- → Is the proposed benefit of the supplement supported by **scientific evidence**?

The last two questions are key. When thinking about using a supplement it is vital to know whether it is safe and, of course, beneficial to use.

In terms of safety, look out for either the **Informed Sport** logo or the **NSF Certified for Sport®** logo, or search their websites for products. This will confirm that the supplement has been tested by an independent third party and is safe to use. Safety means quality assurance, no contaminants; it means that the product is what it says on the label; and it means that there is no risk of breaking doping rules by accident if you are a competitor. All very important.

Next, is there good scientific evidence to support the use of the supplement and suggest that it will be beneficial? There are so many supplements out there with many claims about improving performance, health, aesthetics and much more, but only some have good evidence to support their use.[1] It can feel like a full-time job to sift through all the nonsense and emerge with the supplements that actually do have science backing them up.

The supplements in this chapter are those that have good evidence behind them for use either specifically in climbing or in other sports where the physiological needs are relatable.

Whey protein

Whey protein is derived from milk via a filtering process. It could be argued that whey protein is a food rather than a supplement, but it is included here for completeness as it is purchased and consumed in a similar manner to other supplements. Essentially, using whey protein can be a practical and efficient way to meet your protein targets with minimal fuss (see chapter 3).

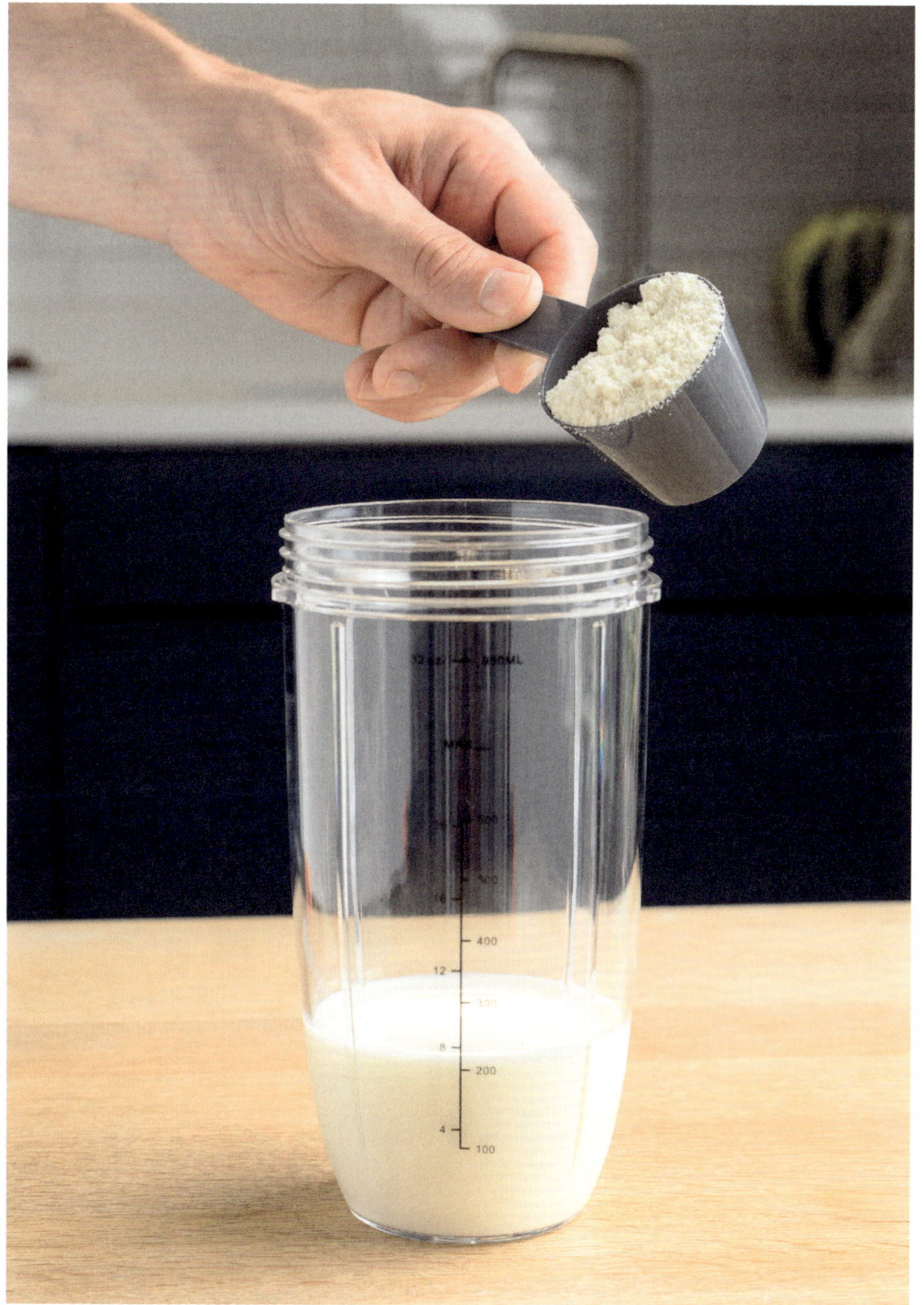

WHEY PROTEIN CAN BE A PRACTICAL, EFFICIENT WAY TO MEET PROTEIN NEEDS; ONE SERVING OF WHEY PROTEIN TYPICALLY CONTAINS 20–30 GRAMS OF PROTEIN.

Whey protein in particular is considered a gold-standard protein choice in terms of its ability to stimulate muscle protein synthesis; it contains all the essential amino acids, has a high leucine content and is easily digested.

But which whey powder, you may ask? There are different versions of whey protein on the market, including isolate, concentrate and hydrolysate. These are similar in that they have all the essential amino acids, but there are some key differences to consider.

Whey isolate: the purest (most filtered down) form of whey with a high protein content (usually above 90 per cent), low carbohydrate content and a low lactose content. This is the most expensive version.

Whey concentrate: this version is less processed/filtered so has a lower protein content per serving and a higher carbohydrate content (from lactose).

Whey hydrolysate: a pre-broken-down version of whey isolate for easier digestion.

If you are vegan or don't tolerate dairy, there are, of course, non-dairy versions such as pea, rice, hemp, soy and various blended combinations. When looking at these, consider the overall protein dose, whether it contains the full spectrum of essential amino acids and the leucine content per serving.

One downside to using whey protein – or any protein powder – is cost. Supplements like this are not cheap and using them regularly will incur costs that could be avoided by using food to meet protein needs instead. But, for many people, 'time is money', and the practical convenience and time-saving benefits make it worth the cost. Of course, there is a middle ground where protein powder is used more occasionally while food is the main source of protein the rest of the time. This also means that the benefits of whole foods – other macronutrients, micronutrients and fibre, and so on – are still gained most of the time, but in particular windows you can benefit from a quick, easily digested protein hit.

Creatine monohydrate

Creatine monohydrate is one of the most researched supplements out there and, as such, it comes with a high level of scientific backing for its use in sports performance.[2] There are also potential benefits for recovery, injury prevention and cognitive function.[3]

What does it do?

Taking a creatine monohydrate supplement increases muscle creatine stores which means more available creatine for use in the phosphocreatine (PCr) energy system (see chapter 1 for a recap on energy systems). This is the system that provides energy for repeated high-intensity muscle output. Think top-end strength and power; necessary both when climbing and when training for climbing. Alongside the immediate benefit, consider the result of being able to push harder each session on long-term training adaptations. Creatine supplementation may lead to greater lean mass as well as strength and power gains over time, provided the training stimulus is there.[4]

Despite there being limited research directly into climbing, there is some that suggests creatine could help with upper body power in climbers.[5] In addition, in his paper about nutrition for bouldering, researcher Ed Gibson-Smith highlights the evidence around creatine and the forearm which could be very relevant to the demands of climbing. In particular, the positive effect creatine showed on sustained maximal grip power as well as increased blood flow to the forearm; both of which could greatly benefit climbing performance.[6]

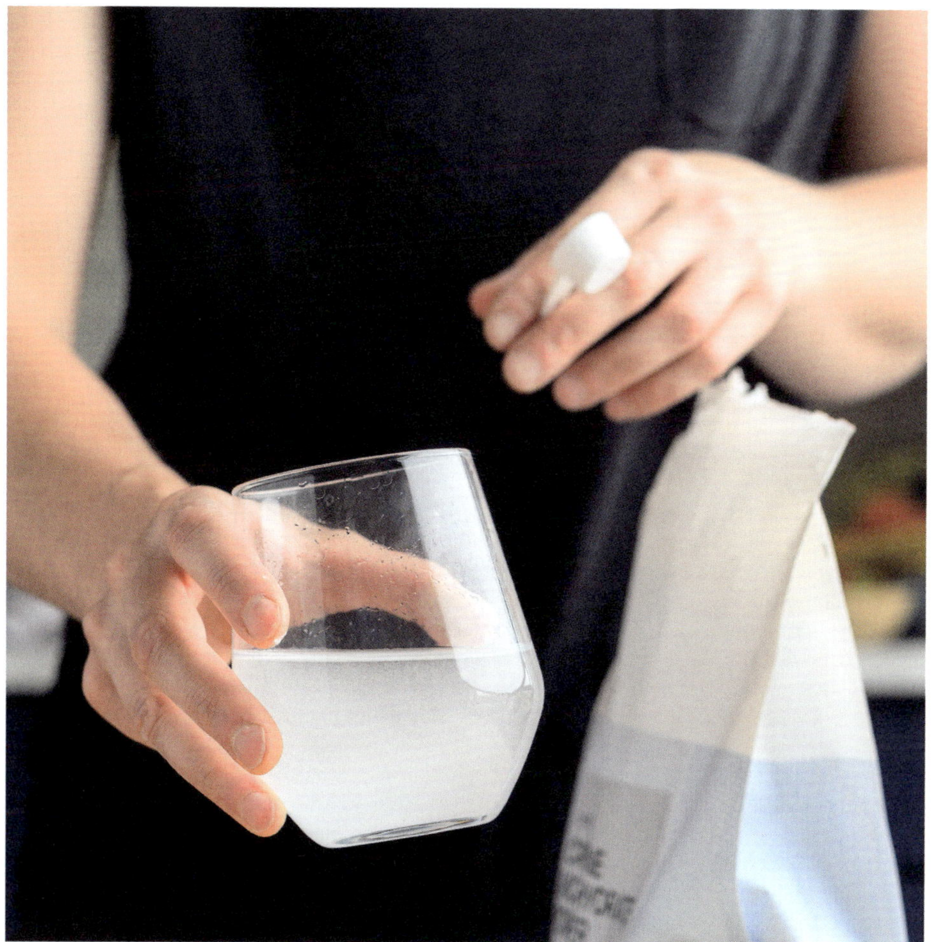

CREATINE MONOHYDRATE ENHANCES THE PCr ENERGY SYSTEM VIA INCREASED MUSCLE CREATINE STORES AND ITS POSITIVE EFFECT ON SPORTS PERFORMANCE IS WELL SUPPORTED BY RESEARCH.

There is some evidence to suggest that creatine supplementation can also help with cognitive function, especially when it is particularly challenged such as during sleep deprivation.[7] This could be a useful nugget for those climbers undertaking multi-day challenges where sleep is minimal or disrupted. Or those balancing climbing with family life – spot the mother of two! Needless to say, climbing is a very cerebral sport, so any improved cognitive function is definitely a plus.

Vegans and vegetarians are likely to be some of the highest responders to the effects of creatine supplementation. This is because foods containing creatine are predominantly meat and fish, and so vegetarians and vegans are likely to have lower baseline levels of muscle creatine stores, and therefore, will experience a greater response when it is added as a supplement.

Are there any downsides?

Something to consider on the 'cons' side of the creatine-for-climbing discussion is potential water weight gain when taking the supplement.[8] While creatine may benefit absolute strength and power, climbing is a weight-sensitive sport and so this is a justifiable consideration. Having said that, despite the idea of creatine-related water retention being widespread, the research is mixed. While there is evidence that creatine may increase water retention in shorter-term studies, there are many studies suggesting no increase to body water over longer periods of time.[9]

For most climbers, the positives gained from increased creatine stores likely outweigh the negatives of any short-term weight gain. Developing the strength side of the strength-to-weight ratio will reap greater benefits over time than trying to minimise body mass gain at any cost. After all, while water weight may feel like useless baggage, lean mass – in the right places – is certainly not. One thing to consider is that any fast weight gain from loading creatine may pose an injury risk, especially to the fingers where small weight increases can have a significant effect on connective tissue load.

Finally, while there is no research that examines the phenomenon, anecdotal reports suggest that some climbers experience increased 'pump' when supplementing creatine. This is something to look out for on a personal basis and, if experienced, perhaps consider using creatine only in phases that focus on strength and power.

How to take it

Historically, creatine was loaded at doses of 20 grams per day for five to seven days initially, but more recent discussion of research suggests that this isn't necessary.[10] As mentioned above, it may be wise anyway for climbers to use a gradual loading dose of 3–5 grams per day to protect the fingers.

Beta alanine

What does it do?

Beta alanine supplementation increases muscular stores of carnosine which, in turn, helps with intracellular buffering of hydrogen ions (the build-up of which plays a limiting role in muscle function). In real terms, this means a boost to sustained high-intensity exercise performance, delayed fatigue in muscles, reduced sense of effort and increased recovery between stints. It has shown small but positive effects in exercise lasting from 30 seconds to 10 minutes.[11]

These kinds of effects could be helpful to both climbing and training capacity for climbing as it is a sport that often requires sustained effort in these time frames. Think about long boulder problems and sustained crux sequences on routes; this is where beta alanine may help to delay the burn.

There has been one study into beta alanine alone for climbing performance specifically.[12] The researchers took fifteen elite climbers and tested their performance in three areas: a campus board exercise, a hard traverse and an easy traverse. They then gave half of them beta alanine and the other half a placebo for four weeks and then retested. The results showed a significant improvement in the campus board exercise and the easier traverse but not the hard traverse. The authors suggest that the effect of beta alanine on the hard traverse was limited by the reduced time on the wall (due to difficulty); essentially, there was not enough time for the build-up of hydrogen ions to be great enough to benefit from the increased buffering effect.

The authors went on to study the effects of beta alanine combined with sodium citrate on climbing performance where thirteen climbers were tested on two bouldering circuits ('hard' and 'easy') to exhaustion.[13]

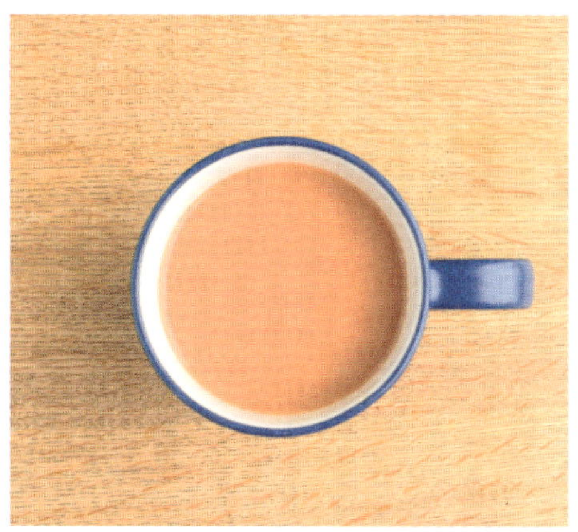

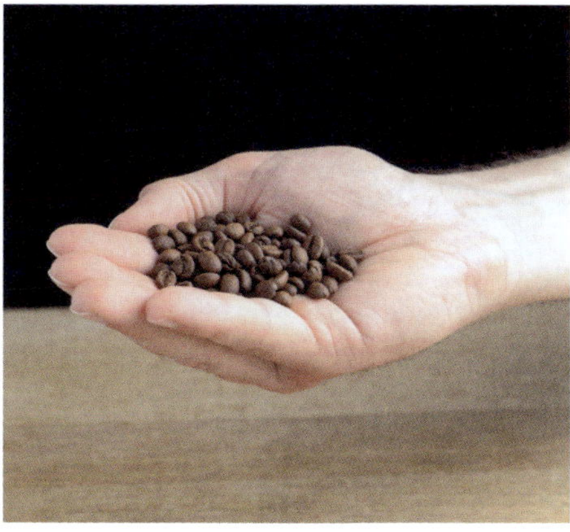

YOUR MORNING CUP OF TEA OR COFFEE MAY BE A KEY PART OF YOUR PERFORMANCE PREPARATION EVEN IF YOU DON'T REALISE IT! CAFFEINE IS A CENTRAL NERVOUS SYSTEM STIMULANT WITH EXTENSIVE RESEARCH TO SUPPORT ITS USE IN SPORT.

Climbers in the intervention group – those given beta alanine and sodium citrate together – performed better on both circuits.

While some research, as mentioned above, suggests that beta alanine will aid buffering from 30 seconds upwards, other research specifically into climbing seems to suggest 60 seconds upwards.[14] Either way, there are plenty of instances in climbing where an improvement in efforts in the 1–10 minutes range would be highly beneficial and this appears to be something that beta alanine (with potential co-ingestion of sodium citrate) can offer. Having said that, these are just two studies into climbing specifically; more research would be helpful in determining if, how much and in which scenarios beta alanine can improve climbing performance.

Are there any downsides?

Many people who take beta alanine experience a strange tingling sensation. This is harmless but nonetheless a bit weird and can be off-putting! The dose can be split up and spread over the day to reduce this. Interestingly, the researchers in the study that looked at beta alanine and climbing performance did split the dose as part of their protocol to avoid participants guessing whether they had received the intervention or the placebo.

How to take it

The general recommendation for beta alanine supplementation is 65 milligrams per kilogram of body weight split into doses over a day, for 10 to 12 weeks.[15] Although both studies that saw an improvement in climbing performance specifically were only four weeks long, so the benefits may be seen sooner.

As an example, for a climber with a body weight of 65 kilograms, the beta alanine dose would be approximately 4 grams a day in four doses of roughly 1 gram spread out evenly throughout the day. If taking sodium citrate as well, the study suggests co-ingestion of 0.6 grams a day to be effective.

Caffeine

What does it do?

Commonly found in coffee, tea, chocolate and some sports drinks, caffeine is a central nervous system stimulant with extensive research to support its use across a wide range of sports. Caffeine increases alertness, reduces perceived effort, improves muscle endurance, reduces reaction time and improves overall neuromuscular function.[16]

Again, there is little specific research into the use of caffeine in climbing, but, from looking at research in other sports, it is reasonable to suggest it would be helpful, physically and mentally. There was one study in 2013 that looked at the effect of caffeine in climbers.[17] The researchers measured pull-up power output, pull-up repetitions, hand grip and climbing time. They found that the caffeine group performed better than the placebo group in the number of pull-up repetitions and overall power output, dominant side hand grip and climbing time, but not in the single pull-up power test.

Are there any downsides?

Caffeine can cause a few issues in some people. Tolerance to it is quite varied so it is worth proceeding with caution if you are not used to using it. Caffeine can negatively affect sleep, for example. It has a half-life – the time taken to eliminate half the dose from your system – of five to seven hours, so even an afternoon coffee may, in some people, affect night-time sleep.[18] This alertness, of course, may be the exact reason it is used, but being mindful of timing is crucial. Caffeine can also cause increased heart rate, diarrhoea and a feeling of jitters; if this is you then consider having a bit less, spacing it out or not using it.[19]

Another, less-discussed, downside is the role caffeine can play in covering up symptoms of low energy availability. It's all too easy to use caffeine as a prop while not eating enough. It is crucial that energy from food is supporting any climbing and training first and foremost. If your sleep is good but you still feel like you *need* lots of caffeine to get through your sessions, consider adding more food, specifically carbohydrates, and reducing your caffeine intake gradually.

How to take it

A general recommendation in sport is 3–6 milligrams per kilogram of body weight, but lower doses may also have the desired effect.[20] It takes about 60 minutes for caffeine to have an effect. As mentioned before, responses to caffeine are very individual so it is worth starting lower and testing the water, so to speak. Bear in mind that different versions of coffee and tea have varying levels of caffeine in them and it's hard to always know exactly what you are getting. For example, with coffee this is affected by numerous things such as grams of coffee beans used per serving, type of bean and brewing style.

Nitrates

What do they do?

Nitrates are found naturally in foods such as beetroot but can also be used in concentrate as a supplement – often beetroot juice concentrate. Nitrates are converted in the body to nitric oxide which can increase the dilation of blood vessels with positive effects on blood flow, muscle oxygenation, exercise economy, muscle damage and, potentially, sporting performance.[21]

There are thousands of studies on nitrates as an ergogenic – performance-enhancing – aid with very mixed results. Some show good effects, others nothing. A recent systematic review and meta-analysis dives into this research to try and untangle what seems like a confusing area and determine if using nitrates is worth it.[22] The authors surmise that nitrates, when used effectively – correct dosage, timing, etc. – offer a clear 3 per cent performance-enhancing effect in healthy young men. Three per cent is not to be sniffed at. Women are highly underrepresented in the research on nitrates so, for now, it cannot be touted as effective for us.

But, hold your horses ... Of course, almost all this research applies to other sports. The one study that looked into climbing found no effect from nitrate supplementation.[23]

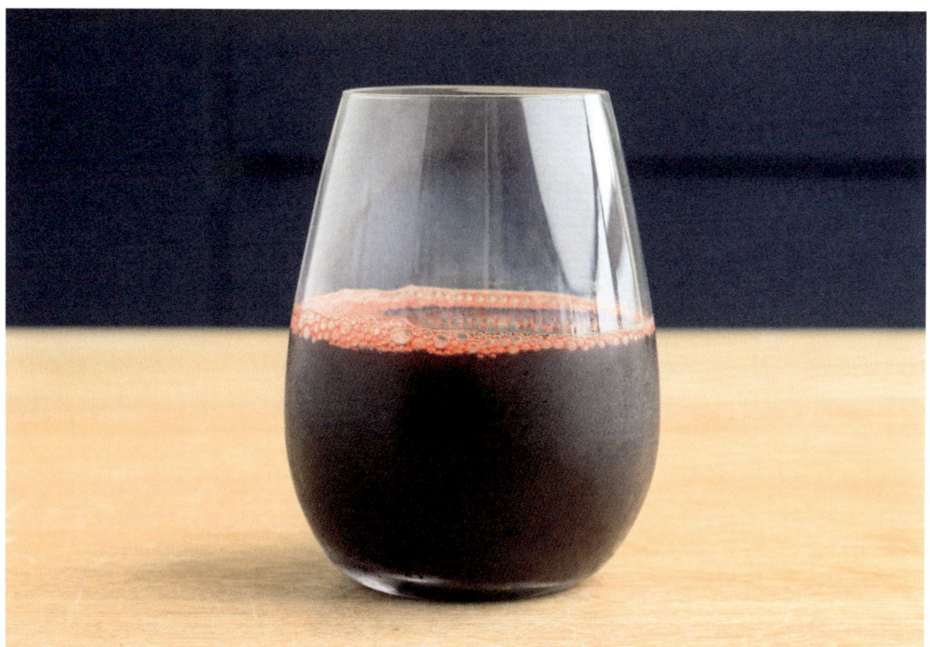

WHEN USED CORRECTLY, NITRATE SUPPLEMENTS MAY OFFER A CLEAR (AND IMPRESSIVE) 3 PER CENT PERFORMANCE-ENHANCING EFFECT FOR SOME PEOPLE, BUT THE JURY IS STILL OUT FOR CLIMBING SPECIFICALLY.

This 2023 study by Berlanga et al. looked at climbing-specific neuromuscular tests such as half crimp strength, isometric hand grip strength, pull-ups to failure, countermovement jumps and squat jumps following nitrate ingestion in male sport climbers.

So, could it be a useful supplement for climbing? The jury is still out. With broader research suggesting a positive effect, one study (with only ten participants) isn't enough to take it off the table, but we also can't yet confidently say it will help climbing performance.

Are there any downsides?

One potential downside to this supplement is that it is unclear whether antioxidants such as these may blunt or affect training adaptation when taken long-term.[24] Other than this, there aren't really any downsides, other than cost. Even so, you could choose to increase your dietary intake of nitrates via foods like beetroot and, to a slightly lesser extent, leafy green vegetables. So, unless you really don't like beetroot, there isn't too much to say about the downsides.

How to take them

According to the 2020 systematic review and meta-analysis by Senefeld et al., the most effective way to gain ergogenic effects from nitrates is with a dose anywhere from 5.1 up to approximately 25 millimoles per day, 2 to 3.5 hours before starting exercise. Take it short-term to avoid any risk of blunted training adaptation.

New Zealand blackcurrant extract

What does it do?

Many fruits contain micronutrients called polyphenols which are known to produce anti-inflammatory effects and improve vaso-dilation, blood flow and muscle oxygenation, which, in a similar way to nitrates, may produce improvements in sporting performance.[25]

New Zealand blackcurrant extract has a high polyphenol content (specifically four anthocyanins) and has shown performance-enhancing effects across a few different sports, including climbing, as well as a beneficial effect on muscle damage and recovery.[26] The study into climbing looked at pull-ups, hang time and climbing time (to exhaustion in three bouts). New Zealand blackcurrant extract had no effect on pull-ups, showed a trend for higher hang time but, most notably, had a significantly positive effect on climbing endurance.[27]

Having said this, despite showing improved muscle oxygenation to the forearm, more recent research into this supplement in climbers did not produce improvements in forearm performance.[28]

So, is it worth it? Time and more research will tell, but it's something for climbers to consider and keep an eye on the evolving research.

Are there any downsides?

Like nitrates, one potential downside to this supplement is the question mark over whether antioxidants might have a negative effect on training adaptation when taken long-term.

How to take it

Based on Potter et al.'s 2020 study into climbing performance that showed an increase in performance, climbers should take 600 milligrams a day for seven days to achieve performance effects. Take it short-term to avoid any risk of blunted training adaptation.

Collagen

What does it do?

Collagen is a key part of connective tissue found in ligaments, tendons, cartilage and bone. Exercise (loading) is known to increase collagen synthesis which, in turn, creates stiffer and denser tissues that are stronger.[29] But can supplementing one's diet with collagen – along with loading exercise – help create even stronger connective tissue or help with injury repair?

There is data to suggest that supplementing with collagen (plus vitamin C) will increase collagen synthesis, may help to reduce joint pain and functionality, and *might* help with tendinopathies.[30] Some data even suggests that vitamin-C-enriched collagen supplementation may help with rate of force development due to stiffer connective tissue offering greater force transfer, although this study was in the lower limb so it is a jump (pun intended) to extrapolate this to climbing.[31]

The research is limited and varied when it comes to the efficacy of collagen as a supplement for sports.[32] It is certainly not a panacea for all tendon-related issues and it's possible that it is totally ineffective. But, given that it comes with few downsides or risks, it could be worth thinking about during injury rehabilitation, for example.[33] Due to the high load placed on connective tissues and the prevalence of tendon injuries in climbing, it would be great to see more research on this.

Are there any downsides?

Collagen is an incomplete protein, meaning that it doesn't contain all the essential amino acids to maximise muscle protein synthesis (see chapter 3 for a recap on proteins). Don't replace habitual protein intake with just collagen as it doesn't support muscle protein synthesis (and the resulting training adaptation) as effectively as complete protein sources like whey.[34]

How to take it

Take 15 grams of collagen with 50 milligrams of vitamin C one hour before training, for three months.[35]

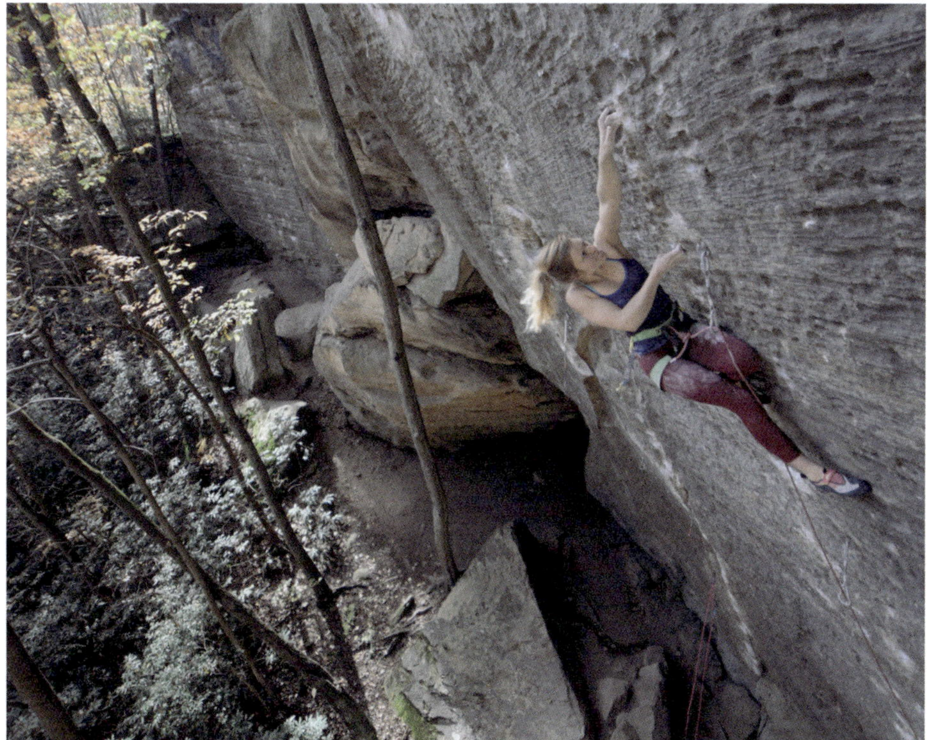

THE AUTHOR ON *LUCIFER*, RED RIVER GORGE, USA. © JAMES TURNBULL

KEY TAKEAWAYS

- Supplements may be used to further enhance performance, training or recovery.
- Before adding a supplement, consider whether the basic aspects of your nutrition and training are optimised, whether the supplement's claims are evidence based and whether it is safe to use.
- The majority of research into most supplements is not specific to climbing, however research into sports with similar demands is useful to consider.
- Supplements that may be worth considering for climbing include whey protein, creatine, beta alanine (plus sodium citrate), caffeine, nitrates, New Zealand blackcurrant extract and collagen.

WHAT CAN I DO?

- Consider the questions at the start of this chapter about whether you are meeting your basic nutrition needs.
- Think about your preferred discipline of climbing and the energy systems that are dominant for you.
- Consider which supplements from this chapter might have a beneficial effect on your training or performance and experiment with using them one at a time.

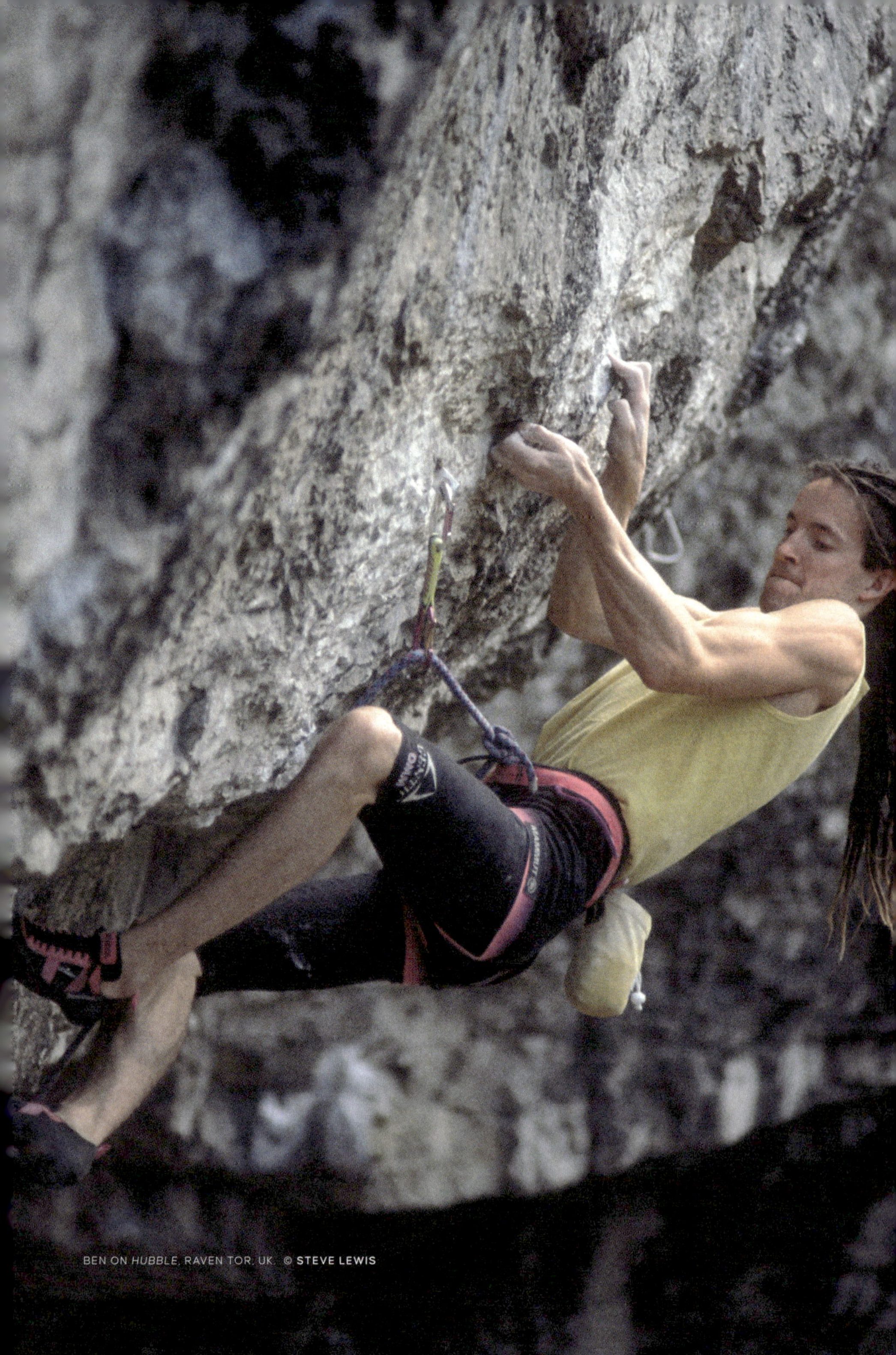

BEN ON *HUBBLE*, RAVEN TOR, UK. © **STEVE LEWIS**

BEN MOON NUTRITION OVER TIME

Ben is one of the best-known climbers in the world. In 1990, at the age of 23, he climbed *Hubble*, the world's first F9a, and 25 years later he climbed *Rainshadow* (F9a). Apart from a short gap when his daughter was young and his business was booming, Ben has been a high-performing climber for over 40 years. Here, he shares his insights and experiences with food and nutrition over time.

I moved to Sheffield in 1983 when I was 17 and started to climb full-time. Like many of my peers, I was on the dole, fully focused on climbing and trying to become a professional climber. Back then in the mid-1980s, training for climbing was booming. I lived and trained with other climbers like Jerry Moffatt, Martin Atkinson and Mark 'Zippy' Pretty; we all had a deep psyche for pushing our bodies and getting as strong as we could for climbing hard. We had all sorts of training books lying around with different approaches to try and different theories to help get us strong.

The food culture among climbers in the 1980s and 1990s was a mixed bag. I don't think much thought was given to nutrition in a supportive or performance-fuelling sense back then. It was more about being light, and, for some people on the scene, that meant eating as little as possible. I have personally always had a good relationship with food; I have a body composition that is naturally helpful for climbing and it doesn't really fluctuate much. As a result, I never felt the need to manipulate it at all, but, of course, climbing is weight dependent and many climbers wanted to be as light as they could. Needless to say, disordered eating was prevalent; people were watching their weight and counting calories. They were performing well but, of course, it's not sustainable. I knew one climber who would sometimes just eat an apple for the whole of an active day and this was seen as a win. Sensible sports nutrition hadn't yet gained traction in our culture back then. Nowadays, despite more knowledge, I think that there is still a difficult balance for climbers to strike when it comes to food and nutrition. This is especially visible in the competition world. Things have changed a lot since the 1980s and 1990s, but some of the age-old issues clearly persist.

Back then, I didn't think about how my diet and my climbing interacted as such. Apart from getting enough protein (mostly through eggs), I didn't consider what I ate as part of the picture of my performance. Having said that, I think I did have a pretty healthy food intake so maybe I was ticking the necessary boxes without realising it. I've loved cooking for as long as

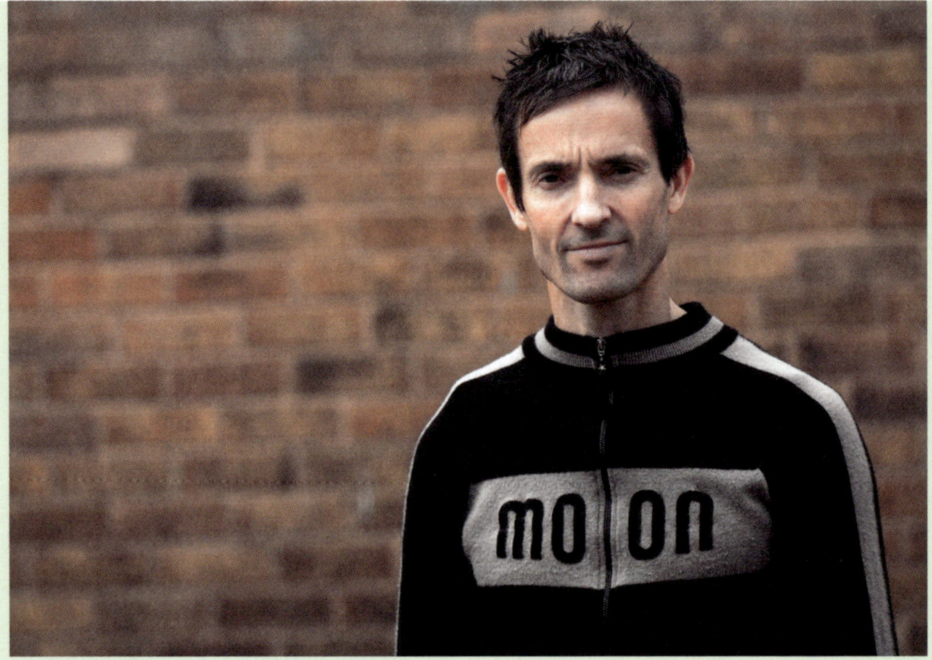

© JOHN COEFIELD

I can remember and I think that has always had a positive influence. Cooking from scratch with good, wholesome ingredients is important to me and this is something that I have always tried to do. My mother was a great cook and this must be where my love and culture of home-cooking came from.

Not long before I moved to Sheffield, my brother and I decided to become vegetarian. We had watched a documentary about abattoirs and found it pretty disturbing; it was enough to take meat off the menu for me for almost ten years. During that time, I used to cook a lot of things like lentils, pulses, wholegrain rice and eggs. I was known in my friendship circle in Sheffield for my vegetarian kedgeree; I made a lot of that. I remember in the late 1980s/early 1990s when I was competing more, I started to eat meat again but this was because of convenience rather than any nutritional goal or tactic. It was simply harder to manage abroad as a vegetarian at the time. I don't remember feeling any different when I started to eat meat again; it certainly didn't make any standout change as far as I can remember.

Fast forward to 2015 when I climbed *Rain-shadow*. One of the things I did during that time was to eat less bread. I can't remember the exact reason for it now, but I ate pancakes for breakfast so it wasn't about removing carbohydrates. I was also vegetarian again and I remember using protein shakes during that time. Who knows if those things played a role in me being able to do the route, but they were things I introduced to help me feel ready for the route and to recover as well as possible. My crag snacks were things like hummus and oatcakes, as well as home-made flapjacks that I made with molasses. Flapjacks make pretty good crag food in my mind; lots of energy, carbohydrates and sugar to keep you going. And tasty of course. It's hard to know what helped and what didn't ... but I did do the route.

As I've become older, especially in the last five years or so, I have noticed my top-end strength declining and my training has really changed to reflect that. I do more weights and board climbing

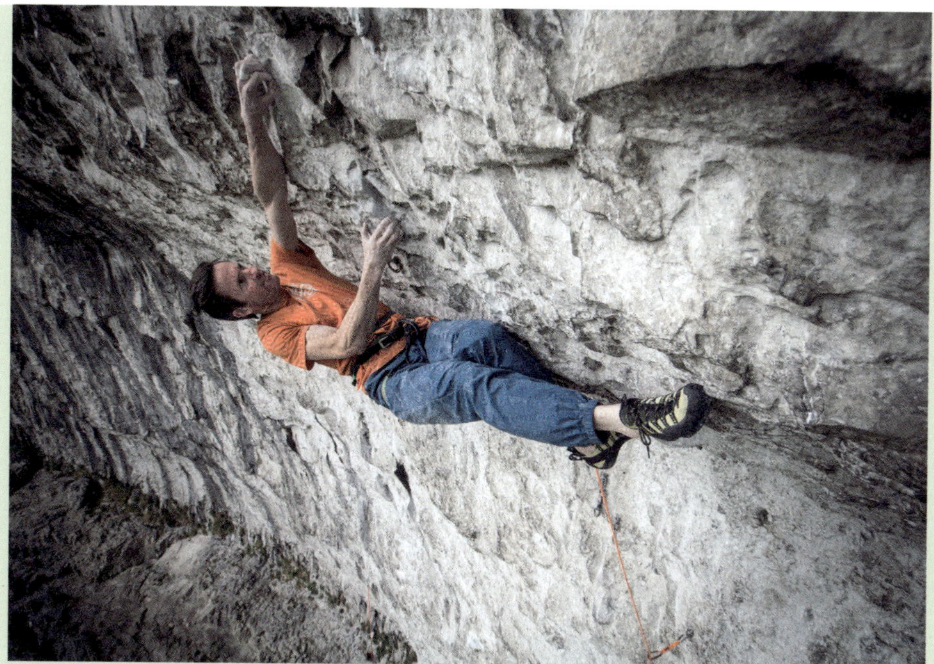

BEN ON *RAINSHADOW*, MALHAM COVE, UK. © **STEVE LEWIS**

and I try to think about getting even more protein in my diet; I've come back to the protein shakes while also trying to have bigger portions of food-based protein in meals. I'm still not really eating meat; I'm predominantly a pescetarian for environmental reasons. Nevertheless, protein is probably still the main thing I focus on as well as making sure I get enough calories overall. I eat regularly and quite a lot actually: often breakfast, a second breakfast, post-training meal and then an evening meal. This is partly because I also run a lot now, which makes me pretty hungry!

Running has taught me a lot about nutrition. I never used to eat before runs or close to climbing sessions because I thought it wouldn't make me feel good. Recently, I started to eat more before bigger runs as I was concerned about running out of energy and actually I didn't get any adverse symptoms and I felt much better for it. I've brought this across to my climbing and I often eat meals closer to climbing sessions than I ever would have in the past. Running has also taught me the importance of remembering to eat after sessions and I have tried to take that learning point over to my climbing too. The running world is very clued up on this stuff and it's interesting to step into a different sport to see how they do things. I'm 59 years old now and as time goes on I certainly see nutrition as more of a tool for climbing performance than I used to.

PART 02

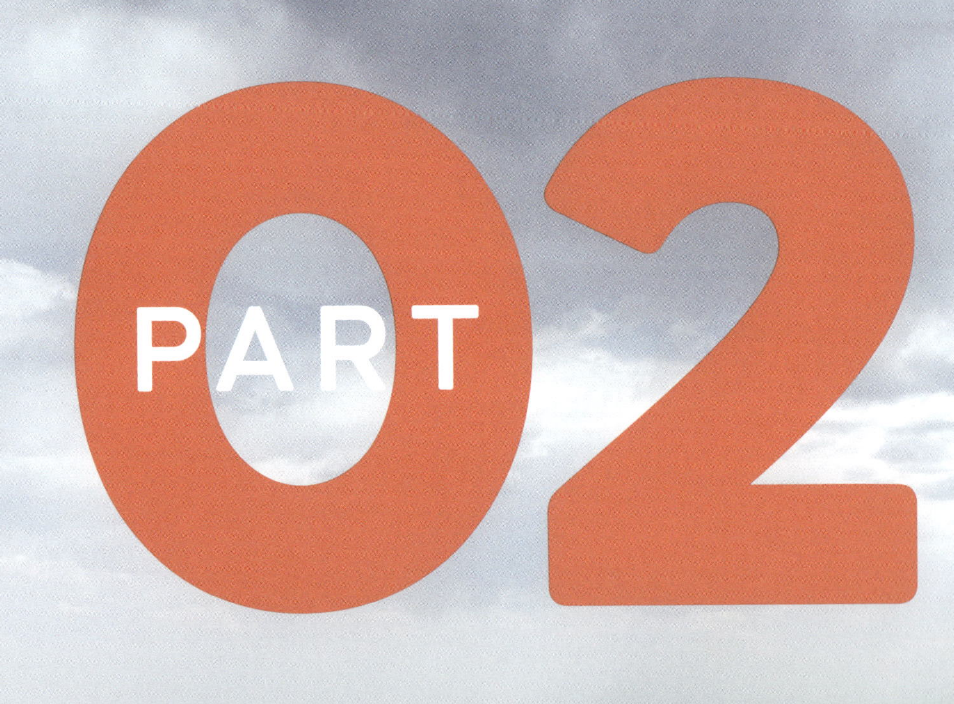

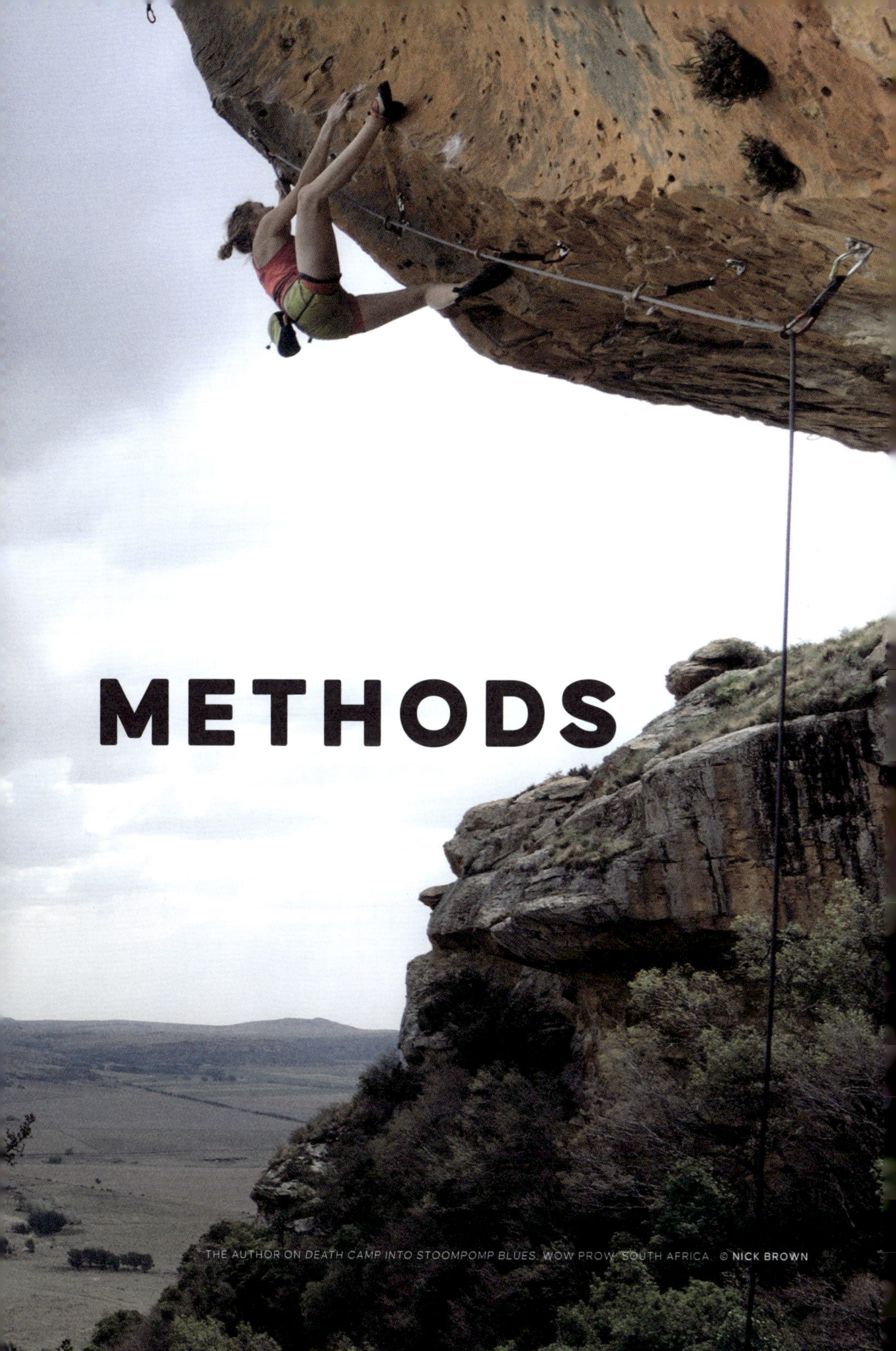

METHODS

THE AUTHOR ON *DEATH CAMP INTO STOOMPOMP BLUES*, WOW PROW, SOUTH AFRICA. © **NICK BROWN**

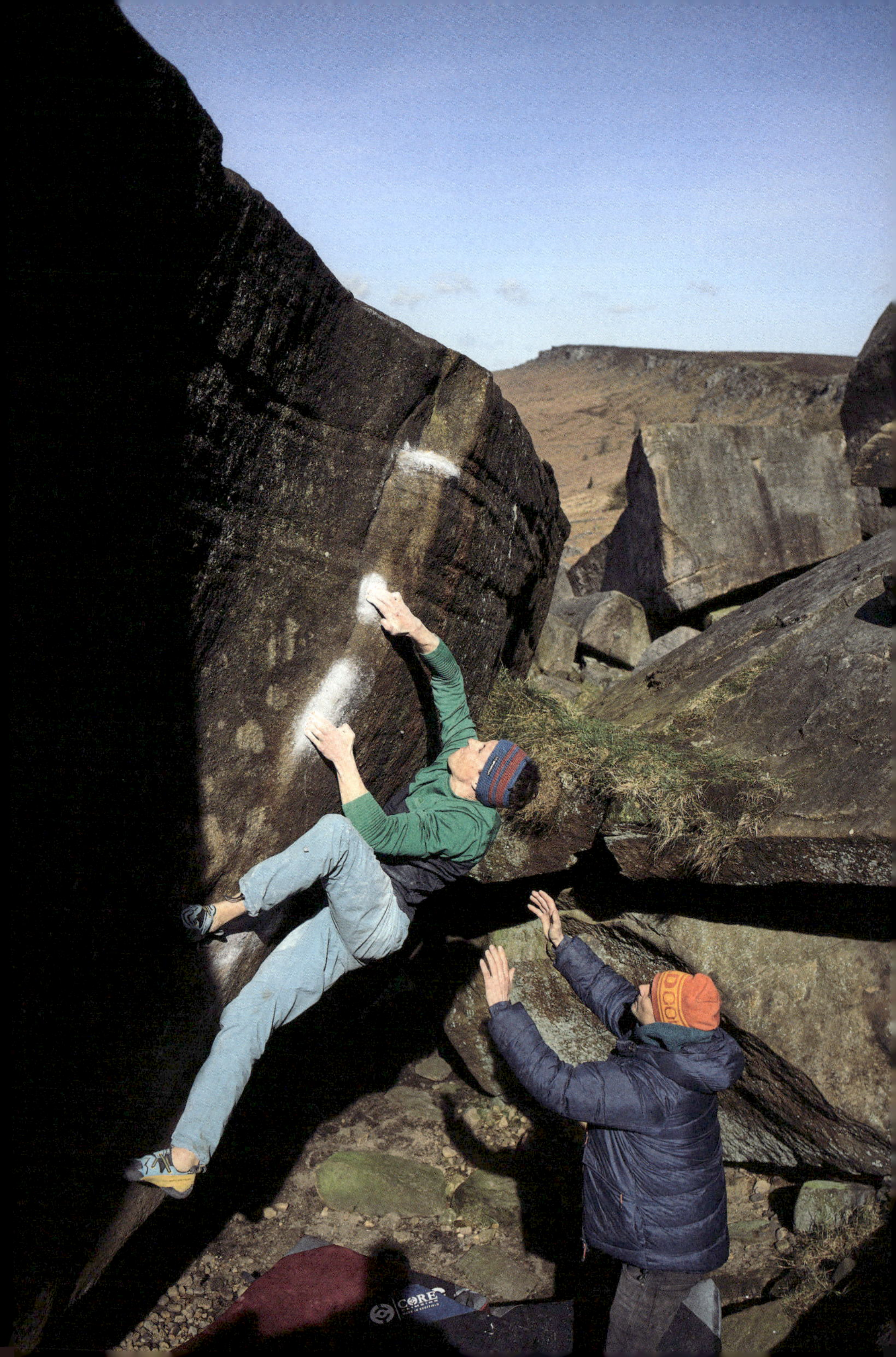

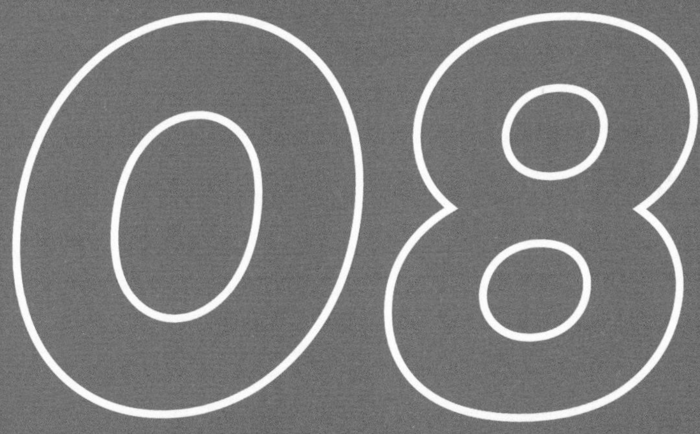

CRAG NUTRITION

FOR BOULDERING, SPORT CLIMBING, AND TRAD AND MULTI-PITCH CLIMBING

STIAN CHRISTOPHERSEN ON *BRAD PIT*, STANAGE PLANTATION, UK. © **JOHN COEFIELD**

Within climbing there are many disciplines, each with a unique set of nuances to consider when it comes to nutrition. For example, depending on the discipline, the length and intensity of effort – and therefore dominant energy system use – will vary and there will be different practical considerations to think about. This chapter will look in more depth at the practicalities of nutrition for bouldering, sport climbing, and trad and multi-pitch climbing. Understanding how to flex your nutrition strategies around practical scenarios and varying needs is crucial to implementation. At the end of the day, there is no point in perfect nutrition if it means staying at home to achieve it!

Bouldering

Bouldering sits firmly in the category of high intensity. It is a strength and power-focused discipline with some power endurance thrown in for good measure on longer boulder problems. While it is a whole body activity with input from most muscle groups, performance is often limited by the forearms which are a relatively small muscle group. This means that, while carbohydrate is very important, intake does not need to be super high to be optimal.

When we boulder outside, we remain on the ground between attempts and are therefore able to eat with more ease at times that suit our hunger and energy demands relative to rope-based disciplines. As with all types of climbing, it's important to consider the demands of the crag approach which, in some cases, can be very tough.

Key nutritional considerations for bouldering

→ Adequate carbohydrate intake (3–5 grams per kilogram of body weight) over the day.
→ Pre-session carbohydrate intake of 1 gram per kilogram of body weight, ideally one to four hours before climbing.
→ In-session snacks (if session is longer than 90 minutes) that contain at least 30 grams of carbohydrate. If sessions are longer (three to four hours), plan for multiple snacks and include some protein-based foods.
→ Post-session recovery meal that has a focus on protein (0.3 grams per kilogram of body weight) and carbohydrate (approximately 1 gram per kilogram of body weight).
→ Aim for continued protein portions of 0.3 grams per kilogram of body weight every three to four hours throughout the day.
→ When training for strength gains, a slight energy surplus may be beneficial for gaining lean mass.

Source: Smith et al., 2017.[1]

EXAMPLE DAY:
BOULDERING

7 a.m. Breakfast: porridge oats with whey protein, honey and nut butter.

9 a.m. Bouldering session starts.

10.30 a.m. Within session snack: banana and/or oatcakes.

12 p.m. Bouldering session finishes.

12.30 p.m. Lunch: wholegrain pasta with olive oil, chicken and vegetables.

3.30 p.m. Afternoon snack: protein shake and wholegrain toast with nut butter and an apple.

7 p.m. Dinner: salmon steak, wholegrain rice and vegetables.

9 p.m. Pre-bed snack: Greek yoghurt, oats, flaxseed and berries.

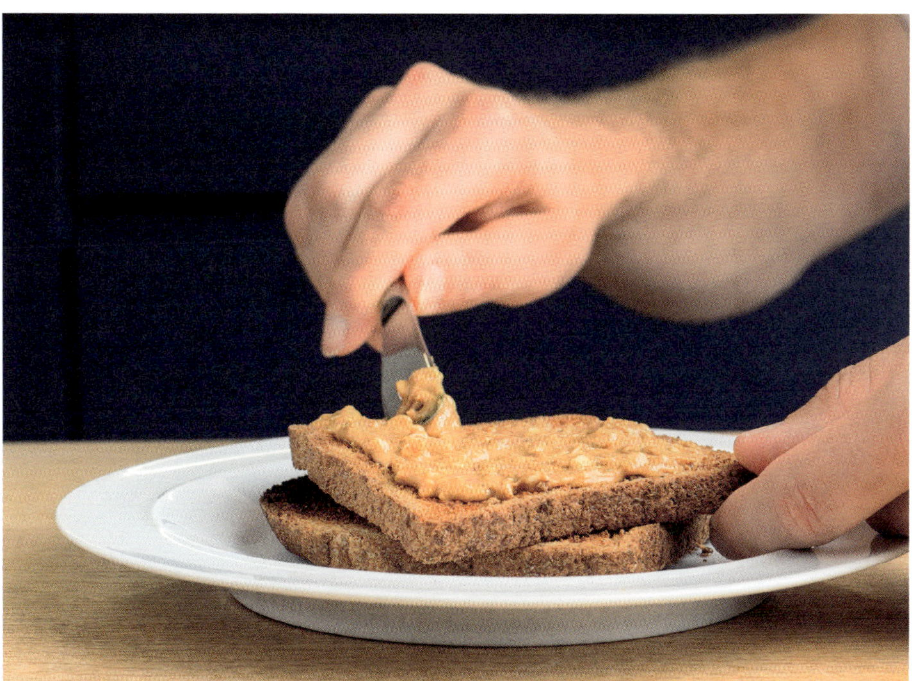

WHOLEGRAIN TOAST WITH NUT BUTTER MAKES A GREAT AFTERNOON SNACK AFTER A MORNING BOULDERING SESSION.

Sport climbing

Sport climbing is similar to bouldering in that it is high intensity and requires both strength and power. However, with sport routes being longer, sometimes up to 50 metres long, it has much more of an endurance component to it as well, both anaerobic and aerobic. This means that, again, carbohydrate is king (and queen!). While sport climbing is still often forearm limited, it relies on longer sustained efforts and often multiple attempts over a day. A higher intake of carbohydrate will benefit performance on sport climbing days so this should be your top priority.

Unlike boulderers, sport climbers will spend a lot of time on a rope. If it is a redpoint it may be quite short, but working goes or onsights can be pretty long. Plus, when back on the ground, belaying duties call, so it is a little trickier to make sure that nutrition doesn't get sidelined. Sessions are often longer too, with full days being spent at the crag. With these kinds of days, it is possible for appetite to be suppressed so it may be beneficial to do some mechanical, planned eating. This means that, for example, each hour (or thereabouts) plan on having a snack, even if you aren't super hungry. This is something to experiment with over time.

As with bouldering, consider the added demands of the walk-in. For example, the uphill walk-in to Céüse in France can take the best part of an hour.

Key nutritional considerations for sport climbing

- Adequate carbohydrate (5–7 grams per kilogram of body weight) over the day.[2]
- Pre-session carbohydrate intake of 1 gram per kilogram of body weight, ideally one to four hours before climbing.
- In-session snacks every one to two hours that contain 30–60 grams of carbohydrate.

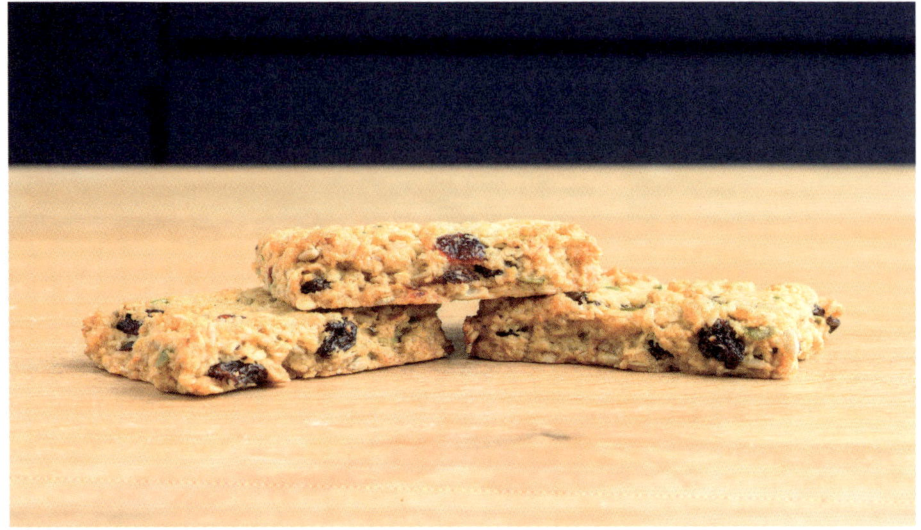

FLAPJACKS ARE GREAT CRAG FOOD: PLENTY OF FAST-ACTING AND SLOWER-RELEASE CARBOHYDRATE, EASY TO CARRY AND TASTY!

- Plan for multiple snacks throughout the day and include some protein-based foods, such as nuts.
- If a 'lunchtime meal' is preferred, consider grazing on it over the day rather than having one bigger meal.
- Think of this as drip-feeding your system throughout the day: try to have something to continually top up with whenever you get the chance, for example in between your time on the rope and belaying duties.
- Consider lower-fibre foods during the climbing day to reduce the load on your digestive system.
- Maintain hydration by drinking often and monitoring urine colour; add electrolytes if needed.
- Eat a post-session recovery meal that has a focus on protein (0.3 grams per kilogram of body weight) and carbohydrate (approximately 1–1.5 grams per kilogram of body weight).
- If time allows in the day, have an additional recovery snack with 0.3 grams of protein per kilogram of body weight before bed, two to four hours after the initial recovery meal.

EXAMPLE DAY:
SPORT CLIMBING

7 a.m. Breakfast: banana pancakes made with eggs, banana and flour, and berries (see page 157).

10 a.m. Snack: oats and Greek yoghurt with peanut butter.

11.30 a.m. Lunch: rice and tuna mix.

1 p.m. Sport climbing session starts. Drip-feed snacks as able between climbing/belaying, at least every 90 minutes; more often if hungry. Times below are examples.

1.30 p.m. Snack: oatcakes.

3 p.m. Snack: energy bar and a handful of nuts.

4.30 p.m. Snack: wrap with chicken and avocado.

6 p.m. Snack: oatcakes.

7 p.m. Snack: banana and a handful of nuts.

8 p.m. Sport climbing session finishes. Whey protein shake.

9 p.m. Dinner: lentil curry with vegetables and wholegrain rice.

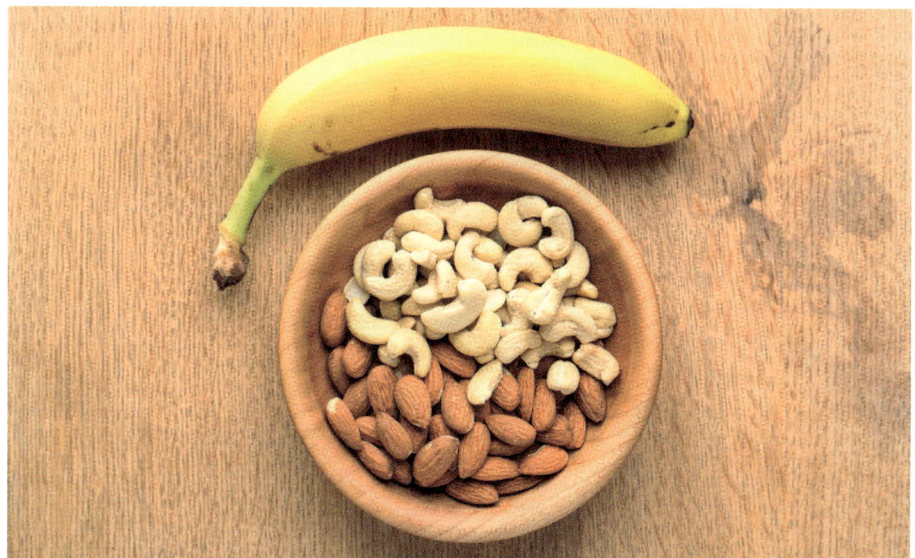

BANANAS ARE A GREAT SOURCE OF CARBOHYDRATE WITH A MEDIUM BANANA OFFERING APPROXIMATELY 30 GRAMS – JUST DON'T LET IT GET SQUISHED IN YOUR BAG!

Trad and multi-pitch climbing

Trad and multi-pitch days can be long days, or even multiple days if you're sleeping on a wall. This kind of climbing can be a mix of high-intensity efforts and endurance on harder pitches, as well as day endurance for multiple consecutive pitches of varying intensity. Again, carbohydrate availability is key for those harder pushes when higher-intensity work is needed. For the lower-intensity parts of the day, the body can utilise fat and/or carbohydrate as fuel.

Multi-pitch nutrition in particular is all about practicality as *everything* that you will eat needs to be carried and accessible. Long days require a drip-feed approach to eating so that you don't suddenly find yourself hungry and burnt out halfway through. Consider snacks that are very portable, have high energy density and that you enjoy eating. Try to remember to eat a little of something each hour or so to keep your energy topped up. Snacks can be a combination of carbohydrate, fat and protein, but try to avoid higher fibre to ease the load on your digestive system. It may be worth having a high-carbohydrate day the day before – i.e. carbohydrate loading – to ensure that you have optimised your glycogen stores. As always, don't forget to consider the demands of the approach.

Key nutritional considerations for trad and multi-pitch climbing

- → Consider carbohydrate loading in the days before a big day (see page 24).
- → Adequate carbohydrate (5–7 grams per kilogram of body weight – or more if able) over the day.
- → Pre-session carbohydrate intake of at least 1 gram per kilogram of body weight, ideally one to four hours before climbing.
- → In-session snacks every one to two hours that contain 30–60 grams of carbohydrate; think about portable, high-energy foods such as sweets, bars or bananas.
- → As with sport climbing, you may take a 'lunch meal', but split it over a few snack breaks.
- → Plan for multiple snacks throughout the day and include some protein-based foods, such as nuts.

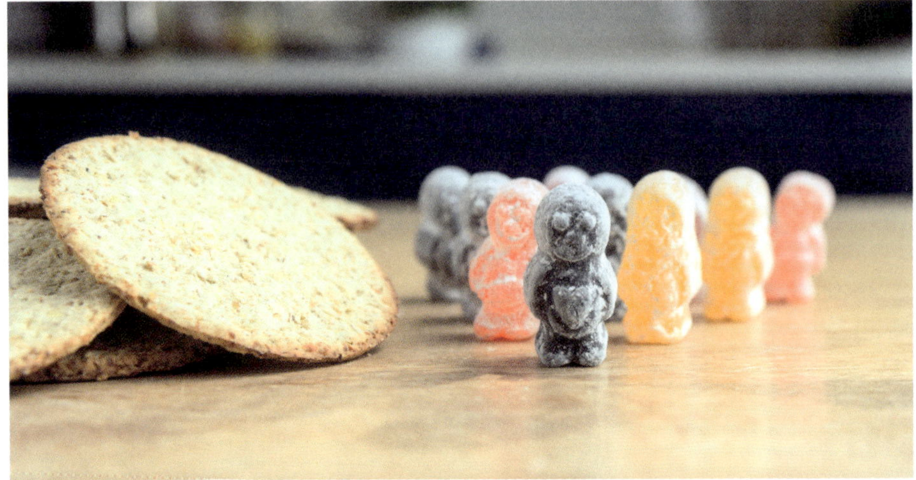

THE BEST FOODS FOR QUICK ENERGY AREN'T ALWAYS THE 'HEALTHIEST'. KEEP AN OPEN MIND WHEN IT COMES TO PERFORMANCE FUEL.

- Think of this as drip-feeding your system throughout the day: try to have something to continually top up with whenever you get the chance, for example at a belay.
- Consider lower-fibre foods during the climbing day to reduce the load on your digestive system and allow for higher carbohydrate intake.
- Pick foods that you like and which are easy to carry – keep it simple.
- Maintain hydration by drinking often and monitoring urine colour; electrolytes are a good idea for longer days such as these. Adding juice or having a carbohydrate-based drink can be a good way to get extra energy in.
- Eat a post-session recovery meal that has a focus on protein (0.3 grams per kilogram of body weight) and carbohydrate (approximately 1–1.5 grams per kilogram of body weight).
- If time allows in the day, have an additional recovery snack with 0.3 grams of protein per kilogram of body weight before bed, two to four hours after the initial recovery meal.

EXAMPLE DAY:
TRAD/MULTI-PITCH

6 a.m. Breakfast: porridge (can be instant if needed) with nut butter.

7 a.m. Trad/multi-pitch day starts. Drip-feed snacks as able between climbing/belaying, at least every 90 minutes; more often if hungry. Times below are examples.

8 a.m. Snack (after walk-in): bar and a handful of nuts.

9.30 a.m. Snack: oatcakes and some jelly babies.

11 a.m. Snack: peanut butter and jam sandwich.

12.30 p.m. Snack: protein bar.

2 p.m. Snack: oatcakes and some jelly babies.

3.30 p.m. Snack: peanut butter and jam sandwich.

5 p.m. Snack: bar and a handful of nuts.

6 p.m. Trad/multi-pitch day finishes. Whey protein shake or bar.

7.30 p.m. Dinner: spaghetti bolognese with cheese (or freeze-dried meal if multi-day adventure).

9 p.m. Pre-bed snack (if single-day outing): Greek yoghurt, oats, flaxseed and berries.

Altitude

Of course, all of these climbing disciplines could be performed at sea level or at altitude. Altitude has systemic effects on the body: increases in sympathetic nervous system activation, and higher respiratory rate, cardiac output, blood pressure and heart rate.[3] This is all to do with reduced oxygen availability and the body's response to acute and/or chronic hypoxia.

The intensity of this effect depends on the level of altitude: 500–2,000 metres above sea level is considered low altitude; 2,000–3,000 metres as moderate; 3,000–5,500 metres as high; and over 5,500 metres as extreme.[4]

Of course, a key part of managing altitude is appropriate acclimatisation, but there are added considerations for nutrition and hydration (for hydration considerations see page 68). If you are planning for a particular trip which involves climbing at altitude, consulting a dietitian may be wise.

Key nutritional considerations at altitude

- A key part of nutrition at altitude is managing energy intake to minimise negative energy balances and associated weight loss.[5]
- Carbohydrate is the preferred fuel source at altitude due to a shift in respiratory exchange rate and as such, carbohydrate intake should be prioritised to meet these needs.[6]
- Exact amounts of carbohydrate depend on altitude level and intensity of exercise, but research suggests that it could be up to 80 per cent of intake.[7]
- Ideally, protein intake should not drop below 1.3 grams per kilogram of body weight to protect against muscle mass loss.
- Fluid needs are higher at altitude.
- Ensure iron levels are replete before starting a trip involving altitude and consider supplementation during the trip (consult a dietitian for advice on this).
- Focus on eating antioxidant-rich foods during a trip at altitude rather than taking supplements.[8]

KEY TAKEAWAYS

- Different disciplines within climbing require different nutritional approaches due to varying demands such as length and intensity of effort and practicalities.
- Flexibility in approach is key to success; it doesn't need to be perfect.
- Bouldering is higher intensity, with usually shorter sessions with higher food availability (because you are on the ground more).
- Sport climbing is more endurance based with high-intensity sections. Practicalities include managing intake around time on the rope and belaying duties.
- Multi-pitch climbing is the most endurance based of the three but can also have very high intensity demands at times. Practically, it is also the most demanding as the climber must carry all their food and water.
- With all disciplines, don't forget to consider the demands of the approach – this can be draining and require extra energy and carbohydrates.
- Altitude brings another layer of complexity to any climbing day with implications for energy intake, carbohydrate intake, hydration and potentially iron levels.

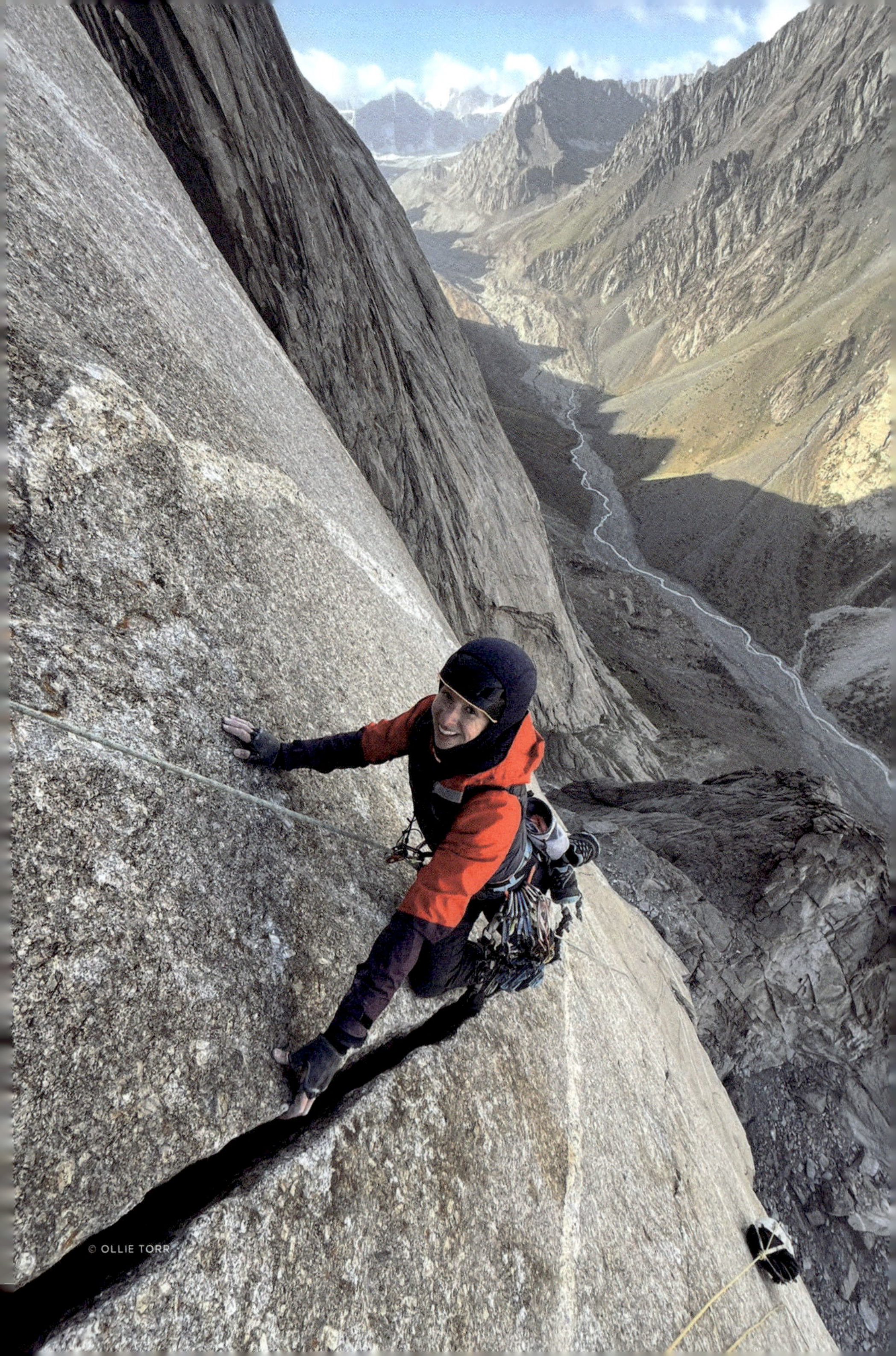
© OLLIE TORR

MADDY COPE
ADVENTURES IN KYRGYZSTAN

Maddy is an experienced and accomplished climber with many hard sport and trad ascents to her name. In 2024, she went on a month-long climbing trip with her partner Ollie to the notorious granite walls that are deep in the Karavshin Valley of Kyrgyzstan. Here, she shares her experience with food and nutrition on their adventure.

Our climbing trip to Kyrgyzstan was different to anything Ollie and I had done before. It took planning on a whole new level, and it gave us an unrivalled experience of true wilderness. The climbing in Kyrgyzstan is often referred to as a 'Russian Yosemite', but, in my experience, it was starkly different. The huge multi-pitch granite walls, a mixture of single- and multi-day climbs, were among the most stunning I have seen and climbed on, but, unlike Yosemite, they also had a remoteness that created a very different kind of adventure. This made logistics much more complex as the topos were few and far between, any amenities like shops were multiple days' travel away and the sense of isolation on the walls was far more intense.

To get to Kyrgyzstan, we flew to Istanbul and then on to Osh. From Osh, we drove for a couple of days on increasingly off-road terrain through military zones and checkpoints before we left the jeeps and walked with horses (to carry our bags) for eight and a half hours. This got us to base camp, at an altitude of about 3,000 metres in the Kara-su Valley. From base camp, most of the climbing was one to four hours' walking away, with climbing summits in the 4,000-metre range. We did a mixture of day trips, some trips where we slept the night before at the base of the climb to maximise daylight hours, and then some multi-day trips where we slept on the wall.

Food was interesting. We were in a large group and the most efficient way to manage food for us – and many people who travel to this valley – was to hire a cook. This was done as part of a package through our 'fixer' who arranged lots of things for us from border permits to transport. The cook provided meals each day and we let them know in advance which meals we would be at base camp for and when we would be away climbing and not need the provision. We had no control over the food or the nutritional components of it.

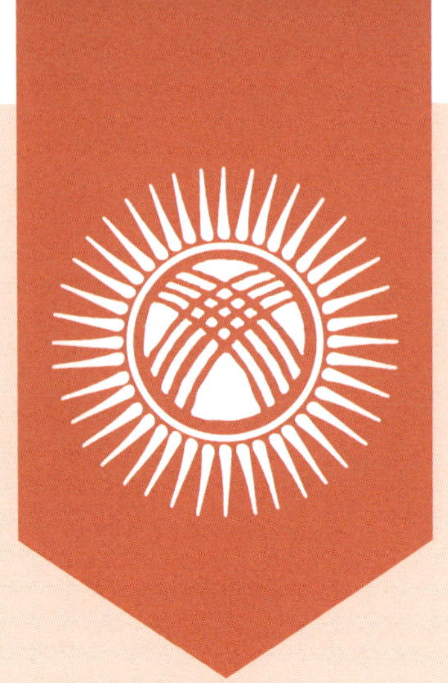

The food was predominantly meat-based stews with plenty of cabbage. Getting enough fibre and protein was not an issue! I usually eat – and feel good from eating – lots of carbohydrate, especially around my climbing, and this felt a little lacking for me in the main meals. Alongside the main meal there were always plenty of sweet treats like wafer-type biscuits, chocolates and Nutella to snack on, and this is probably where I made up my carbohydrate intake, albeit in the form of refined sugar.

In the valley there were freshwater springs and this was where we got our drinking water. We treated the water using a filter pump to minimise the chance of getting ill (other people used things like tablets). On climbing days, we usually took five to six litres with us for a 24-hour period, which probably wasn't enough given the altitude and the heat on some days, but, as any big wall climber will know, it's a balance between what you need and what you can carry and haul. We had some really cold days too and on these I found it particularly hard to drink enough. One of my top tips is to always carry a chapstick as dehydration feels worse with cracked lips!

The meals provided by our cook were not super easy to transport or take on a wall, so we decided to opt for our own snacks and meals that we had brought from the UK on climbing days that took us away from base camp. Breakfast was always the same: it had to include a cup of English tea of course, and we opted for a pack of sweet ginger oatcakes each – basic, but they go down well dipped in tea.

After many years of climbing I have learned that, for me, eating on multi-pitch climbs has to be both mechanical and logistically easy. There is no point having a bagel with me if it's at the bottom of my bag and I can't reach it easily; it will just sit there as I get more and more hangry. Belays are a busy time and place; lots of sorting of ropes and gear. I need my food to be easily accessible as well as quick and simple to eat. I also know from past experience that I need to eat regularly regardless of hunger, otherwise I find myself losing focus, feeling emotional (*hello, big wall tears!*) and not functioning very well overall. So, for me, bars are the perfect answer once the climbing has started. We took a mixture of CLIF bars and Chia bars and we each consumed between four and six over a climbing day. They may be a bit boring to eat after a while, but this was outweighed by ease, convenience and calorie density. They fitted nicely into my jacket breast pocket so, at a busy belay, it was a simple task to eat. Don't get me wrong, it's a lot of bars and, by the end of the trip, I was ready to not look at one for a long time, but they served a really good purpose. We also had backup snacks of sweets, trail mix and the like, but I knew from past experience that surviving on just those wasn't ideal for me. They worked as a morale boost when we needed them. I know many people take more 'real food' options and make it work – everyone's a little different in their approach to these things.

In the evenings away from base camp we used freeze-dried meals that we had brought with us. Not only are these calorie dense and light to carry, they are warm, which is important to me at the end of a climbing day. I know many climbers who wouldn't take a Jetboil with them on a wall, but, for me, the morning tea and the evening hot meal

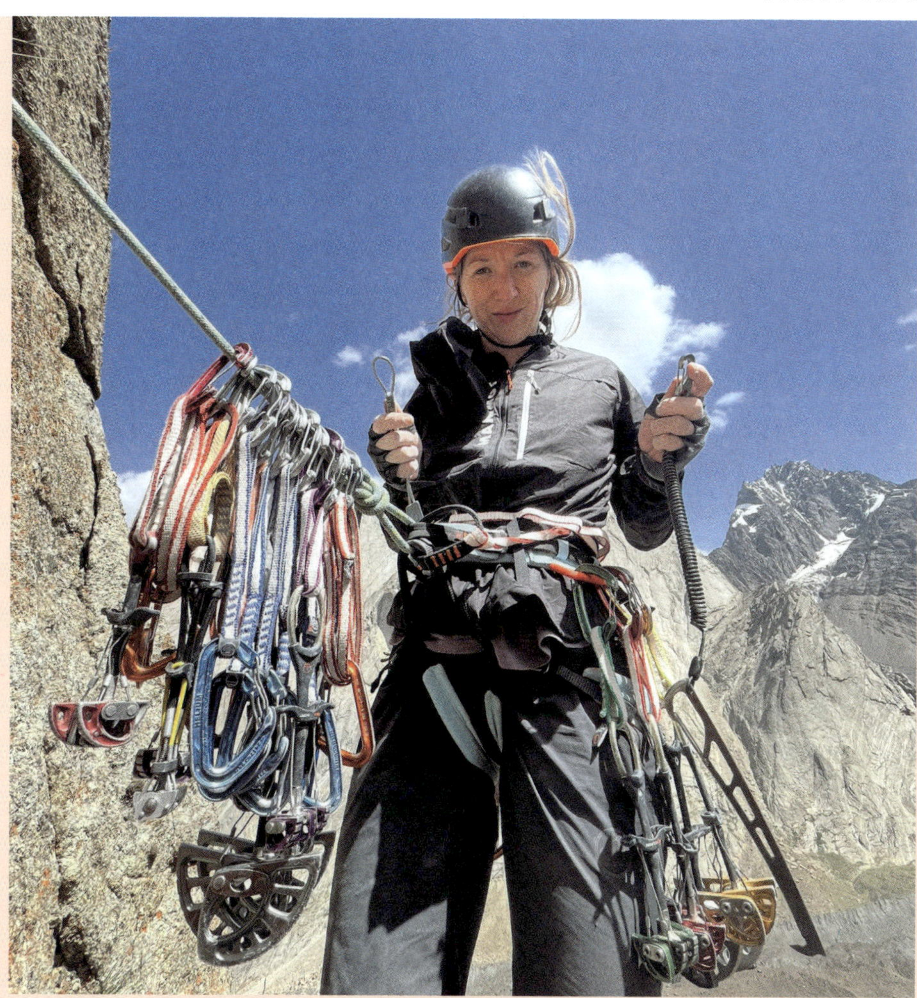

© OLLIE TORR

are key components for maintaining my sanity.

Did we get enough food in to support us nutritionally given the high output and conditions? Probably not quite, but we minimised the deficit as much as we could. Climbing days are busy, it's logistically hard to eat enough and you also need to carry it all. Over the month-long trip I lost two kilos and, despite the fact that I am already lean, this didn't seem to upset my body too much. My period arrived on time which I use as a marker for how well my body is coping with stress and overall load. Interestingly, I also didn't feel too tired after this trip – as I have on other trips – and I think this was down to a dramatically decreased overall allostatic load. Yes, we were hiking and climbing, hauling and carrying a lot, but we weren't working, and we weren't looking at screens or dealing with life admin. The headspace and interaction with a truly beautiful and wild place definitely did me good. But I was glad to eat something that wasn't meat stew or a bar when we got home!

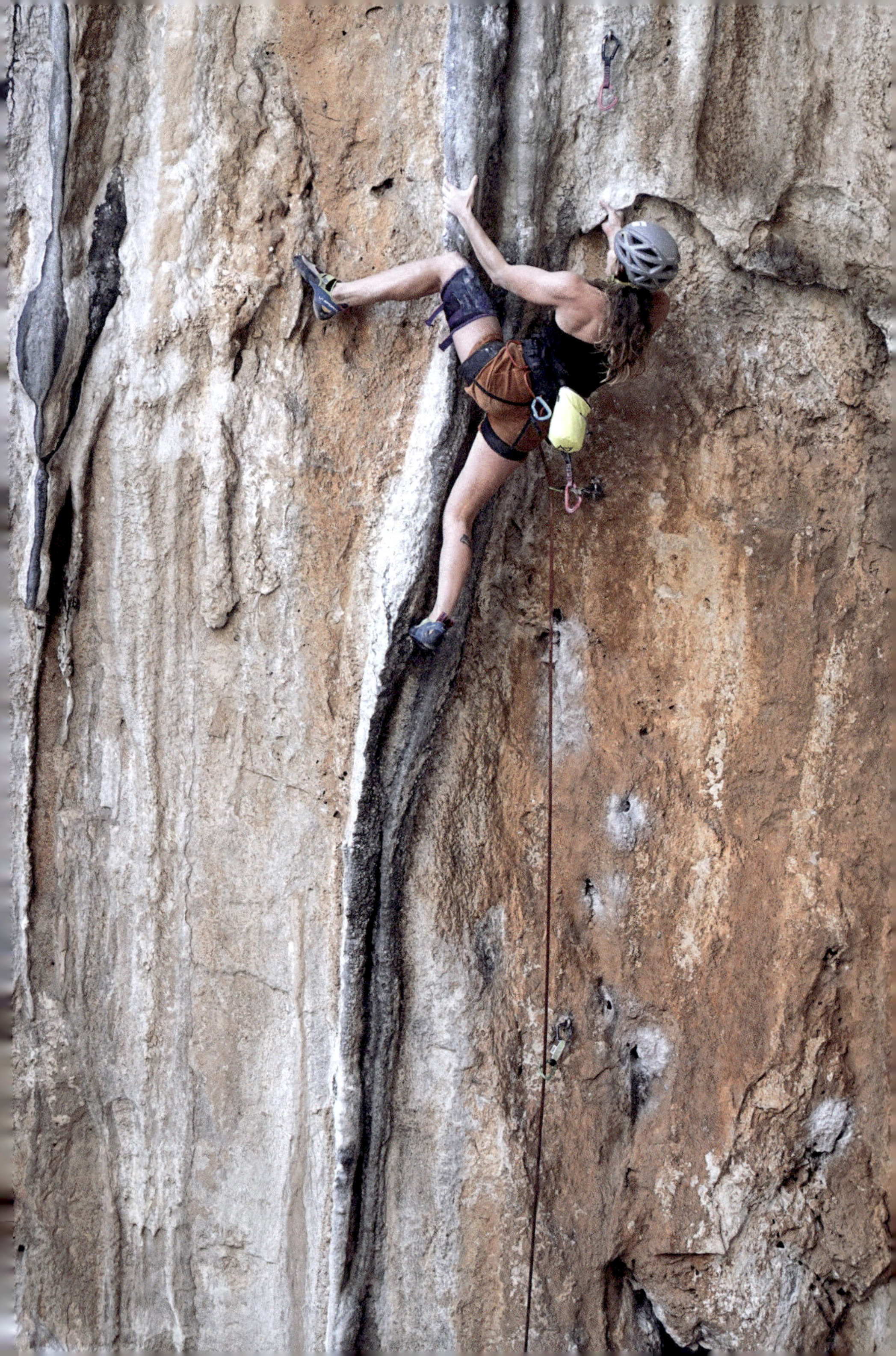

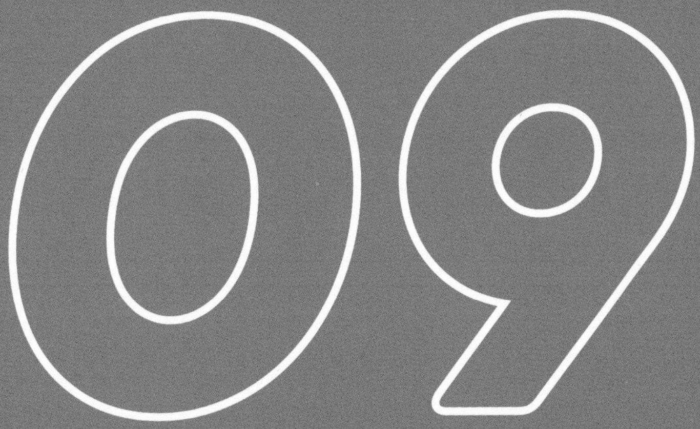

THE FEMALE CLIMBER

SHOULD WOMEN EAT DIFFERENTLY?

ALISON KAPLAN ON *RÜZGAR*, DATCA, TURKEY © **KEITH SHARPLES**

As female participation in climbing grows and flourishes, it begs the question: *Should women climbers be training and eating differently?* Female athletes have a lot to potentially contend with: monthly periods, possible contraceptive use, pregnancy, breastfeeding, perimenopause and menopause. All these life stages bring physiological changes that may affect climbing, training and nutrition. So, how and when should women take a different approach?

The short answer is that we don't yet have a full comprehensive picture of how being female affects exercise performance or what a different nutritional approach might look like and how this might vary from woman to woman. This is still a big grey area; more research is needed before any firm conclusions can be drawn.

That isn't to say that, if you are female, everything you have read so far in this book should be disregarded. Not at all. The basics like adequate energy intake, macronutrients, micronutrients and hydration are still key, and actually getting these foundations right should be your priority before anything more specific is done. Once the basics are working optimally, there may be some nuances to consider on an individual level, based on what is currently understood about female hormones and how they interact with exercise and nutrition. One thing we do know for certain is that women have vastly different experiences in all the above mentioned life stages and, therefore, an athlete-specific approach is currently the safest and most evidence-supported way to go.

Exercise and nutrition research in women

Female athletes are still significantly under-represented in sport and nutritional science research, and it is unknown whether the data that exists for men can – or should – be extrapolated out to women.[1] If something hasn't been tested on women, can the results really be applied to them in the same way? Female physiology affects exercise metabolism, thermoregulation, body composition, fatig-ability, recovery and therefore likely nutritional needs too, but there is not a set of guidelines that is appropriate for all women given the huge interpersonal variation and the limited research of varying quality.[2]

There is not much direct research when it comes to women in climbing, let alone nutrition research specific to female climbers. Up until 2020, climbing nutrition research either exclusively studied males or did not state the sex of the participants.[3] Since 2020, two papers have included women when studying the dietary intake of elite climbers, and another, by Giles et al., has looked specifically at the body anthropometrics and performance characteristics of female climbers.[4]

Review papers can be really useful in trying to understand new areas of interest

For simplicity and clarity in reading, the terms 'women', 'female' and 'she/her' will be used in this chapter. However, the author and publisher recognise that gender and sex are different entities, that not all individuals identifying as women are biologically female, not all biological females identify as women and that many people who have periods may identify as non-binary or male. The information in this chapter is aimed at any person who finds it useful to their or another person's climbing, regardless of gender or sex.

where information is sparse by connecting the research at any given intersection, for example the physiological demands of climbing and athlete nutrition. There are two review papers that discuss the nutritional demands for climbing in this way, however neither of these has any specific considerations for female climbers beyond highlighting an increased risk for negative consequences of low energy availability.[5] In 2024, I tried to bridge the gap between female athlete nutrition and climbing nutrition by conducting a review into these areas and where they intersect.[6] The review looked at research on female athlete physiology, exercise and nutrition, and combined it with climbing physiology research and nutrition research that exists in climbing and comparable sports. While this paper is not a 'fix all' set of guidelines for women in climbing, it does offer a resource to better understand some of the considerations that female climbers may benefit from.

The best way forward at the moment is to work on an individual basis with an awareness of current scientific information on female physiology, exercise and nutrition, and how these things *may* have an effect. Taking into account life stage, symptoms, training history and preferences will help to build nutritional habits that work for an individual. In this context, the following sections will discuss nutritional considerations during specific periods of the female lifespan and how these may be overlaid on to current nutrition advice for climbers.

Nutritional considerations for female climbers

Before going into more depth on potential nutritional considerations for the different phases in the menstrual cycle, pregnancy, breastfeeding and the menopause, it is worth noting some considerations that will apply all the time. For example, before doing *anything* more specific, it is **vital** that female climbers, like all climbers and athletes, ensure **adequate energy intake** to support both their climbing and basic bodily functions.[7] This is particularly pertinent to mention here as studies that look specifically at female climbers have shown a tendency for inadequate energy intake.[8]

Another area with some specific considerations for female athletes is **micronutrients**, in particular iron, calcium and vitamin D (see chapter 5).

Iron is a key micronutrient for female climbers due to potential menstrual losses. This is why females are advised to have a higher recommended daily intake (which goes down following menopause when they are no longer menstruating). In studies looking at iron in female climbers, both low dietary intakes and low iron measures in the body were found.[9] Vegetarian and vegan female athletes are at increased risk of low iron levels due to reduced dietary intakes of this mineral.

Calcium and **vitamin D** work together to promote optimal bone health, and some preliminary research suggests vitamin D and calcium intake is also inadequate in female climbers.[10] Women are more susceptible to reduced bone density in later life, so taking good care of bone health during their adult years is very important. While calcium intake – from foods such as dairy – itself is key, sufficient energy intake to maintain hormonal function is just as important for healthy bones because oestrogen is a key player in helping the calcium move into the bone.[11]

Female climbers should be mindful of getting enough iron and calcium in their diet. Aim for at least 18 milligrams of iron and 700 milligrams of calcium each day (see chapter 5 for specific advice). For vitamin D, the best way to ensure adequate levels is to supplement daily over the winter months with at least 400 IU.

Menstrual cycle

During the adult years of a woman's life, she will – provided she is not taking contraceptives and is premenopausal – have a menstrual cycle. There are, of course, conditions or times when a menstrual cycle will be disrupted or absent, such as with hypothalamic amenorrhea caused by low energy availability, or polycystic ovary syndrome, or when pregnant or breastfeeding. If a woman is not on contraceptives, or pregnant or breastfeeding, and her period goes MIA, this is a red flag. The monthly bleed is also known as the sixth vital sign and it can be considered a marker of health. Female athletes, especially those in weight-sensitive sports like climbing, are particularly at high risk for low energy availability and the negative consequences that come with it. For more in-depth discussion of this, see chapter 11.

The presentation of the menstrual cycle can vary hugely between women. A 'cycle' usually lasts anywhere between 23 and 35 days and can be broken down into phases in order to understand the hormonal fluctuations that occur. These phases are represented in figure 11 below and consist of the *follicular phase* (which starts with the bleed if the person is not pregnant) and the *luteal phase*. The transition from the follicular to the luteal phase is marked by ovulation. While the hormonal fluctuations seen in a cycle may seem standard, the experiences of women are certainly not. These phases are experienced very differently from one woman to another. As we will discuss further, this is why tracking your own cycle and how *you* feel in each phase can be really important.

There are some nutritional considerations that are specific to the phases of the menstrual cycle.

Follicular phase

This is the phase that starts on day one of bleeding and continues until ovulation occurs. This is often referred to as the 'lower hormone phase', when levels of oestrogen and progesterone are both at their lowest.

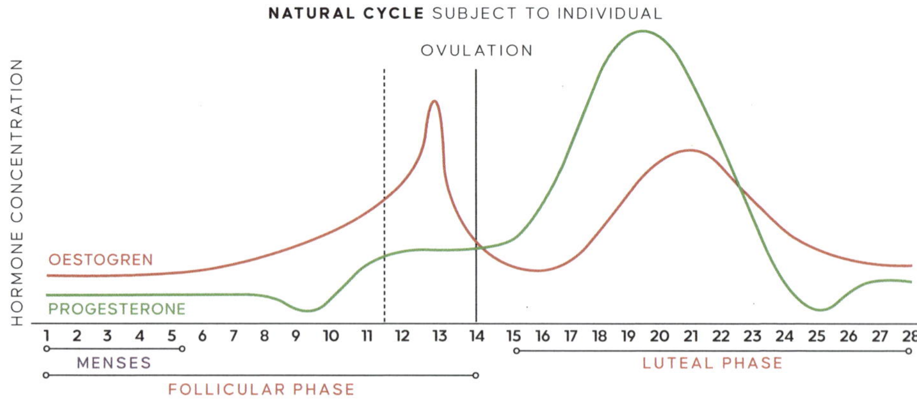

Figure 11: The phases of the menstrual cycle. Adapted from Leslie-Wujastyk and Gibson-Smith, 2024.[6]

During this phase, as the cycle builds towards ovulation, oestrogen rises gradually before spiking when an egg is released. This can be a phase when female climbers feel they perform well and feel good generally. For some, the feel-good comes on day one of the period, for others menstruation is not a pleasant time and only after the bleeding finishes do they get the feel-good vibes.

In this phase, glycogen storage – how the body stores carbohydrate – is lower and therefore it may be beneficial to eat a slightly higher overall intake of carbohydrate (potentially up to 6–8 grams per kilogram of body weight depending on training/climbing demands) when climbing to ensure that the fuel is available when needed.[12] Plus, this means that if it's a feel-good phase, then there is adequate fuel so you can push hard.

Research has shown bigger markers of muscle damage and inflammation in the follicular phase than in the luteal phase, and so it is also crucial that recovery meals are prioritised with adequate carbohydrate and protein.[13]

Luteal phase

This phase starts after ovulation – the release of an egg from the ovaries – and is often referred to as the 'higher hormone phase'. After an initial post-ovulation dip, both oestrogen and progesterone rise before gradually dropping again (if not pregnant). The rise of progesterone helps to build the lining of the womb for any potential pregnancy to implant. If pregnancy doesn't occur then this lining is lost as a period, and progesterone and oestrogen drop. It is this reduction in both hormones at the end of the cycle (if not pregnant) that can result in some of the symptoms associated with the lead up to a period. Many women find that exercise in the luteal phase may feel a bit harder, especially high-intensity exercise. If this is the case, rest assured you are not alone, but if it doesn't sound familiar, that's normal too. As previously mentioned, this is not a one-size-fits-all area.

The energy that the female body requires at rest may be higher in the luteal phase which would suggest that eating slightly more during this phase may be beneficial. However, the data on this is mixed.[14] It is also likely that eating will spontaneously increase during this time anyway – *hello, cravings!* – so this is not necessarily something that needs to be planned in.[15]

Some researchers suggest that the high progesterone in the luteal phase may affect fluid retention, resulting in higher body mass which could affect performance; it is worth being aware of this.[16] In the luteal phase, women typically present with a higher core temperature which is also down to higher progesterone levels.[17] However, most research indicates that these differences in core temperature do not appear to affect fluid regulation or sweat rates during exercise.[18] So, for now, stick to the advice in chapter 6 for managing fluid intake.

In the luteal phase, women will naturally burn more fat as fuel with lower carbohydrate use at baseline. But, this doesn't mean you should eat fewer carbs. As climbing is a high-intensity sport where carbs are key to big efforts, it is important to make sure exogenous carbohydrate is available; this means eating carbohydrate-based snacks, particularly before and during a session.[19] Because women use more fat as fuel at baseline in this phase, it is also crucial that fat intake doesn't drop too low.

One further consideration is that protein breakdown is higher in the luteal phase compared to the follicular phase, and so increased protein intake is a good idea.[20] This could just mean adding an extra serving of protein each day during this phase, or increasing the size of each protein portion slightly.

Premenstrual syndrome (PMS)

PMS is essentially a set of varying symptoms that women experience in the week or so leading up to their period. This can be a rough time for a lot of women and how it is experienced varies hugely. Some women have pretty much no symptoms, whereas others will have disrupted sleep, headaches, period cramps, bloating, lethargy, mood swings or food cravings, to name a few. As mentioned earlier, this is due to the dramatic drop in circulating hormones that happens at the end of the luteal phase. This can obviously have a huge impact on climbing performance.

So, are there any evidence-based things that can help from a nutritional perspective?

The research in this area is limited but there are a few things that may be worth trying. The general advice for menstrual disorders including PMS is to maintain a healthy eating pattern: eating with a focus on fresh, unprocessed foods, and avoiding refined foods, excess salt and alcohol.[21] This is a good place to start before getting more specific.

Some studies have shown that lower levels of calcium are associated with PMS and, in addition, that supplementation with calcium could help with symptoms.[22] A recent systematic review still suggests more research is needed to establish a firm link and to understand supplemental dosing strategies, but keeping calcium-based food intake adequate might be something that could help.[23]

Vitamin D is also a micronutrient that has been studied in relation to PMS and there seems to be a correlation between vitamin D levels and PMS symptoms, as well as some evidence that supplementing with vitamin D at higher doses may help with symptoms.[24]

It's fair to say that both calcium and vitamin D are beneficial micronutrients for female athletes, and, as there is some evidence to suggest that maintaining optimal levels may help with PMS, it is a good place to start if the days before your period are a tough time.

There is also some evidence to suggest that zinc, vitamin B6 and magnesium may help with PMS, although researchers suggest that more evidence is needed before they can be touted as effective treatments.[25] Again, ensuring a varied whole food diet will help keep all these topped up.

***

There is a lot of potential variation throughout the menstrual cycle and every person will have a unique set of symptoms and experiences. Tracking one's cycle can be really helpful to learn more about it, check it is regular and present, monitor patterns, and discover what works and doesn't work on an individual basis. Even if there isn't a solution to times of the month when performance is affected, knowing when these occur could be really helpful when planning trips or redpoint attempts.

What about hormonal contraception?

This is a question a lot of female athletes will have, and rightly so. Hormonal contraception has many benefits, from reproductive control and sexual freedom to management of menstrual-cycle-related symptoms and stability in performance. Being on the pill (or other hormonal contraceptives) can also give athletes control over when they bleed which can be really helpful in planning for performance windows. The downside of any hormonal intervention is that the athlete will not know the status of their hormonal health as clearly as if they did not use it. As mentioned before, having a period is a marker of health, and knowing that it comes regularly is reassuring for many who train hard or climb a lot. Equally, with a natural cycle, any dysfunction can be picked up earlier; the menstrual cycle, when paid attention to, often shows disturbances before disappearing completely. For example, a shorter luteal phase, anovulation or a single missed period during a time of high output and lower or inadequate calorie input. Hormonal contraceptives put a blindfold on this. Even if there is a monthly bleed, it's important to know that this is not a true period; it is a withdrawal bleed that occurs when the person takes a seven-day break from the pill and synthetic hormone levels drop.

Using hormonal contraception is a personal decision and there is no right or wrong answer here. It is situational and person-dependent. But what do we know about nutrition and exercise when it comes to female athletes that do use it?

A meta-analysis headed up by well-known female athlete researcher Kirsty Elliott-Sale looked at exercise performance on the oral contraceptive pill (OCP) versus a natural cycle.[26] They found a slightly lower exercise performance in those on the OCP, but this was a trivial difference and the quality of the studies analysed was mixed. They did note that exercise performance on the OCP was stable over the month, which is potentially very appealing to an athlete. The presence of mixed results and varying quality of studies was echoed in another review that considered responses to training.[27] It is worth noting that some research suggests higher markers of inflammation following exercise in women taking the OCP.[28]

When it comes to nutrition, there is no set of guidelines on whether or how to adapt for contraceptive use. There are so many different types of contraceptives, and the research on the varying effects on exercise and nutritional needs is both scarce and mixed in its findings.[29] For now, nutritional needs should be tailored to the individual based on their needs and experiences, with potentially some extra focus on greater carbohydrate intake around sessions during active pill weeks (due to a reduction in available carbohydrate, similar to the luteal phase), and ensuring recovery nutrition needs are optimised.[30]

Pregnancy and breastfeeding

Pregnancy is a time in a woman's life which puts an increased demand on her body. Continuing to exercise is seen as a very positive step for maternal and foetal health, providing any sport-specific risks are minimised, and many female climbers choose to continue to climb and train right up until they give birth.[31] While eating for two is not necessary, there is an increased demand for energy intake: nothing extra in the first trimester, 350 extra kilocalories a day in the second trimester and 500 extra kilocalories a day in the third.[32] When exercise such as climbing is added on top, it is best that this increased demand comes from carbohydrate as carbohydrate usage increases during pregnancy, both at rest and during exercise.[33]

For women who breastfeed after birth, their calorie intake will also increase. Exact amounts vary depending on how much milk is produced of course, but it is worth knowing that it can be around 400 to 500 kilocalories each day.[34] Calcium needs are also higher; the British Dietetic Association's recommended intake for women who are breastfeeding is 1,250 milligrams. Hydration is also key for nursing mothers, especially if they are exercising

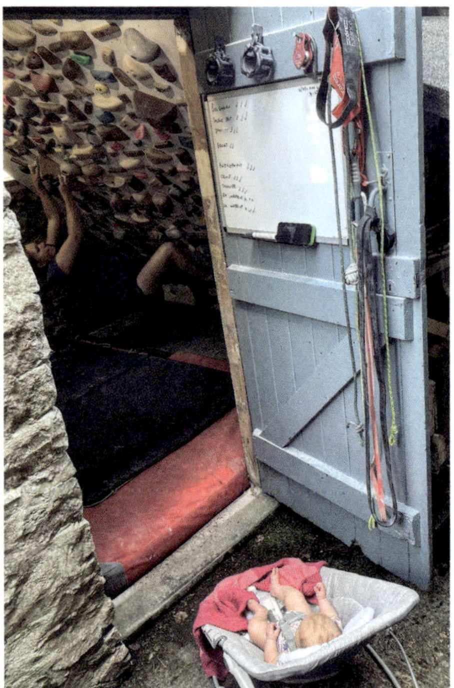

© DAVID MASON

as well. Extreme thirst will likely kick in, especially in the early months – keep water close!

These are times in life to really home in on listening to one's body. Whether it is hunger, thirst or a need for rest, the body knows best. During these phases, focus on eating well with plenty of whole foods, protein, complex carbohydrates, fruit, vegetables and fluids. As pregnancy and breastfeeding are such nutritionally demanding times for the body, it may be worth taking a multivitamin supplement. Check with your doctor or midwife to discuss the best option.

Menopause

Menopause is the point at which female sex hormones reduce dramatically as the ovaries stop producing eggs. Of course, this does not happen overnight, and perimenopause – the transitional phase leading up to menopause – can go on for many years, often starting in a woman's 40s, with menopause being reached in her early 50s. During perimenopause and menopause, there is a lot of hormonal flux, with many symptoms including hot flushes, fatigue, mood swings, anxiety, brain fog, urinary issues and low libido. It can be a really challenging time for many female athletes across all sports.

The decline in oestrogen that occurs with menopause is associated with a reduction in muscle mass, so a particular focus on maximising muscle retention and development is key.[35] This means including resistance training and, of course, optimised protein intake, aiming for the upper end of recommendations (see pages 35–36).[36] The reduction in hormones – and muscle mass – also has implications for bone health, and, as such, meeting energy needs as well as calcium and vitamin D intake is crucial as well as continuing with load-bearing exercise. Climbing is great for this as the muscles pull on the bones in multiple directions and, with bouldering, there is plenty of jumping off and loading of the lower body too.

Creatine may also be especially beneficial for menopausal women as there is evidence to suggest it may positively influence muscle mass, bone health, and potentially mood and cognition.[37]

Of course, hormone replacement therapy (HRT) is something that many women may consider due to some of the possible benefits to well-being, athletic performance and bone protection. Check in with your doctor to discuss if this is a good option for you.

KEY TAKEAWAYS

- → Much of the research into exercise and nutrition is based on male data which cannot necessarily be extrapolated to female athletes.
- → Research specific to female climbers is sparse and currently the best approach is to manage nutrition on an individual basis with an understanding of your specific hormonal profile.
- → Adequate energy intake is essential for female climbers who may be at a higher risk of low energy availability and the negative consequences that accompany it.
- → Key micronutrients for female climbers include iron, calcium and vitamin D.
- → In the follicular phase of the cycle, consider a higher intake of carbohydrate and optimise recovery nutrition.
- → In the luteal phase of the cycle, be aware of a potentially higher energy requirement and higher core temperature. In addition, ensure adequate in-session exogenous carbohydrate intake and increased overall protein intake.
- → Some micronutrients (vitamin D, calcium, zinc, vitamin B6 and magnesium) may play a role in PMS symptoms.
- → Tracking your cycle is a great way to monitor symptoms and adjust nutrition accordingly.
- → If you take hormonal contraception, consider increasing carbohydrate intake on pill-taking weeks and having a focus on recovery nutrition due to the potentially higher inflammatory response to exercise.
- → Pregnancy and breastfeeding both require an increase in energy intake; this should be considered on top of energy needs for climbing.
- → During the perimenopause and menopause, protein intake, overall energy intake, load-bearing exercise, calcium and vitamin D are key areas to focus on to optimise muscle mass and bone health. Creatine may also be particularly beneficial.

WHAT CAN I DO?

- → Consider first if you are optimising your nutrition overall: are you getting adequate calories, macronutrients, micronutrients and hydration to support your body?
- → If menstruating, track your cycle to see how you feel in different phases and experiment with adjusting your nutrition.
- → Consider where you are right now in your lifespan and how nutrition may positively support you: what can you **add** to your intake to optimise how you feel?

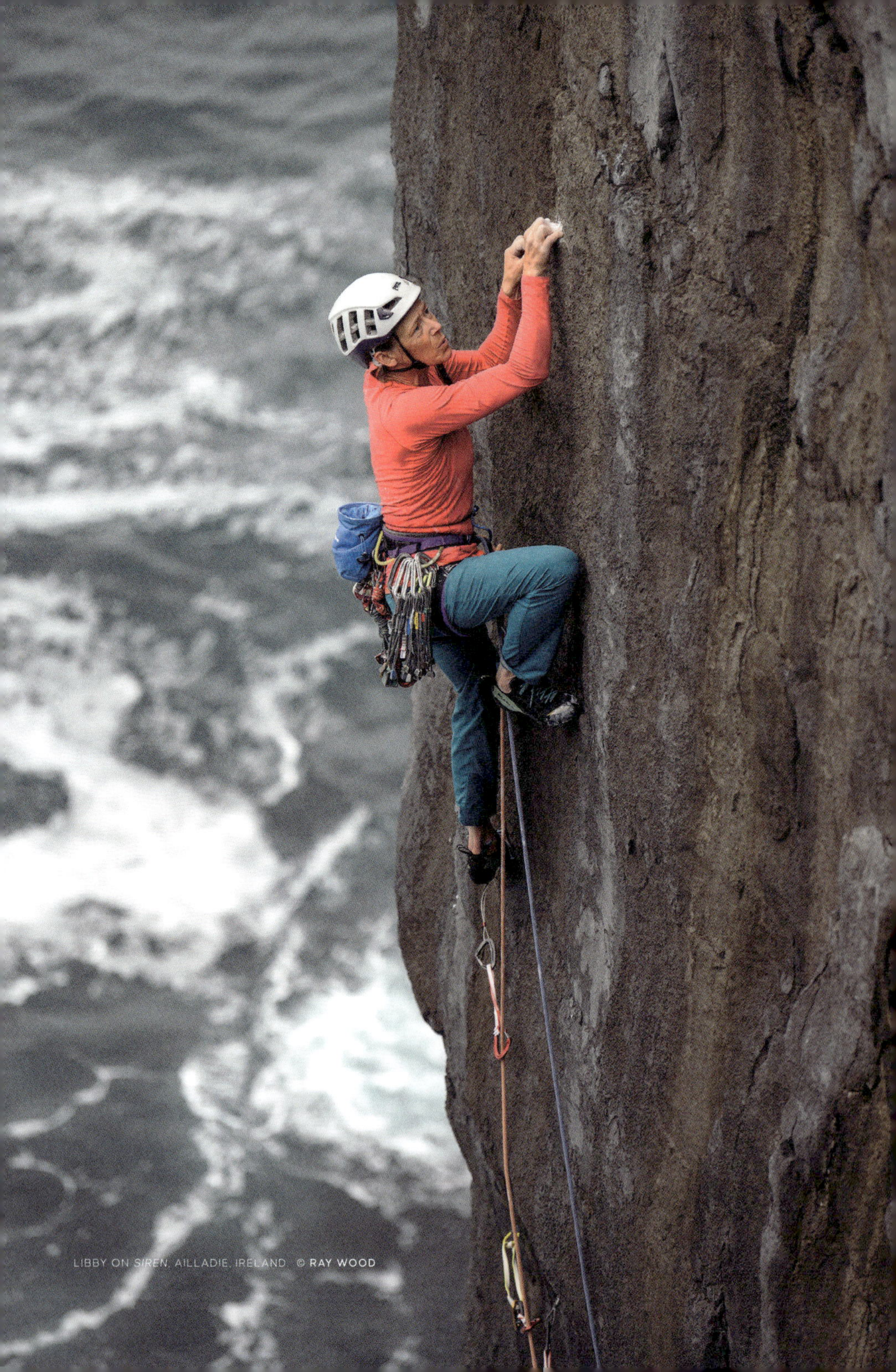

LIBBY ON SIREN, AILLADIE, IRELAND © **RAY WOOD**

LIBBY PETER
NAVIGATING THE MENOPAUSE

Libby is a woman of the outdoors; she lives and breathes being active in the mountains. Having found climbing and alpinism early, Libby has made many notable ascents, including an onsight ascent of *Right Wall* (E5 6a) on Dinas Cromlech in North Wales. Alongside her personal climbing, Libby works as a British Mountain Guide. She teaches climbing and mountaineering skills while taking others on adventures to share her passion of exploration. Libby is now 58 and she kindly shares her journey through the menopause and the nutritional changes she made during this time in her life.

I have always loved walking and being in the mountains, that was my route into climbing – the old-fashioned way, before commercial climbing walls were so widespread. Looking back, I'm quite grateful that they weren't around then – as fun as they are now – because I would have got sucked into that. From the start, I loved everything to do with the outdoors and I got into climbing to enable me to do more adventurous things in the mountains.

Funnily enough, I used to think I was afraid of heights. I'm not really sure where the notion came from, it must have been suggested at some point when I was young. It's amazing what sticks with you. Because of that, before I ever tried it, I thought I would hate climbing. In the last year of school I went abseiling and I was dreading it, but it turned out I had no fear of heights at all – I loved it.

I knew I wanted to work outside so I did a sports science and geography degree, although I quickly realised that climbing was what interested me the most. During my 20s I continued to develop my climbing and mountaineering, as well as work through my qualifications. I qualified as an IFMGA guide in 1996 when I was 30; it was a proud moment – it's a long, tough process. I'm glad I did it all early when I had so much time and energy as well as the confidence of youth. Food and nutrition weren't something I gave a lot of thought to in those days; I was actually really good at being able to go long stints in the mountains without eating much. I would often experience clients having anxiety over taking enough food for

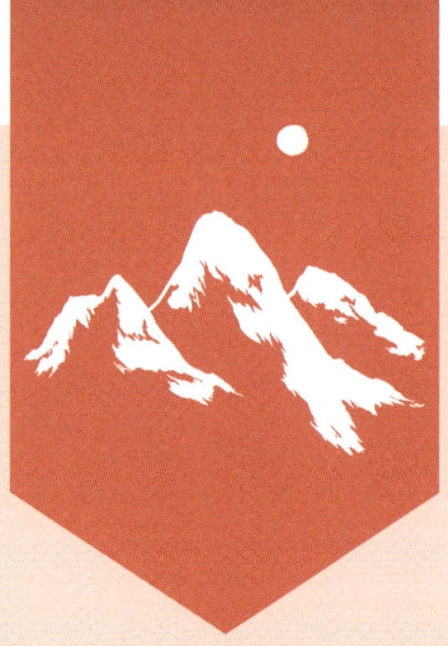

days out or expeditions; this wasn't an issue for me as I knew I could manage without if need be. I know that's not the right way to do it necessarily, but it worked for me.

As a woman in the outdoor industry there is a lot to navigate; the female lifespan is littered with hormonal changes and disruptions. Puberty, menstrual cycles, pregnancy and breastfeeding (if desired and able), and then perimenopause and menopause; it's a lot of ups and downs with few time periods that feel consistent. I had a few years of guiding before I had children and I'm grateful for that. I'm now 58 and the most recent change for me has been the menopause. In some ways I have been lucky – it started for me in my early 50s and the transition probably only took three to five years. I didn't really feel like anything changed for me in my 40s, so in that sense I was fortunate. Three to five years sounds like a long time, but I know women who have suffered through debilitating symptoms of perimenopause and menopause for up to ten years.

My main symptoms were poor sleep, brain fog, hot flushes and muscle loss. I did also have a bad bout of Covid and some other health issues during this time, so, of course, it's hard to separate out what caused what. Poor sleep was the big one for me: I was so tired. I could get to sleep okay but would wake up in the night and be unable to get back to sleep which was very frustrating. I remember feeling absolutely wiped out. It reminded me of my years as a new parent; the sleep deprivation became a new normal but it was a really challenging experience. It impacted both my work as a guide and my personal climbing. My job is physical and there is also a big element of decision making. I hate the feeling of not quite being 'on it' and present, which was part tiredness and part brain fog.

During this time, I also noticed that I could no longer go for long periods of time without food. I really needed to think about regular snacks when I was in the mountains in a way that was novel for me. Sugary things felt unhelpful too; I began to avoid them to prevent the peaks and troughs they caused in my energy levels. I needed slow-release carbohydrates to fuel my days with lots of top-ups to prevent me from crashing out. Suddenly, I had to plan in a way that I hadn't needed to in the past.

Muscle loss is inevitable as we age, but especially so for women post-menopause. The drop in hormones puts us at a disadvantage very quickly and it takes work to hang on to lean mass. I didn't take hormone replacement therapy (HRT) – it wasn't really on my radar at the time, perhaps as I didn't consider my symptoms to be too extreme. I was most aware of the hot flushes and the sleep and I was coping with those. Maybe HRT would have saved or delayed some muscle loss, who knows? However, I did make a conscious effort to increase my protein intake and do some resistance exercise to help with maintaining muscle; these are both things I wish I had started sooner. It's easy to think you're getting enough protein if you eat well, but I did my own research on protein recommendations and calculated the numbers for someone in my position. Turns out it's a *lot* of protein and it can be quite tricky to get it in from a practical perspective. I eat chicken and fish so some of it came from there, as well as nuts and some yoghurt. I dabbled with protein powders but I never really found one that I liked the taste of – I'm not a great fan of milk which makes it a bit more difficult.

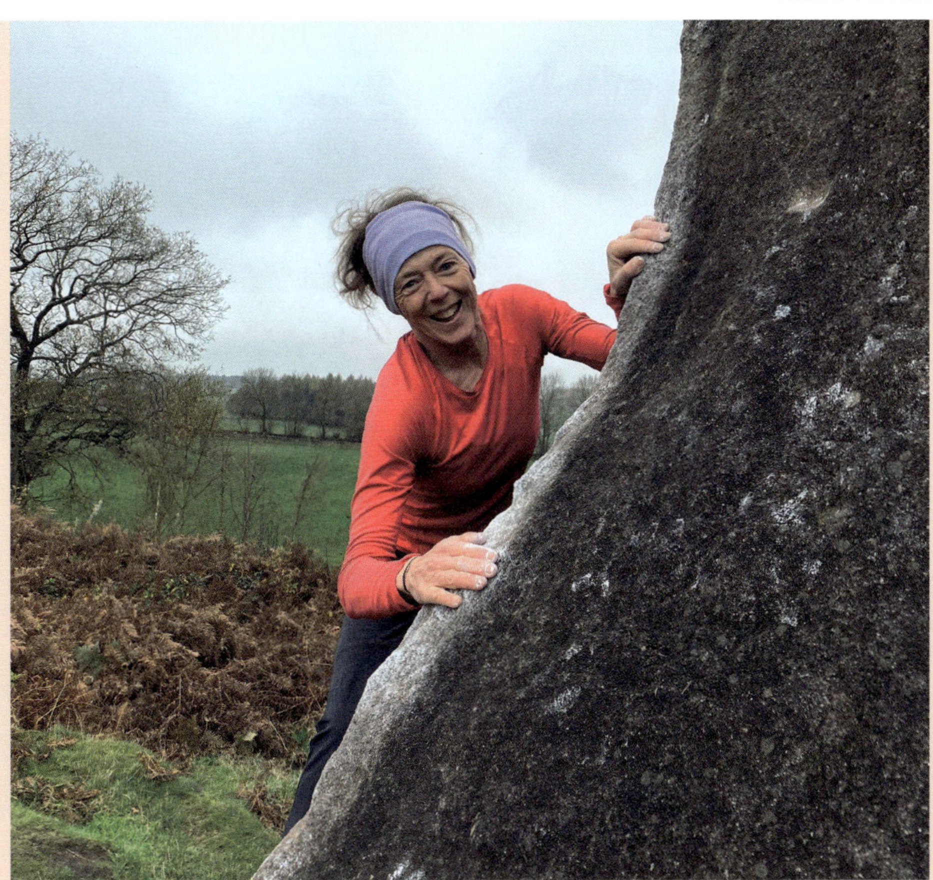

© LIBBY PETER

There are no quick fixes for the menopause, of course – annoyingly, it's something that only time will sort out. All of my interventions were quite reactive rather than planned out in advance. If I were to give anybody advice on this topic it would be to plan ahead: build muscle and get into good habits with nutrition *before* you get to the menopause years. If I knew then what I know now, I would have invested more time on these things in my late 30s and 40s. It's like saving into a bank for your later life, but for your muscles, bone density and energy levels. It'll be much harder to get and maintain if you wait.

Cultural influences can also be a factor in all this. They can play a big role in how we see ourselves, our bodies and, consequently, how we approach nutrition and exercise. I'm glad to see the body-image culture for women changing, especially in sport. The (hopefully) outdated beauty standards encouraging thinness and discouraging muscles is so unhelpful for the long-term health of women and girls. I think broad shoulders and muscles on women are beautiful and I'm glad to see more celebration of this type of physique in climbing. The promotion of muscles in our younger years will have such positive and long-reaching effects on our health as older women. I have two daughters and I hope they both are able to build and celebrate their strength, for now and for later.

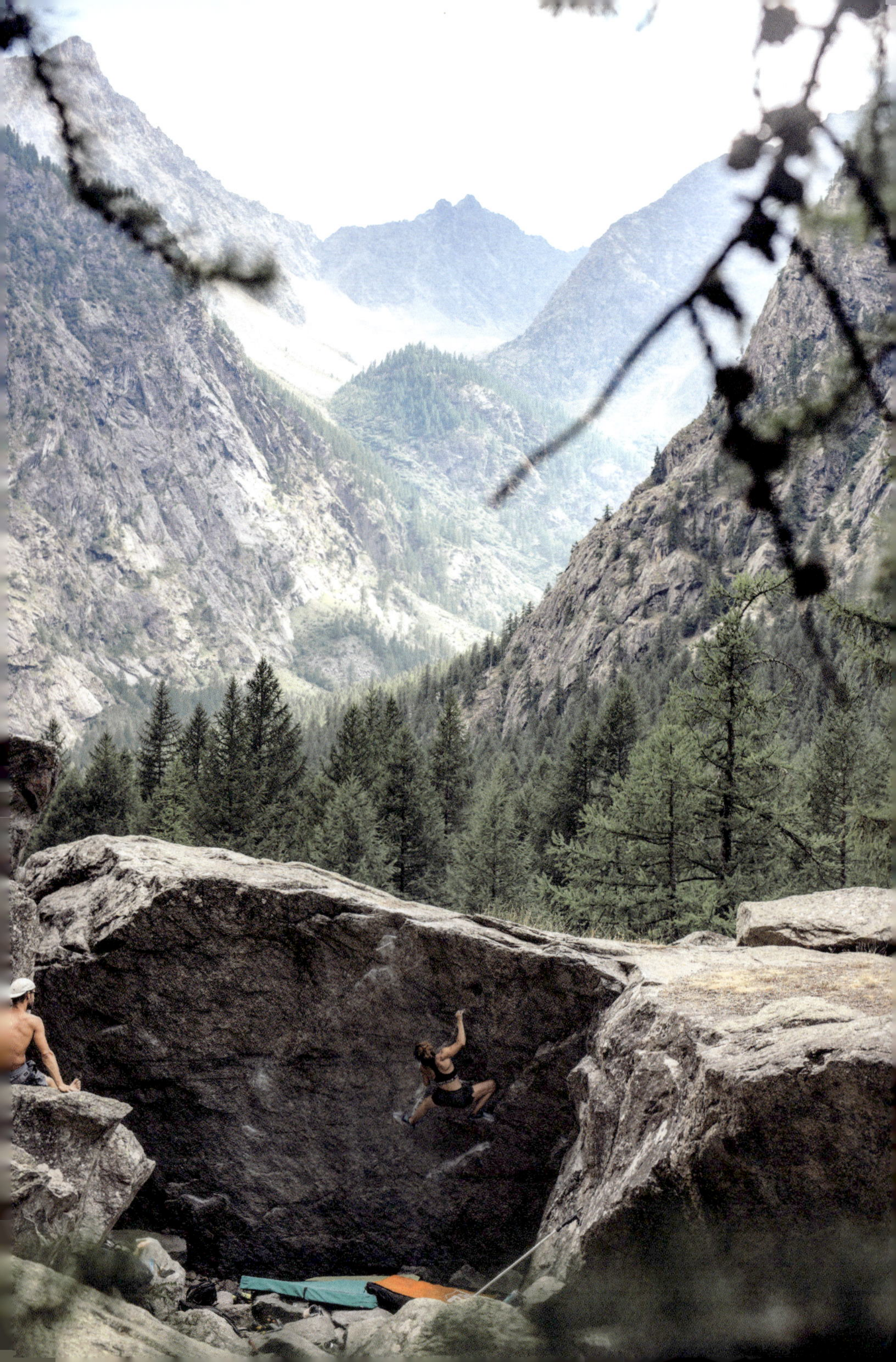

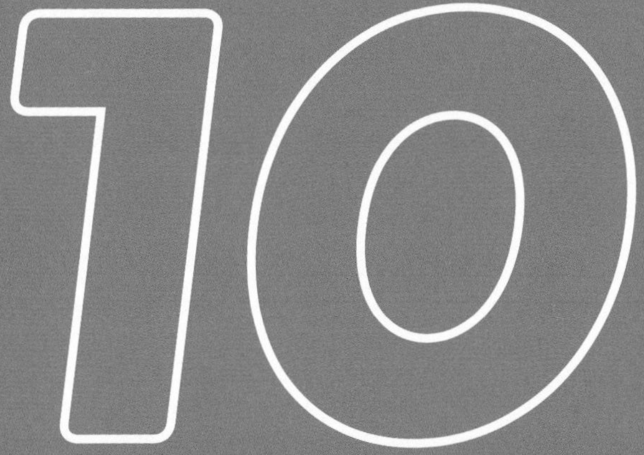

NUTRITION FOR INJURY

MOLLY THOMPSON-SMITH ON *FANTASTIQUE*, AILEFROIDE, FRANCE. © SAM PRATT

Injuries are so frustrating. They often pop up out of seemingly nowhere at the worst possible times. Suffering a setback, having to slow down and doing all the boring rehab can be quite daunting and even demoralising. So, can nutrition help?

Before we dive into what nutrition can do in supporting injury recovery, it's important to mention the best option of all: prevention. As I hope you have gathered so far in this book, supportive nutrition in the form of adequate energy intake, macro- and micronutrients, and proper hydration is key to boosting performance – and, alongside appropriate rest and quality sleep, it can help you avoid injury.[1] Being a robust athlete is particularly important in sports like climbing where falls are a part of every session, and the movement is dynamic, open-chain and there is a tremendous amount of force placed on some parts of the body in lots of different positions. Training and nutrition can be a big part of creating a robust body that is strong, adaptable and not easy to break. Having said all that, none of us can escape bad luck every now and then, so let's talk about nutrition for injury.

Injuries come in many forms, some traumatic and major, some small and niggly. The way nutrition changes during an injury will, of course, depend on the type and severity of the injury. With most injuries there are two distinct phases, the acute stage and the rehabilitation stage. In the acute stage, rest and sometimes immobilisation are necessary to allow for tissue repair. In the rehabilitation stage, movement and strengthening may be introduced in a staged programme which leads towards a return to function and climbing.

A 2023 systematic review on nutritional strategies for rehabilitation of musculoskeletal injuries highlighted some key areas for consideration, including balanced energy intake, a high-protein and carbohydrate-rich diet, strong avoidance of low energy availability, and the potential use of supplements such as collagen, creatine, omega-3 (fish oils) and vitamin D.[2] These areas will be the main focus of this chapter.

Overall energy intake

When we are injured, our aim should be to avoid unnecessary muscle loss and ensure enough energy for tissue repair while also avoiding excess body fat gain.[3] Ideally, nutrition support will help us get enough energy intake to ensure energy balance or even a slight surplus, as this will help to protect against muscle loss while also providing energy for healing.[4] This may seem counterintuitive because a period of injury often requires a decrease in activity and maybe even some immobilisation of the injured body part. However, research suggests that energy expenditure could be up to approximately 20 per cent higher during the early stages of an injury, especially for severe injuries, because tissue repair (in particular muscle protein synthesis) is a high-energy-consuming process and not having enough energy could hamper the process.[5] It should go without saying – but I'll say it anyway – that low energy availability during injury should be avoided at all costs.

Of course, this is a tricky balance as excess energy intake could result in increased body fat which may make the return to climbing feel tougher and add to systemic inflammation which could actually increase the rate of muscle loss.[6] So, what to do? Don't actively reduce your energy intake under the premise of lower activity during injury as your body needs the fuel to fix the injury. However, if body fat starts to increase, consider modifying a little to find the right balance. As with anything nutrition, it's a bit of trial and error.

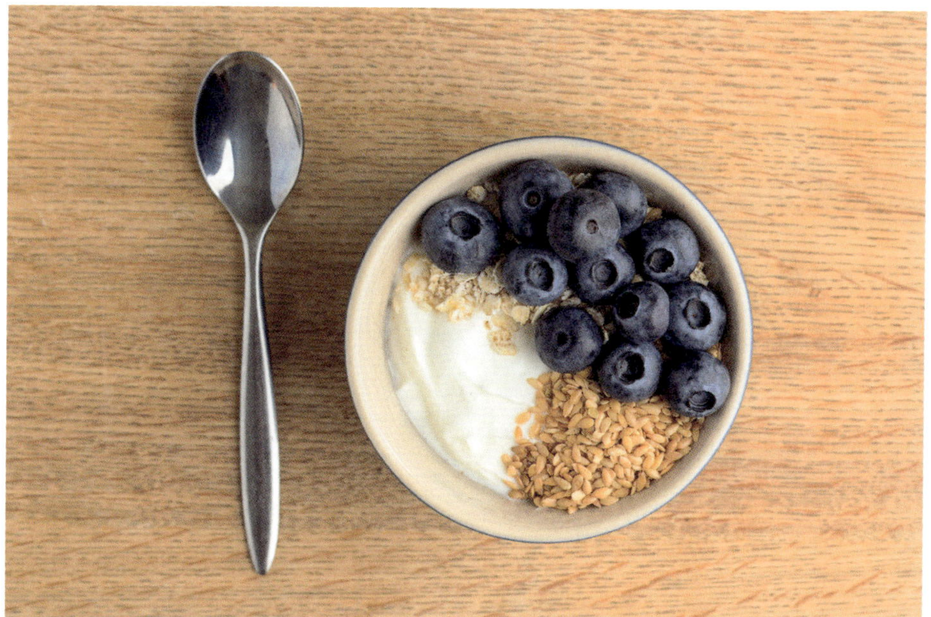

GETTING ENOUGH PROTEIN IS REALLY IMPORTANT IN TIMES OF INJURY AND GREEK YOGHURT IS A GREAT SOURCE, WITH APPROXIMATELY 11 GRAMS OF PROTEIN PER 100-GRAM SERVING.

And remember to listen to your body: appetite is a really useful indicator to listen to and follow.

Protein

During any immobilisation, approximately 0.5–0.6 per cent of muscle may be lost each day, with loss of strength and neuromuscular degeneration as well.[7] In addition to this, periods of inactivity can create a state of anabolic resistance in a muscle.[8] This essentially means that the muscle is less sensitive to amino acids (protein) and requires a greater stimulus for muscle protein synthesis (the building of new muscle).

All those hard-won gains can easily slip away, but prioritising protein above the usual intake is one way to limit the damage. Not eating enough protein during injury can compound the above effects to increase the amount of muscle lost as well as decrease the rate of tissue repair, slowing recovery.

Recommended intakes for injury are in the range of 1.6–3 grams of high-quality protein per kilogram of body weight per day in servings of 20–30 grams spread throughout the day in four to six meals/snacks.[9] High quality means ensuring there is enough (approximately 3 grams) of the particular amino acid leucine which is crucial for triggering muscle protein synthesis and therefore vital when combatting injury.[10] This strategy can include a pre-sleep dose of protein which may also be beneficial to promote muscle synthesis overnight with a greater portion of 40 grams.[11] As an example, this could be Greek yoghurt with peanut butter or a simple protein shake made with milk. Some research suggests that casein is a particularly good choice for overnight protein due to its slow release. Carbohydrate is also your friend in this scenario as it helps to reduce muscle protein breakdown by ensuring that protein is not used for energy, as well as providing energy for and promoting other aspects of recovery.[12]

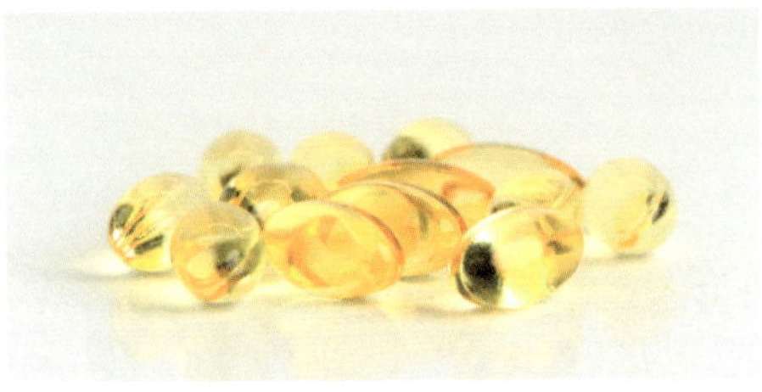

IF YOU DON'T LIKE EATING FISH, FISH OIL CAPSULES ARE AVAILABLE; IF YOU'RE VEGAN, IT IS POSSIBLE TO GET EPA AND DHA FROM ALGAE SUPPLEMENTS.

Collagen

Supplementing with collagen (see page 80) along with vitamin C has been shown to increase collagen synthesis which is often an important part of injury healing and recovery.[13] Research also suggests that it might help with reducing joint pain, increasing functionality and accelerating return to sport which are of course also key to rehabilitation of injuries.[14]

Ideally, collagen should be used prior to loading the tissues for the greatest effect so it may be that this supplement really comes into its own during the rehabilitation stage of an injury where gradual loading is reintroduced. As per the recommendations on page 80, take 15 grams of collagen with 50 milligrams of vitamin C one hour before loading for three months.[15] The vitamin C is considered important due to its role in some of the reactions that create collagen cross-linking. While there is not enough evidence to suggest that taking excess vitamin C is helpful for injury recovery, it is important to ensure baseline needs – covered by the 50 milligrams – are met to ensure normal collagen synthesis.[16]

Creatine

Creatine is another supplement that may be helpful during injury. Creatine is very well researched and helps to support the PCr energy system which is used in high-intensity muscle contractions (see pages 4–5). Inactivity, for example when we are injured or a body part is immobilised, has been shown to reduce muscle mass and strength but also, specifically, reduce muscle creatine stores.[17]

Research suggests that when we are injured and our muscle contractile function is compromised, supplementing with creatine can increase these stores and consequently improve physiological adaptations to rehabilitation.[18]

Creatine is found in foods such as meat and fish, but to optimise creatine stores, supplementing with creatine monohydrate is recommended. A programme of loading at 20 grams a day for five days followed by a dose of 3–5 grams a day is ideal during times of injury.[19]

Omega-3 fatty acids (fish oils)

Omega-3 fatty acids – aka fish oils – are touted to be beneficial in sport in general.[20] They are potentially helpful during periods of injury for reducing muscle loss and inflammation, however this is debated.[21] Acute inflammation can cause pain, swelling and loss of function in the initial stages which may be helped by the use of omega-3s – specifically EPA and DHA – if it becomes prolonged.[22] However, it is also argued that the inflammatory response is a necessary and natural part of injury and blunting it could slow down the healing progress. These conflicting ideas are the basis for some controversy over whether omega-3s should be used in injury recovery; more research specific to injury recovery is needed.[23]

Another consideration is that taking fish oils long-term may improve sensitivity to amino acids, combatting the anabolic resistance mentioned on page 38 that can occur with injury.[24] This could prevent or lessen muscle loss but, again, more research is warranted.

Having a higher intake of omega-3 relative to omega-6 fats may be the most prudent advice at the moment.[25] Omega-3 fats include things like salmon, nuts, seeds, olive oil and avocado, while omega-6 fats are found in processed meats, fried foods and vegetable oils.

Vitamin D

There is a wide array of research that demonstrates the role of vitamin D in bone health, muscle function, adaptation to exercise and injury risk.[26] Low vitamin D status may also delay muscle strength recovery after injury which suggests that avoiding deficiency during times of injury is crucial.[27] There is some mixed evidence on this topic as well, so more research would be beneficial to allow for specific dosing protocols to emerge.[28] At this time, ensuring that levels are not deficient should be your main focus.

As discussed in chapter 5, vitamin D is not primarily absorbed from food. It is synthesised in the skin from exposure to sunlight, with only 10–20 per cent derived from dietary sources. Foods that do contain it include salmon, eggs, red meat and fortified foods. In the UK, supplementation is advised at 400 IU over the winter months, but for an injured climber the best option would be to measure vitamin D levels and supplement accordingly.

* * *

There are many other nutrients that potentially play a role in healing, although, for many, this is through their antioxidant properties which combat inflammation. Inflammation in injuries is still a controversial topic.[29] Therefore, it is best at the moment to focus on a food-first approach to most vitamins and minerals unless a measured deficiency is found.[30]

KEY TAKEAWAYS

- → Supportive nutrition can play a big part in helping you stay injury free; prevention is better than cure!
- → Nutritional strategies will vary depending on the type and severity of the injury.
- → Balanced energy intake and the avoidance of low energy availability are important to ensure adequate energy for tissue repair and healing.
- → Protein intake should be high and good quality to minimise muscle loss. Adequate carbohydrate also supports this.
- → Supplementing with collagen and vitamin C as well as creatine may aid recovery.
- → Supplementing with omega-3 fatty acids may play a positive role in injury recovery but the evidence is mixed. Aim for a higher intake of omega-3 relative to omega-6 fats through food intake.
- → Ensure vitamin D levels are not deficient.

WHAT CAN I DO?

- → Be proactive about your nutrition during times of injury.
- → Make a plan for how you can use nutrition to support your body at this time.
- → Consider whether you are tempted to reduce intake and be reminded of all the support your body needs to work on healing your injury – the last thing you want is to slow things down!
- → Increase your protein intake and consider supplements such as creatine and collagen, depending on the injury.

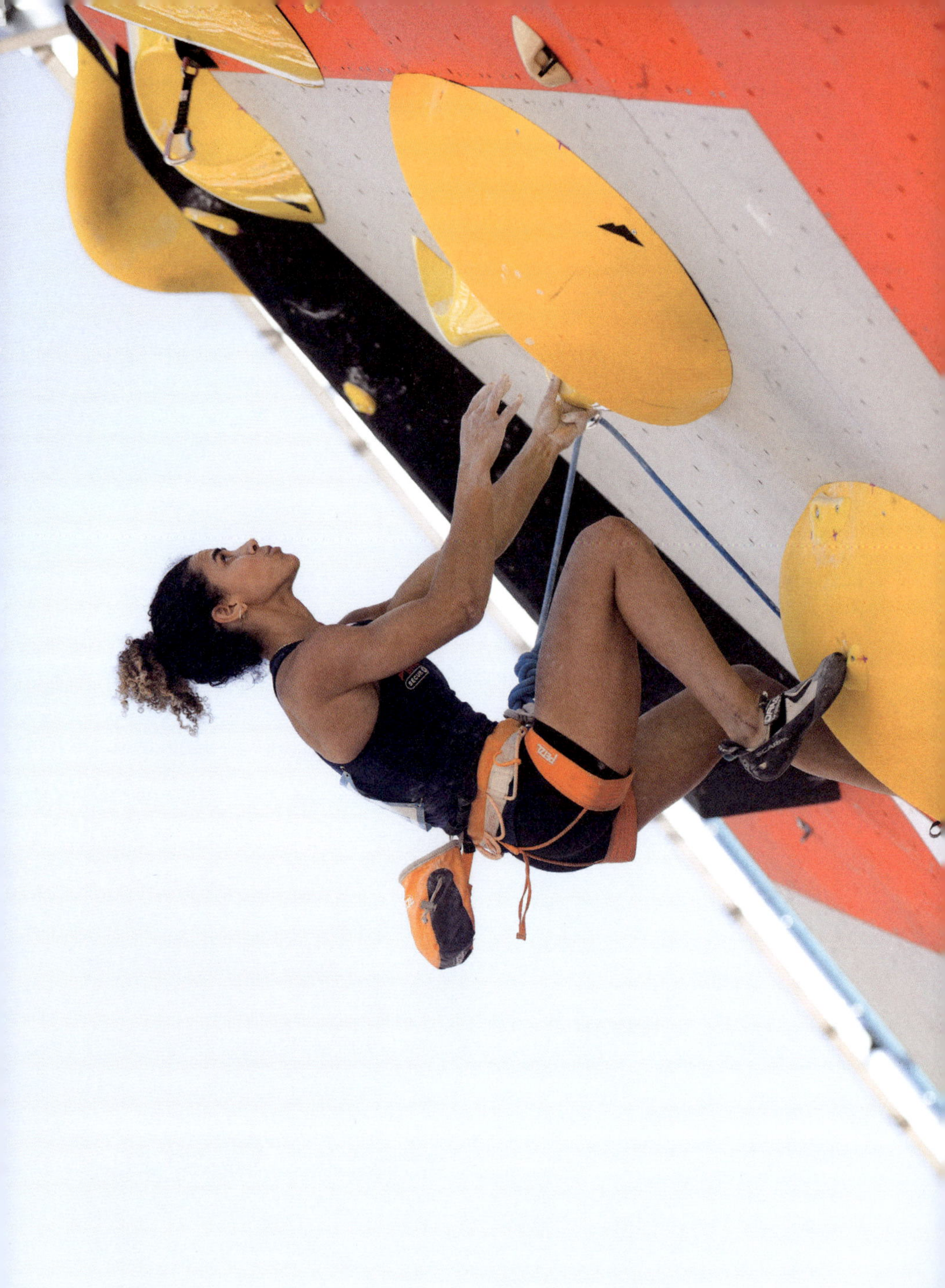

© SAM PRATT

MOLLY THOMPSON-SMITH
COMING BACK FROM INJURY

Molly has long been a household name in UK climbing and, as an Olympian since Paris 2024, she is an internationally known athlete. Despite her obvious talent and skill as a climber, things haven't always been easy for Molly. She has had more than her fair share of injuries, surgery and comebacks. Here, Molly shares her approach to nutrition during one of her most challenging injuries.

I wasn't even supposed to go out climbing that day. I was getting ready to travel to Jakarta for the next lead climbing world cup, followed by a long-awaited trip around Malaysia with my mum who had just retired. But the weather was great and some friends were heading out bouldering on the grit so I went to meet them. My shoes were in my bag but I wasn't planning on using them, I was just going to hang out. Except when I got there, they were trying *Suavito*, a stunning compression climb. I had tried it before, but it is quite high with a very committing last move and we had only had two pads last time. This time there were lots of pads, lots of spotters, good conditions and high psyche. It seemed like the perfect opportunity to have another go.

Fast forward half an hour and I am lying on the mats looking at my foot which is now at a right angle to my lower leg. I really went for it on the last move, but the top wasn't as positive as I had expected and I came off fast at an odd angle. Sam, my partner, pushed me on to the mats but one of my legs got caught in the process and so I landed with all my weight on the other leg. Multiple fractures and a full dislocation. Mountain rescue came and gave me gas and air under the boulder while they manually re-aligned my ankle before taking me to hospital. As injuries go, I knew this wasn't going to be a quick recovery.

It was three weeks before I had surgery to internally fix a plate with screws and an additional pin, and I sat on the sofa for almost the whole three weeks. This was when I first

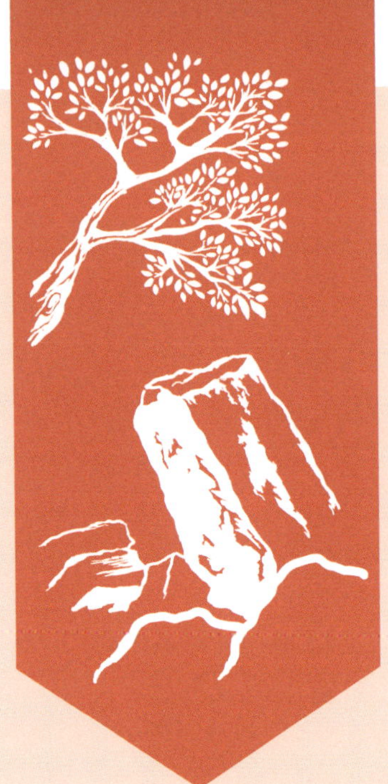

started to consider proactive nutrition. My surgery had to wait until the swelling had reduced and this took longer than I expected, and I wanted to do everything I could to speed things along. One of the hardest parts of this phase was how incredibly reliant I was on other people. I needed help with absolutely *everything* and that was tough. Food wise, it meant that someone else was shopping, cooking and preparing food for me. Even going to the bathroom was agony, not to mention a logistical nightmare.

Even so, I did as much as I could with my nutrition to support the acute recovery phase. I ate lots of foods containing antioxidants like vegetables and fruit which helped with the inflammation, as well as high-calcium foods and protein. I also opted for high-fibre foods where possible to help offset some of the constipation caused by the regular painkillers I needed to take following the injury. Alongside this, despite not having much of an appetite, I made sure to eat intentionally and regularly to keep up my energy intake. When you're sitting on the sofa all day and not feeling hungry, it can feel counterintuitive to do this, but I knew that there was a lot of invisible, energy-expensive work going on in my body. I was tired and cold all the time and, even though I was consciously trying to eat enough, I still lost weight. This happened surprisingly quickly and a lot of it was muscle atrophy, both on the affected limb and in the rest of my body.

After the surgery, with plates and screws holding my ankle together, the next phase of recovery started. I had a boot on and was non-weight-bearing for a period of time before I could start to use the foot and work on getting strength and function back. I tend to gain muscle quite easily, but I knew that the rehab work would require good supportive nutrition to optimise and speed up the process. Plus, I was still so tired and adding in more activity just exhausted me more. So, I made sure I was getting a good amount of carbohydrate, protein and micronutrients, as well as keeping my energy intake as high as possible to support muscle gain. Muscle growth needs extra energy and I was told I couldn't progress further in my rehab until I could do a calf raise ... so I needed to regrow some semblance of a calf muscle! I also added extra things to my diet like calcium and vitamin D supplements, some whey powder to sneak in more protein and some collagen powder too. I'm not usually a fan of powders and I like to take a food-first approach, but in this instance it worked well for me to add these in. I would mix the powders into my baked-oats breakfast so I didn't have to taste them!

It all felt quite mechanical as my appetite still wasn't normal, but I knew, from my study of nutrition, that it had to be done. I was really grateful at this point that I had studied nutrition in the past as it gave me the confidence to commit to more food intake at a time when it might be tempting to eat less. The last thing anyone wants after time out from an injury is to return 'out of shape' with a negatively altered body composition. I get that and I felt it strongly at the time, but not

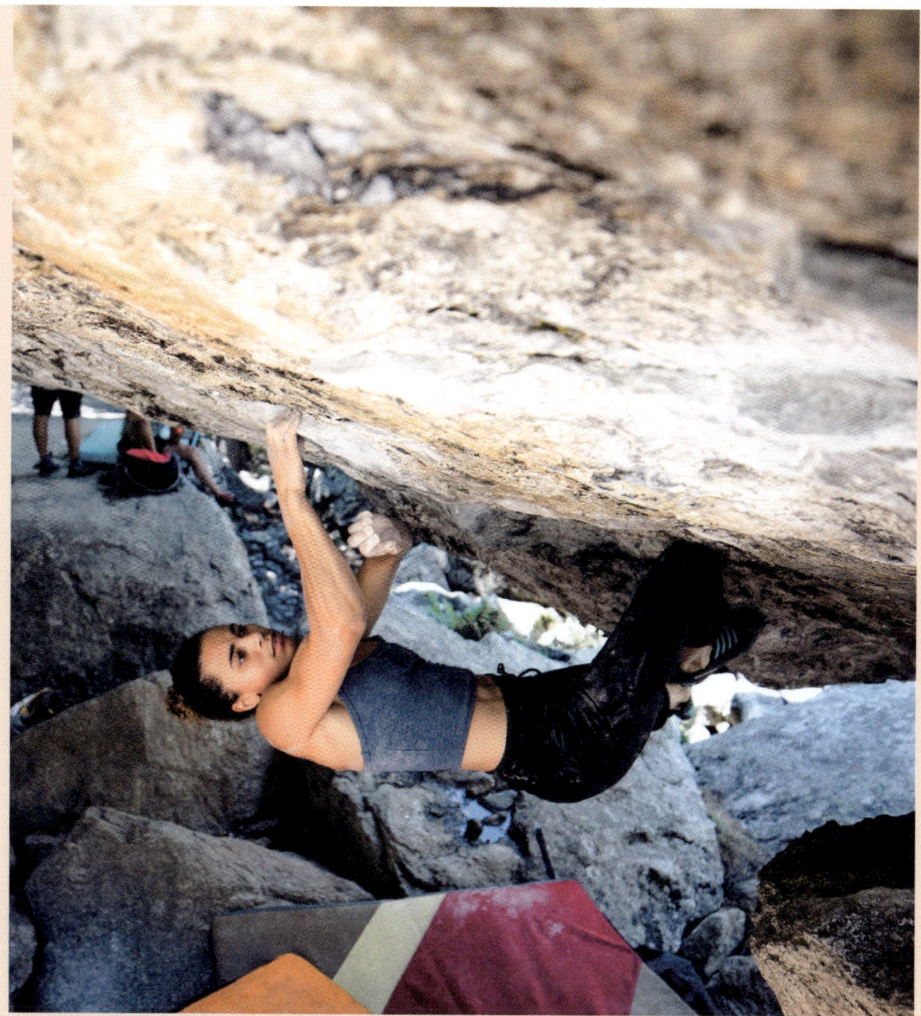

MOLLY ON *SICAPLAF*, AILEFROIDE, FRANCE. © **SAM PRATT**

eating enough would have slowed things more and made all my rehab efforts less effective. As I did more and more rehab and training my appetite came back and suddenly the hunger was intense. It was nice to feel that again and to be active, even if a lot of it was still rehab focused.

Did my approach to nutrition help my recovery? I think so. It also made me feel like I was actively doing everything I could at a time when I felt quite helpless and uncertain. That alone had psychological value, but I do think that optimising nutrition at times of serious injury is a task worth taking on for physiological gain too. It's hard to comprehend what the body is able to heal from, and I like to think I gave my body a helping hand.

My ankle isn't perfect – there were and are more surgeries to come – but after three months I climbed again, and eight months later I was competing at a bouldering world cup and in 2024 I became an Olympian.

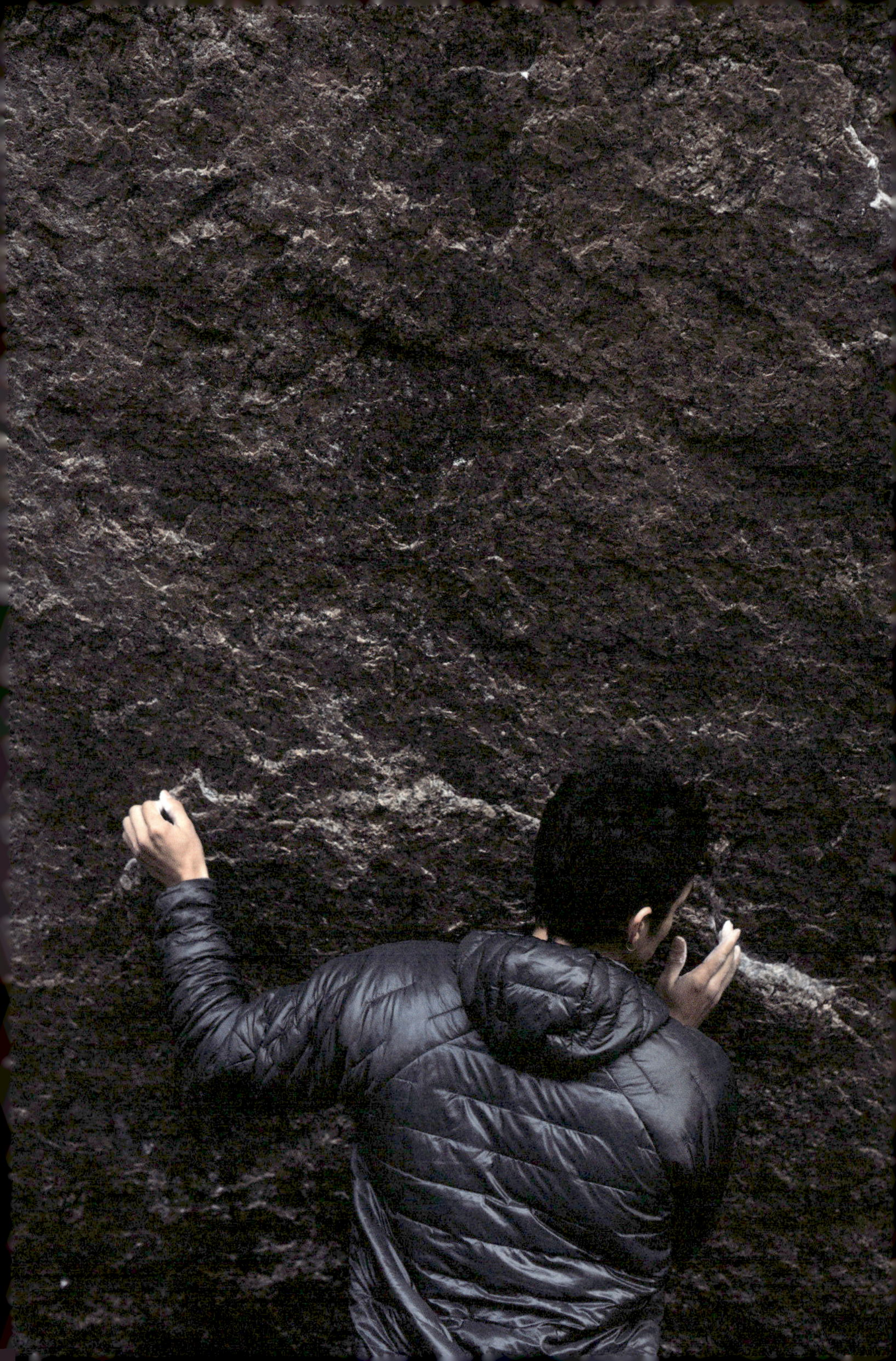

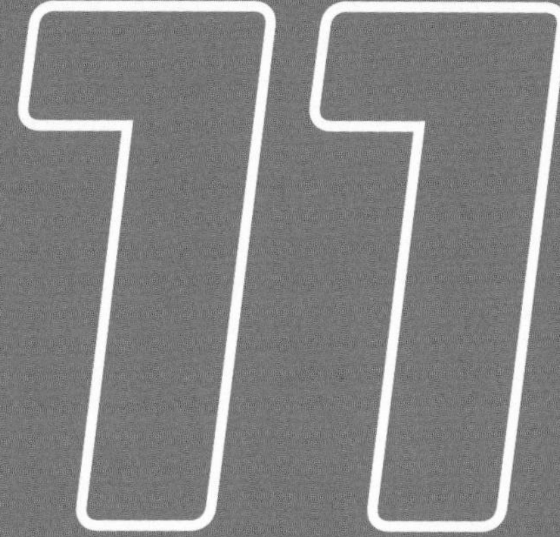

WEIGHT LOSS AND CLIMBING

IS LIGHTER BETTER?

© SAM PRATT

Is it wise to lose weight for climbing?

There is no getting away from the fact that climbing is a weight-sensitive sport. It literally involves lifting our body weight and carrying it up a rock face, and a lighter body requires less effort to carry. Our fingers take a huge strain and it's not surprising that climbing has developed a culture of 'lighter is better', with climbers idolising the thin, ripped physique. A 2023 study of competition climbers found that 46 per cent of male and 38 per cent of female climbers had intentionally tried to lose weight to perform and, of those, around 76 per cent reported using practices described as concerning, such as dehydration, vomiting or the use of laxatives.[1] This is really worrying and underlines the need for more information and education in climbing around weight loss because, like many things, the reality of weight – and losing it – is more nuanced than it may at first appear.

To begin with, scale weight is a very basic data point; one crucial consideration is that it includes muscle mass as well as body fat. Weight can also be lost and gained without flux in fat or muscle; hydration, fibre and salt all affect absolute weight. Manipulating weight alone is a blunt tool because it does not consider all the factors that contribute to a scale reading.

Really what climbers are searching for is the optimal strength-to-weight ratio rather than a lower absolute weight. The key here is to remember that this optimal ratio may not come at the lowest weight. For example, scale weight will go up after effective training periods as muscle is (hopefully) gained and, despite an increase in absolute weight, strength-to-weight ratio may also improve as the weight that is gained helps on the strength side. Equally, weight may reduce if muscle is lost, and the strength-to-weight ratio could worsen. Of course, these scenarios can be played out with fat loss and gain too, and this type of weight is less helpful to carry. But bear in mind that a certain amount of body fat is necessary to be healthy and that this threshold will be different for different people – *hello again, genetics!* It is also difficult to control what kind of weight is lost and, invariably, when dieting there will be some muscle lost as well as fat.

So, in theory, a climber could be at a higher or lower weight with the same strength-to-weight ratio in both situations. The clincher is that if the focus is on strength gain through supportive nutrition rather than fat loss through dieting, there is more potential moving forward. Eventually, fat loss will stall and then there will be nowhere to go. On the flip side, building muscle and the benefits that come with that approach open many more doors. The ultimate goal is a body composition – the distribution of muscle mass and fat mass – that gives an optimal strength-to-weight ratio on the wall while also maintaining health – both mental *and* physical. The tricky part here is that this looks different for different people, with modifying factors including age, sex and genetics.

Of course, in some situations, it may be beneficial to lose some fat mass, for example in the build-up to a peak performance to maximise your strength-to-weight ratio, or for improved health. There are ways to do this in a sensible way, ideally with the support of a dietitian or nutritionist.

Practical considerations for body composition change

If body composition change feels necessary, a useful method is to periodise nutrition across the year to reflect this.[2] Don't try to maintain 'fighting weight' all the time; consider the times when it's important to be at the most optimised strength-to-weight ratio and when it is less important. For example, a competition climber might aim to be leaner for the competition season but then regain fat mass for the training season. This is a much more sustainable approach for the body to handle and it means that nutrition is always tailored to the athlete's current situation. As mentioned before, ideally this would be managed with the help of a dietitian or nutritionist to ensure it is sport specific and maintains health and performance.[3]

The fundamental principle of weight loss is to create a calorie deficit, but there are many different methods for achieving this. For example, the deficit could be taken from different macronutrient categories, depending on the needs and existing habits of the individual. Adherence is also a key factor to consider: is the chosen method sustainable for the desired time period? For example, it may be easier, more manageable and therefore more successful to sustain a smaller deficit.

Being in a calorie deficit means the body is in a catabolic (breaking down) mode which makes it very hard to gain muscle mass at the same time because building muscle is an anabolic (building up) process. So, ideally, not too much time – especially during a training block or performance block – should be spent in a calorie deficit. It is also crucial to make sure that the deficit is not too extreme and does not last for too long as this can backfire and really mess with health and performance (see the section on REDs on page 128). To help retain muscle mass, a loss of no more than 0.5–1 kilogram per week is ideal, with protein intake at the higher end of the recommendations for climbers (see pages 35–36).[4] Exactly how much of a deficit and for how long is very individual, and dependent on many things including body composition goals, health status, current body composition, age, sex and much more. This is why it is best to do this kind of thing with qualified support.

Creating a calorie deficit is also trickier than it sounds. All calculations to estimate energy needs (see chapter 1) are just that: estimations. Measuring output in climbing is also very hard to do accurately. Equally, measuring food intake, whether using an app or weighing things out, is also an estimation. So, deciding how much food is needed in any numerical and quantifiable way is layer after layer of estimation.

Tracking food intake to implement a deficit also has other downsides. It can create a hyper-focus on food and calories which is unhelpful and potentially dangerous. Having said that, it can also – if used short-term and with a healthy perspective – give an insight into the energy content of food, which may create some opportunities for change that are easy to implement. For example, simple swaps of higher- for lower-calorie options, or reducing consumption of foods like fizzy drinks and cakes that are high in calories but confer little other nutritional benefit. Tracking may help with noticing habits that aren't helpful, for example, under-fuelling in the day that leads to eating past fullness in the evening. Here the key is to fuel more effectively in the daytime which, as well as making the day feel more productive and energetic, may help stave off overcompensation later on. Small hacks like this can make a big difference.

There are some other things that can help support a calorie deficit phase. One of these is maintaining high protein intake as this helps with feeling full and will also help to protect against losing muscle mass (although this still may happen).[5] High intake of whole foods, fruit and vegetables also helps with feeling full due to the higher fibre content, and keeping intake of these high will also help ensure micronutrient needs are met. While it may be tempting to

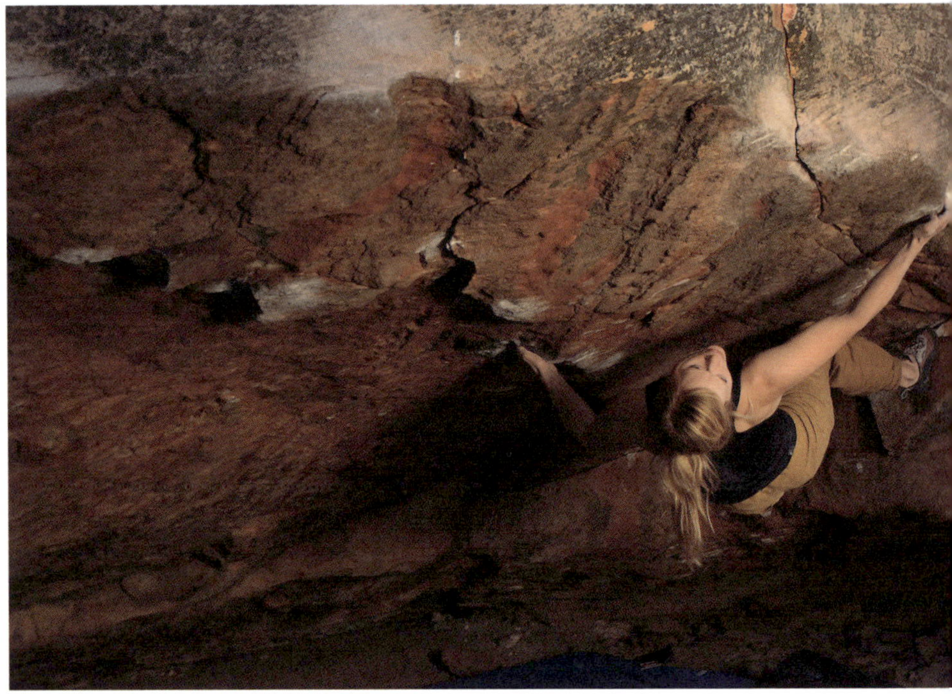

THE AUTHOR ON *THE VICE*, ROCKLANDS, SOUTH AFRICA. © DAVID MASON

heavily reduce or cut out carbohydrates, please don't! The initial drop in weight from cutting out carbohydrate is from associated water loss, not actual fat loss, and carbohydrate is key for climbing performance and training.

In an ideal world, weight loss would not be a part of a climber's nutritional strategy. It could be argued that focusing on supportive nutrition while climbing and training is the best way forward with the most sustainable long-term results. Often, with this approach, a sport-specific body composition develops anyway over time. But, like any weight-sensitive sport, it would be naive to ignore this aspect of nutrition, especially at an elite level. Marginal gains in elite sport are hard won and some periodised body composition change may be appropriate, but it will usually also be strategised and monitored by qualified dietitians or nutritionists.

So, why all the caution? Let's dive into what can happen when attempts at weight loss go wrong.

When it all goes wrong: REDs

What is REDs?

Relative energy deficiency in sport (REDs) is a term used to describe the condition of an athlete who is suffering symptoms underpinned by chronic problematic low energy availability and/or low carbohydrate availability. Essentially, REDs is what can happen when a person chronically underfuels, although other factors such as genetics, overtraining, illness, stress, behaviours and sleep can play a part. The human body is not infallible and it must adapt to survive.

Energy availability is how much energy the body has each day for basic bodily function, before considering the energy required for exercise. The body will prioritise fuelling for exercise, which means that if there is not

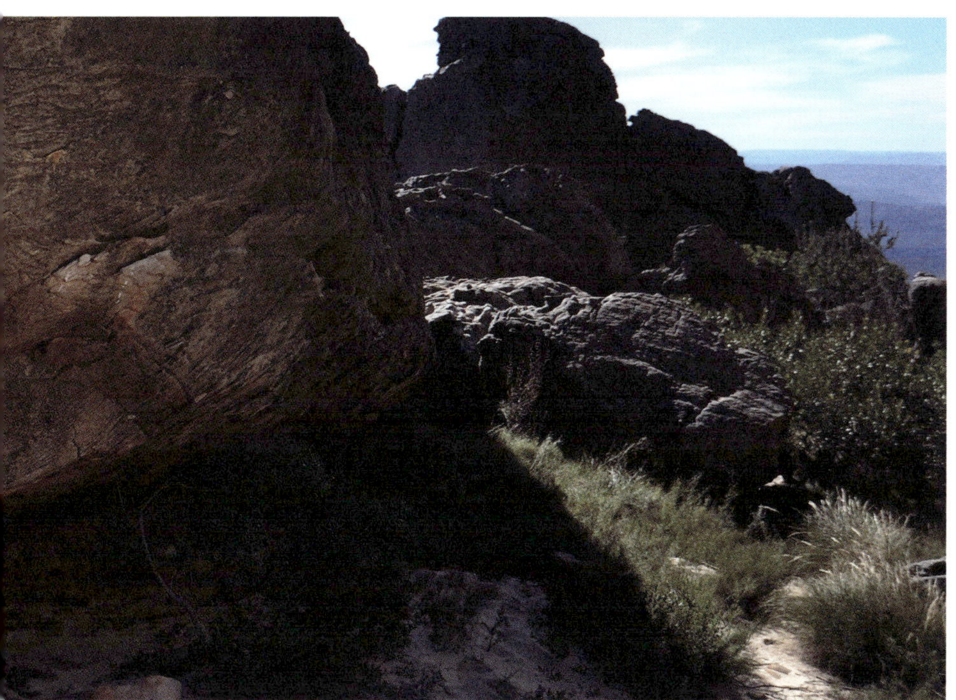

enough overall energy intake to cover this and its basic needs, it is the basic needs that suffer. This means that the body will begin to downregulate things like metabolic rate and hormone production in order to save energy. Liken it to a phone being put on battery saving mode. This can be tolerated in short bouts (coined 'adaptable low energy availability' by Mountjoy et al.), but in the longer term it becomes problematic and leads to REDs which can have serious implications on health.[6]

This is what happens when, over time, the body does not receive the support it needs. It is, in fact, a clever system: not enough energy essentially means a lack of safety, and the body responds by shutting down systems that are not absolutely key to survival. This has a major impact on many bodily systems and can dramatically affect both health and performance.

Interestingly, a state of REDs is not always accompanied by a low body weight or a certain body composition. This can feel counterintuitive as one might expect that not meeting energy demands would result in weight loss. However, over the long term, the body is very clever and metabolic rate has been shown to be reduced in those with symptoms of REDs.[7]

To fully understand REDs, it is important to understand the concept of energy availability and how it is defined. As mentioned above, this is the energy left over once exercise energy needs have been accounted for. It can be represented as an equation where it is measured relative to fat-free mass:

$$\textbf{Energy availability (EA)} = \frac{\text{energy intake (EI) - exercise energy expenditure (EEE)}}{\text{fat-free mass (FFM)}}$$

The research thus far has provided thresholds of energy availability under which there is likely to be dysfunction for an individual. Interestingly, these vary with sex: male athletes appear to be able to manage much lower energy availability levels without dysfunction than their female counterparts. For female athletes this threshold is less than 30 kilocalories per kilogram of fat-free mass, whereas for males it is less than 9–25 kilocalories per kilogram of fat-free mass, although there is a large potential for inter-individual variance.[8] This is quite a stark difference and explains, in part, why for so long this was seen as a female issue and why it seems to present more widely in women.

Historically, it was in fact called the 'female athlete triad' – a condition affecting female athletes that comprised low energy availability (with or without disordered eating), bone mineral density degradation and menstrual dysfunction.[9] In 2014, the International Olympic Committee released a consensus statement that renamed and expanded on the female athlete triad.[10] It brought together evidence and clinical understanding which suggested that the concept of the female athlete triad was a bit too narrow. The condition was renamed as REDs to include male athletes and encompass a wider set of symptoms and dysfunctions. This was then further updated with consensus statements in 2018 and 2023 to give a fuller picture of what is now considered REDs.[11]

Symptoms of REDs

REDs can present differently for different people; below are some of the symptoms that can arise:

→ Impaired reproductive function: in female athletes this presents as menstrual dysfunction and low libido; in males it can present as low libido and/or decreased morning erections
→ Impaired bone health
→ Impaired gastrointestinal function
→ Reduced immunity
→ Urinary continence issues
→ Mental health challenges
→ Impaired cardiovascular function
→ Sleep disturbances

In terms of performance decrements, below are some signs and symptoms that may occur:

→ Decreased endurance performance
→ Decreased power performance
→ Decreased training response
→ Decreased recovery
→ Decreased cognitive function
→ Decreased muscle strength
→ Reduced motivation
(Mountjoy et al., 2023)[12]

It is worth emphasising that REDs is a diagnosis of exclusion and it does not, as yet, have a single definitive diagnostic test. It is an area where a lot of confusion and misdiagnosis can occur due to the large array of symptoms. It needs the attention of an experienced clinician, blood tests and other tests to exclude other pathologies. If you are concerned you may be heading towards a state of REDs or feel that your relationship with food is disordered, please seek the help of a qualified professional.

Many things can contribute to ending up in a state of REDs. It could be excessive training in an attempt to get better at climbing and restricted food intake in an attempt to lose weight, or it could be unintentionally not meeting energy demands. Either way, for climbing as a sport, moving towards a culture that promotes positive, supportive nutrition and axing the narrative that lighter is better is an important movement. Because, yes, climbing is a weight-sensitive sport but lighter certainly isn't always better.

KEY TAKEAWAYS

- → Climbing is a weight-sensitive sport but weight loss and/or body composition change is more complex than it may appear.
- → Strength-to-weight ratio is a more useful perspective than absolute weight.
- → Attempts at body composition change should ideally be done with the help of a qualified dietitian or nutritionist.
- → The core principle of weight loss is creating a calorie deficit; there are different methods for achieving this.
- → There are risks to dieting, including a hyper-focus on food, muscle mass loss, reduced performance/energy levels and REDs.
- → REDs is a complex syndrome that can occur when low energy availability is problematic and chronic.
- → REDs has many negative performance and health outcomes.
- → Lighter is not always better.

WHAT CAN I DO?

- → Take some time to critically consider your core beliefs about body weight and climbing.
- → Are these beliefs serving you, your climbing performance and your well-being?
- → Are there any shifts in your thinking that might serve you better over the long term and perhaps give you space to perform better overall?

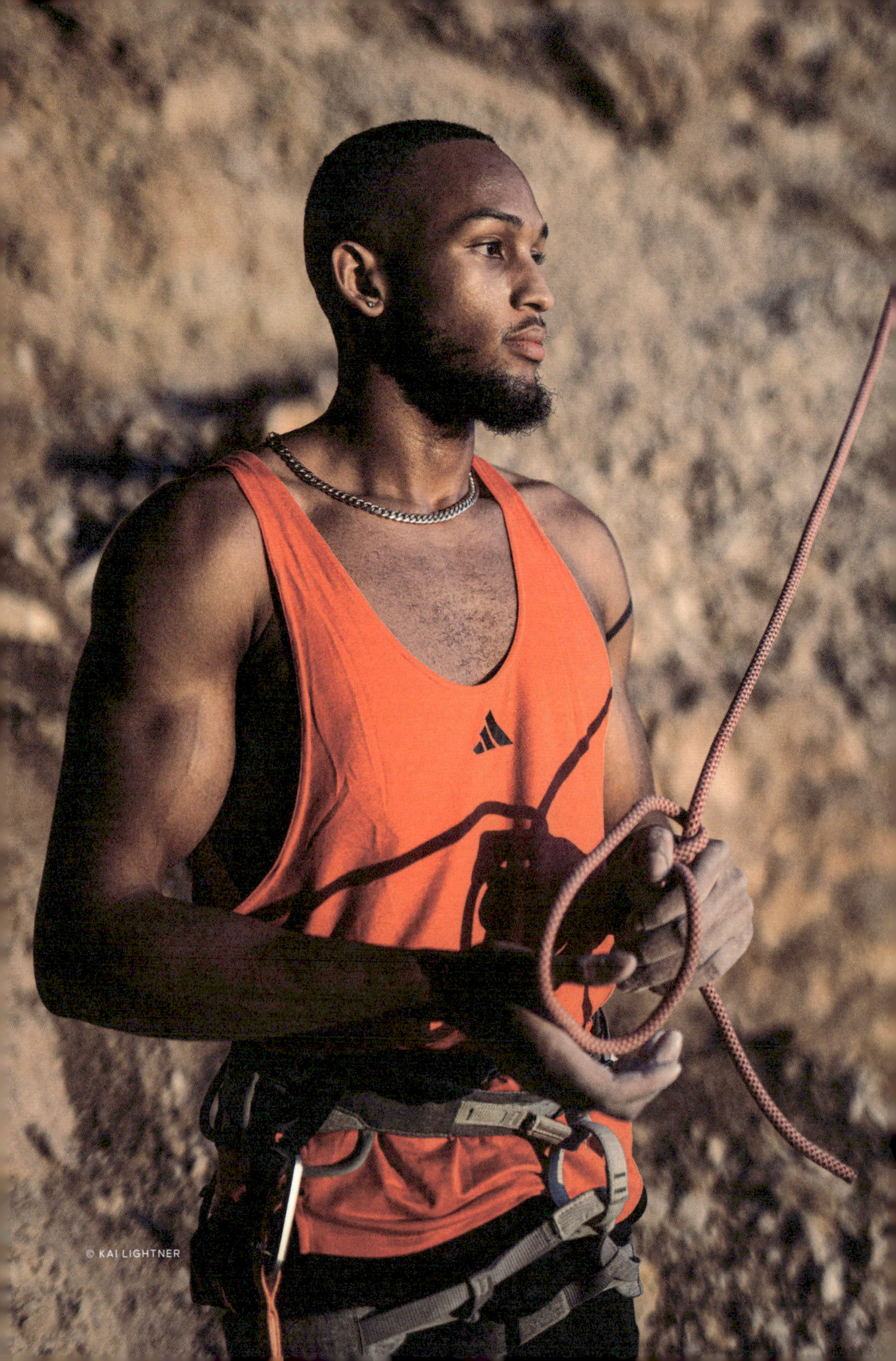

KAI LIGHTNER
TWO VERSIONS OF SUCCESS

As a youth athlete, Kai was unstoppable. With ten youth national championship titles, two open national titles, five youth world medals and six pan-American titles, he was no stranger to success. But behind the medals there was a lot more going on: a young person whose drive to be the best was becoming his undoing. Now, as a 25-year-old man, Kai looks back with perspective and wisdom on that time and the role that nutrition played. He shares his then and now; his two very different versions of success.

It's no surprise to me now that as a child growing up with ADHD, I instantly loved climbing. For those of us that are neurodivergent in some way, activities like this can be extremely positive and enticing. Climbing is made of patterns and puzzles, and, if things like that hook you, it's easy to get drawn in. From the start I loved the laser focus it required, the problem solving and the minute details of body movement. I could get lost in the dance of climbing; little shifts in my body here and there would unlock a climb and that was hugely satisfying. I never wanted to leave the gym. There was always something new to learn, an adjustment to make or a skill to pick up, and that made climbing particularly fascinating to me. I loved climbing so much, from the first minute I tried it. I was also really determined and competitive; I was so stubborn, always wanting to get to the top of the wall. I never thought that any challenge was too big or too hard and I saw no reason why I shouldn't be at the top. I cried a lot; there was a lot of passion.

Like many inner-city black kids, I grew up without a whole lot of resources. My mom was a single mom on a teacher salary and she did her best, but we ate a lot of basic food that probably wasn't super nutritious. Things like TV dinners, microwave meals and fast food. It was what she could afford and, to be honest, we didn't think about nutrition too much back then, even when I started climbing. My diet probably wasn't as good as most of the other kids competing at my level, but I made up for it with hard work, adrenaline and passion. Those things can outweigh a lot of other factors.

From the start I was pretty good, and I won a lot of titles and medals. But in the background I felt like I was on the clock and running out of time. I come from a family of tall people: my dad is 6 foot 9 and my mom is 5 foot 9. Despite what an outsider may think, being tall isn't the best thing for climbing. Most top climbers are actually quite small but with long arms, and this allows them to stay light but still have the necessary reach. From a really young age I was made aware that size and weight mattered in climbing. People often commented on my size and even said to me that I would outgrow the sport, that I wouldn't continue to be good for long. For my age I was already quite stocky and it seemed like everyone thought that as soon as I hit puberty I would grow super tall, get too heavy and I would be finished. I internalised a lot of what I heard from the people around me. Despite having a lot of talent, it felt like the writing was on the wall already; it was all going to get difficult.

So, I felt like I was working against the clock. People were watching my weight, what I ate and how much cardio I did. It felt like I had to do my part as well. I was trying to battle against my genetics and stay as light as I could for as long as I could. It was the one part I could have some control over since getting tall wasn't negotiable. Controlling my weight seemed like the only way I might keep up my success in this body that was sentenced to be unfit for hard climbing. What I was doing also wasn't unusual, it seemed like everyone was doing it back then. I remember being in isolation for my first adult competition final when I was 13 and sitting with all my idols; all of them openly talking about what they had and hadn't eaten to stay light. It was everywhere, normalised and accepted.

I don't think one individual thing hit me more than another, but they all culminated in a bigger message to my young mind – that weight matters. And everyone is doing it, it comes with the territory of climbing. So, I worked hard at staying light, I didn't eat snacks or junk food, and I kept cutting out things where I could. The restrictions increased more and more as time went on. It was so incremental that I don't think I ever realised how unhealthy it had become. Also, it paid off: I was performing better than ever, and I felt light and strong on the wall. It made me wonder how much more I could lose and how much I could gain in performance from doing so. It spiralled to a point when I was barely eating. There was fear and anxiety around everything – my training, my performance and my food.

A turning point for me was when I was around 13 or 14 and I started having odd health issues like acid reflux, stomach problems and weird pains in my body. One day my mom came to get me early from school. She said that we were going home but it soon became clear that we weren't. We pulled up to the doctors and my mom took me in for an evaluation. They tested a bunch of stuff, and not only was I seriously underweight, I was close to liver failure and was low on many nutrients and fluids. I felt so exposed and – honestly – embarrassed. It's so hard to see the damage when you're in the eye of the storm, and I was only doing what I thought everyone else was too. When I looked in the mirror, I saw the same old person.

The next few years were a tricky balance to strike; I wanted to keep performing but I also knew I had to eat enough to stay healthy. I did my best with my mom's support to make some changes. I started to eat more and gain a little

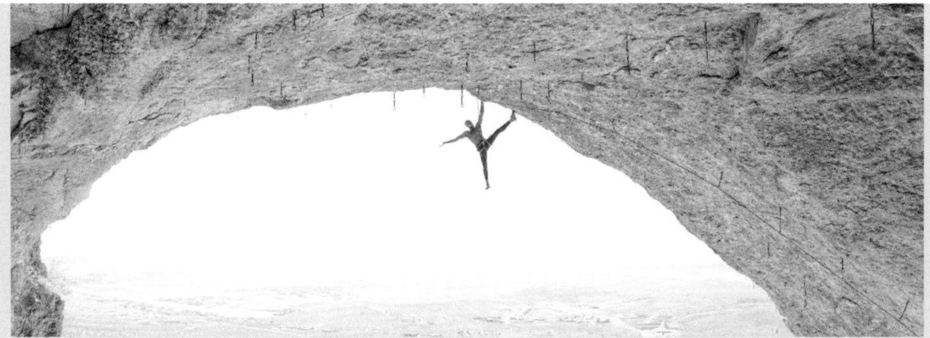

© KAI LIGHTNER

weight, but I also thought that if I wanted to keep climbing well I couldn't eat too much. As I got taller, the fear set in. I walked what felt like a tightrope through those years; it was a constant battle. I still had goals and people still expected me to win; I held so many titles at that point and I didn't want to let them go. I was managing to do it, but it felt costly to my mental health and my body felt tired.

At 18 I retired. It was actually the year of the first ever Olympic qualifiers for climbing and everyone expected me to try but I just didn't have it in me. My body was exhausted and starting to break down. I was mentally tired and losing the love for it: burnt out. I stopped competing and climbing altogether because I just couldn't muster the effort for it all any more. It was all just too stressful. I went to college and I realised what a normal life could be like: seeing friends, going out, eating normally. It took this complete removal from my climbing world to realise how abnormal my habits had been and how unbalanced my life was before. This time away allowed my body to have a break and to grow and develop properly. It was probably the best decision I've ever made.

It was a few years before I started to dip my toes into climbing again. When I did, it was purely for leisure. I remembered that outdoor climbing had always been a peaceful place for me compared to competing; it's less pressured, the rock isn't going anywhere. So that's what I focused on. I remember early on my mom and I went on a trip to Santa Linya and to begin with I had to fight my way up 5.13a (F7c+), but by the end of the trip I was sending 5.14c (F8c+). It was all still there and, importantly, it was there in my body as a built, 6-foot-2 man. Maybe it was possible to find a healthy space to push myself again? There were still so many things I wanted to do, and I wanted to rediscover the joy that I used to get from climbing.

Climbing became my focus once more, but I swore to myself that I would only keep going if I could do it in a healthy way. It became a challenge; could I get back to my top level and stay healthy? I didn't want to lose the love of climbing again. I'm in a much better place with food now, I eat healthily in general but I also don't restrict myself on things like dessert or sweets. In training, I really focus on the strength side of the strength-to-weight ratio and I do everything in a way that feels sustainable. When I was younger, I could climb forever without getting pumped but I would often hit moves that I didn't have the power for. Now I feel stable and powerful; I can do hard moves and I have a high level of power endurance. I'm performing at my best again just in a different way and I have a much more balanced life at the same time. I'm definitely more well rounded as a climber physically and also a lot less anxious; climbing well or not no longer feels like life and death.

It's hard to believe in yourself when you don't see people like you doing the thing you love. I am back to being a full-time professional climber and I hope that other people can read my story or see me climbing and know that it's possible to be a top climber in a taller, heavier body.

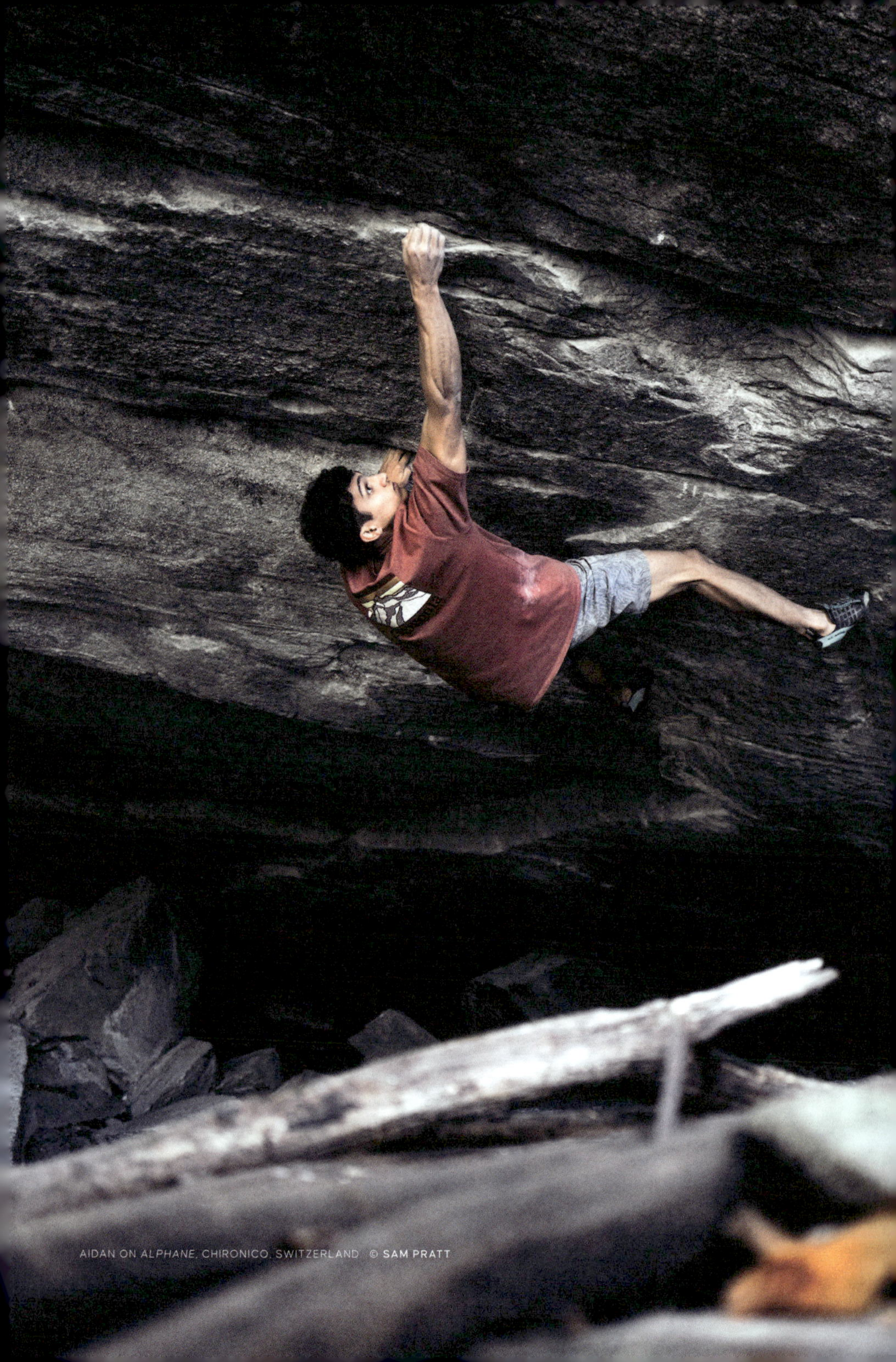

AIDAN ON *ALPHANE*, CHIRONICO, SWITZERLAND © **SAM PRATT**

AIDAN ROBERTS
ELITE PERFORMANCE AND WEIGHT

Aidan is currently one of the best professional boulderers in the world. He is no stranger to finding and projecting new lines and he has pushed hard climbing to the limit both at home and abroad. Aidan shares his insights into how nutrition played a role for him on his first ascent of *Arrival of the Birds* (Font 9a) in Ticino, Switzerland.

Before I did it, it was called the Midnight Project; a face of rock that sits on the hill above the famous *From Dirt Grows the Flowers* boulder in Ticino. I went to Ticino in the spring of 2022 for the first time and I saw this boulder early in the trip. It's tall, blank and unassuming; river-polished, slick rock that has just enough features on it to be climbable. It's also really dense rock and the holds are created by gas bubbles that have left these slot-like rounded crimps. The nature of the holds requires a high angle of flexion in the fingers for them to stay in place, with only three fitting in each one. The feet are poor and very far to the sides, so a lot of force goes through the fingers. As a result, the moves require slow precision and steely digits. I was instantly drawn to it – this is my forte, the style of climbing that suits me best. To find a project that felt so very hard in my specialism was exciting and also humbling. It was intimidating from both a skin and injury perspective because it was so very intense on the fingers. I tried it that first trip and split my skin very quickly. There were subsequent sessions where I could barely get established on the moves. Every move was hard and it wasn't possible to have a light session on it. It was all or nothing every time I pulled on.

Trying this boulder was a pivotal time in my climbing; I worked on it over a few seasons and I feel like I changed a lot as a climber during that time. It was a bit of a roller coaster to be honest. From 2022 onwards I would try it with increasing focus in the shoulder seasons, spring and autumn. Between those trips I would come home for about three months to reflect, re-evaluate and train. It became a repeating cycle and each time I got back from trying it I would think about how I could be better, how I could eke out another one or two per cent in my performance. I had to decide what to focus on in terms of skill development which meant some neglect elsewhere; I was getting less well rounded as a climber, but I got more and more specialised in the area that was already my style. Everything was planned out and then reviewed in a very intentional way. The more energy I invested, the more rewarding I found it, but it also became all-consuming.

Of course, I did all the usual things to try and progress through training, but, in this particular case, it was clear that my body weight would play a part in how hard it felt to climb these moves. Climbing is, of course, always affected by weight to some degree, but especially so on climbs like this that are so finger intensive and require such slow precision. My initial weight drop actually happened by accident. I was on a climbing trip over the winter in 2023 and it was really cold; I must have been burning more energy than I realised to keep warm. When I got home, I felt really good on the rock; it was quite stark. This really brought weight manipulation to the forefront of my mind when I thought about the Midnight Project.

I became more intentional around reducing my weight with a planned strategy around controlling my food intake in the lead-up to my next trip. I'd had support from a nutritionist in the past so I had a decent grasp on how I should approach it. I knew I needed to create a deficit to further lose body weight, but I wanted to ensure I didn't compromise my energy and strength while I did this. A tightrope if ever there was one. The key for me was to reduce energy intake without reducing carbohydrates and protein, and timing my food intake quite strictly around my training sessions so that I always had available fuel and recovery food at the best times. I had a lower fat intake which allowed me to create a deficit while boosting the other two macronutrients to maintain my energy, performance and recovery. Fats are important for health of course, but they are also the most calorie-dense macronutrient so this approach helped me to reduce my energy intake in the short term. I've always been vegetarian and so my high protein intake was made up of things like eggs, 0% fat Greek yoghurt and protein powders to try to minimise muscle loss.

Along the way I made some quite conscious decisions around social food situations in order to keep control of my strategy; this sounds severe, but it felt necessary to maintain my trajectory, and performance was my priority at this time. I felt good in my training sessions, I was making progress and my weight was also coming down. I assume over a longer time frame it would have reduced my work capacity in some way, but I knew that my skin would never outlast my work capacity on the Midnight Project so it wasn't an issue I was concerned about.

I felt amazing on the rock when I went back to Ticino in the spring of 2024. My fingers felt strong and I could move slowly and precisely between the holds. I sent the Midnight Project, thereafter *Arrival of the Birds*, quite quickly. However, I did notice feeling tired and a bit disconnected outside of my climbing sessions. It was like I put all my energy into my climbing, and the other parts of life were where the fatigue and energy deficit showed up. My mind felt slower and I noticed that I didn't engage as much as normal with some things. I was aware that I was testing the bottom limit of where my body was happy, bordering on pushing it to an unhappy place. I had a really performance-focused mindset at the time so, even though I was aware of how it was playing out, I was okay with it. It felt like a sacrifice I was willing to make to perform at my best in those short moments on the rock. At that point in time each day was judged on how much it paid into my performance.

After I did it, I had planned to bounce back to eating in a less controlled way and for my weight

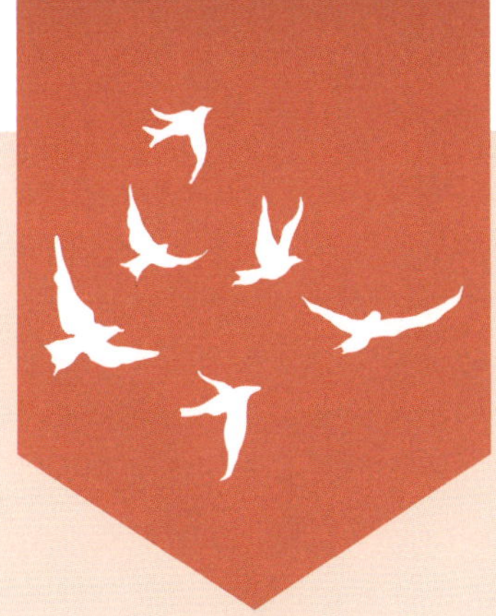

to increase again. This did happen but much more slowly than I thought it would. I was surprised to find my mind clinging on to some of the controlled behaviours I had developed and, even though I knew rationally that it wasn't sustainable, I found it hard to let go of the improved performance that came with being lighter. I guess what I'm saying is that, in the aftermath, despite the calculated approach, a degree of irrationality crept in. This was really interesting and not something I expected.

I went back to my reflective process as I could sense the potential for burnout. Having climbed the hardest boulder of my life I needed to re-evaluate what I wanted from the next phase of my climbing. I decided to redirect my climbing goals towards going on adventures and connecting with people and places. That shift helped me to gradually let go of some of the more controlled behaviours that had become normal for me. This doesn't mean hard climbing has gone out of the window, of course not. That will always be part of what I love and care about within climbing, but I don't want it to be all-consuming all of the time. The mindset and behaviours I had developed to climb *Arrival of the Birds* weren't sustainable.

So, when the next hard, fingery project comes along, will I manipulate my body weight again? Yes, I think I will, and I don't regret having done it for *Arrival of the Birds*; optimal body composition is part of elite climbing performance, that fact can't be escaped. I learned a lot from this experience and I'd like to think that next time I would be more prepared for the nuances of the process, both during and after. This time around I underestimated how irrationality could creep in and next time I would try to accommodate for that. I would aim to have more flexibility generally and also have some accountability from others in place. There is a weight range where my body is happy and I can push the lower limit of that range for top performance peaks, but not forever. I think that periodising nutrition to achieve an optimal weight for specific performance peaks is the ideal. Just like a training plan, this can be done for specific time frames with monitoring and feedback processes in place. I guess, just like training, it takes some trial and error to get the strategy and balance right.

It goes without saying that there is a healthy discussion to be had around weight and climbing. It can be an extremely polarising subject and, for many, a difficult conversation. Will all boulders feel easier when lighter? Definitely not, but some will. While I absolutely agree that it's important to promote health in sport and to discourage unhealthy nutritional practices or disordered eating, the weight-sensitive nature of climbing can't be completely ignored. It would be naive to say weight isn't a factor in climbing, especially at the top end and in particular styles. Where weight loss for performance meets health is a hard intersection to navigate, but we can't just say climbers should never lose weight as a blanket rule. It's more complicated than that and it can be done in sensible ways. I think there is a growing opinion that having a desire to manipulate one's body weight for climbing performance is bad or shameful; it's become demonised. This can create dangerous situations where people feel unable to communicate about it; they may do it anyway in secret with little support and perhaps dodgy methods. Of course, it's not always wise or necessary to lose weight, it's situational. But, if appropriate, it doesn't need to be a case of indefinite dieting without any nuance; there are smart, pragmatic ways to do it.

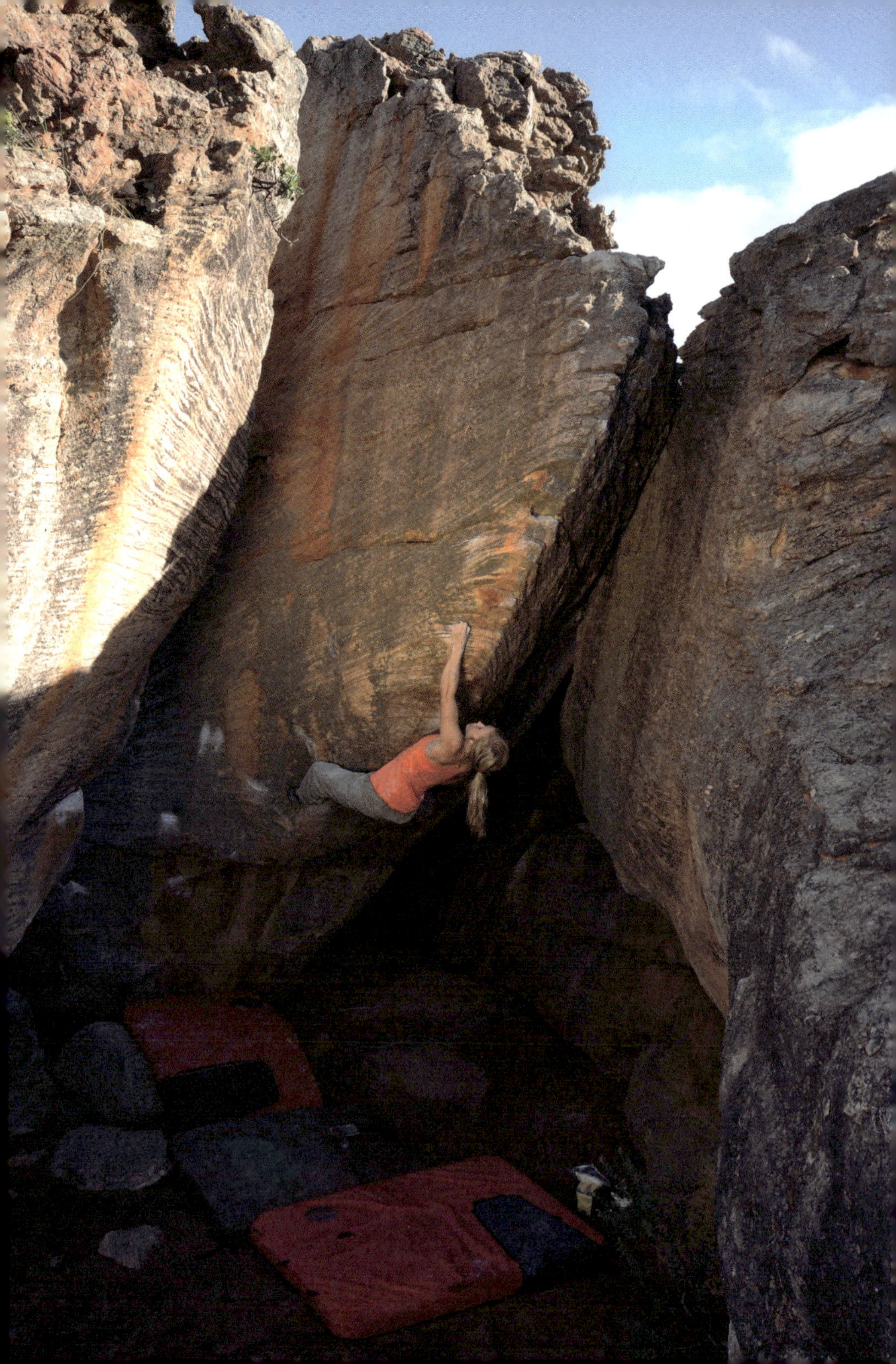

12

CAN CLIMBERS EAT INTUITIVELY?

THE AUTHOR ON *BARRACUDA*, ROCKLANDS, SOUTH AFRICA © **DAVID MASON**

What does your mind conjure up when someone talks about *intuitive eating*? For many, this phrase translates to, 'eat whatever you want, whenever you want'. And while this is not exactly incorrect, it is misleading in its lack of nuance. The idea of following intuition around food, if only lightly understood, may create fear around lack of control for many people, invoking desires for indulgence and overeating of less-nutritious foods. However, the framework as it will be laid out in this chapter will hopefully add some depth to the concept of eating intuitively and what it really means to live and breathe this approach in its entirety. It's a fascinating topic and – in my opinion – a truly worthwhile and liberating framework to connect with. Where intuitive eating intersects with sport is also hugely interesting, even more so in weight-sensitive sports where body composition plays into performance. Can these two areas of nutrition coexist for climbers and what would that look like?

What is intuitive eating?

Intuitive eating as it is known today is a framework for eating that was created in 1995 by two American dietitians, Evelyn Tribole and Elyse Resch.[1] It integrates emotion, rational thought and instinct around food choices while being firmly centred in self-care and weight inclusivity. The practice of intuitive eating is based around ten guiding principles that help a person become attuned to their body and disentangle themselves from the established rules or beliefs around food and body image that are ingrained in many people from cultural influences.

The intuitive eating framework is backed by research that shows an association between using this approach and improved body image, reduced disordered eating, improved diet quality and improved emotional functioning.[2] According to a 2023 survey, most dietitians report using the intuitive eating model in some capacity with the athletes that they work with, especially in cases where under-fuelling may be an issue.[3] One of the joys of the model is that, from the ten principles, there is no set order, and one or some of the principles may be most useful to an individual while others may be less pertinent. It is a framework that can be really flexible to the person and what they need to create a more fully functioning relationship with food and their body.

It is worth mentioning that the intuitive eating model, while extremely helpful to many, is not something that can be effectively used straight away in individuals who are suffering from eating disorders. In these cases, hunger and satiety cues are dysregulated and cannot be relied upon initially for managing adequate food intake. Later on in the rehabilitation process, the intuitive eating framework can be a key part of the recovery approach, but only once weight restoration has occurred and the body's signals are more functional. As always, in the case of clinical eating disorders, it is crucial to work with a dietitian as part of a multidisciplinary medical team.

The ten principles of intuitive eating

1 Reject the diet mentality

This is a big one that sits at the heart of intuitive eating. To be able to fully embrace the intuitive eating way, rejection of diet culture is key. This means turning your back on the idea that the perfect 'diet' is out there, putting a stop to any conscious or subconscious search for a way of controlling what you are eating that will make you or your life feel better. Whether it is calorie counting, intermittent fasting, low carb, ketogenic or simply general ideas around 'good' and 'bad' foods, these preoccupations will not serve you in your journey to becoming an intuitive eater. The creators of intuitive eating go one step further: they encourage generating some anger towards diet culture – see diet culture as the destructive force that it is and be angry about the negative impact it can have on the physical and mental well-being of many people.

2 Honour your hunger

This principle requires what can be very deep work on developing your interoceptive awareness. Interoceptive awareness is the ability to be aware of and respond appropriately to internal body sensations or emotions. Honouring hunger sounds simple, but it can be far from it for many people. For a start, the biological sensation of hunger shows up in different ways for different individuals. For some of us it may be a gnawing sensation in our stomach, for others it might be feeling light-headed, headaches, grumpiness or lethargy. There are also different levels of hunger, from slight sensations to extreme hunger (see figure 12). Try to notice hunger – and act on it – earlier on if possible. Leaving hunger to get to extreme levels can often result in compensatory overeating and overfullness. Acting early also reinforces a sense of respect for the sensations that the body is sending and it builds trust in both directions; the mind trusts the body to communicate its needs and the body trusts the mind to respond. Adhering to this principle is foundational in terms of keeping the body biologically fed with enough energy which, in turn, can have profound effects on mental wellness and your psychological relationship with food. Bear in mind this may take a substantial amount of practice if hunger is dysregulated.

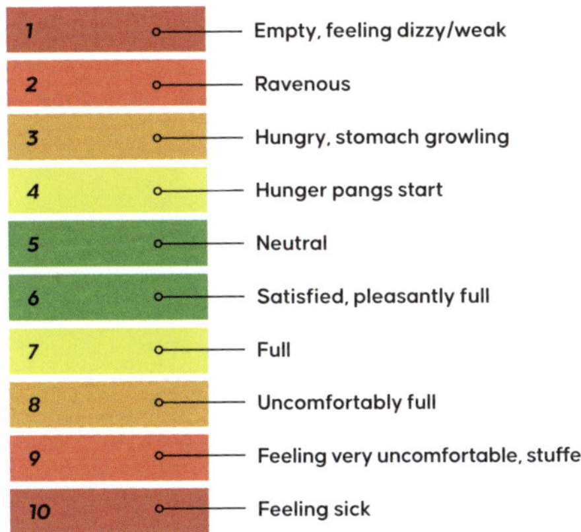

Figure 12: Hunger and fullness scale. Adapted from Tribole and Resch, 2012.[1]

3 Make peace with food

This principle is about giving yourself unconditional permission to eat in any and all circumstances. That means there are no good or bad foods, no forbidden foods, and no food or eating that deserves a feeling of shame or guilt. This internal shift makes food a friend not an enemy; it turns a battle into a collaboration. Instead of always thinking *I should eat this* or *I shouldn't eat that*, thoughts can turn to *What would I like to eat right now?* or *Which foods would make my body and/or mind feel good now?* If food choices feel difficult or counterproductive, let curiosity rather than shame take the lead. Ask questions about what is going on. Denying certain foods in a restrictive way inevitably leads to more craving for that food and, often, when it is eaten, it is done so in a way that may feel frantic or out of control. When all foods are allowed, with a genuine lack of judgement, foods or eating patterns that may in the past have held huge power, no longer do. This is a truly liberating principle.

4 Discover the satisfaction factor

This principle, as described in the title, is about discovering or rediscovering *satisfaction* in food and eating. It sounds simple but it is a facet of the eating experience that is often not given enough importance. Bringing satisfaction, both physical and emotional, to the forefront inherently changes some decisions that might be made around food, for the better. It's easy to feel like one 'should' or 'shouldn't' eat in a certain way or eat certain foods. Coming back to the basics of desire and satisfaction can be hugely rewarding, and, when uncomplicated, they can line up with hunger and fullness, nourishing food and a relaxed mindset. It brings the love and enjoyment back to the eating experience, adding a dimension that is so central to how humans connect. Food and eating are an important part of shared experience, connection and culture among humans. Sometimes diet culture, and a desire to control or restrict eating and/or look a certain way, can take the joy out of the wonderful ritual that is eating. Reconnecting with and giving importance to satisfaction can be a simple game-changer for many. Eating what you really want in that moment, in an environment that is conducive to enjoyment, is truly a pleasure and sets a precedent within the food relationship for inclusion and validation of desires. Often, eating what is really wanted results in eating to comfortable fullness rather than eating more – potentially past comfortable fullness – to make up for a satisfaction gap.

5 Feel your fullness

This is another principle – like *2 Honour your hunger* – that requires you to develop your interoceptive awareness. As with hunger, it is about paying close attention to how your body is feeling and responding appropriately. Refer to figure 12 again to consider the fullness side of the eating experience. The body will send signals that hunger is no longer present, it will notify the brain with symptoms when comfortable fullness is passing by and it will cry out when beyond this point. It may be helpful to integrate pauses within a meal to assess how full you are and how your body is feeling. It's okay to leave food. The clean-plate mentality is deeply ingrained in many of us and of course food waste is not ideal, but most things can be saved and eaten at a later date if desired. Don't treat your body like a rubbish bin that has to clear up unwanted food. This is a great principle to experiment with. Try stopping at different points and seeing how you feel. Explore the different sensations. You can always come back and eat more if you decide you are not yet comfortably full. You have full unconditional permission to do that.

6 Challenge the food police

The food police represents the voice in your head. The one that has certain rules or behaviours it expects around food and gives you a hard time if you don't comply. This voice in the inner psyche develops over time for many people as a result of diet culture, body image expectations, performance expectations and many other individual factors. The first step in this principle is to *notice* the food police voice. Notice if there is even a slight voice that pops up when you go to consider seconds or are choosing a pudding. Do they pipe up when you feel extra hungry on a rest day? Or maybe when you go to a buffet-style dinner? What is leading your decisions around food and how deeply internalised is the voice that represents diet culture? Once noticed, the food police lose their power. Slow things down and take time to challenge the thoughts that attempt to control these moments and consider if the voice has any value. It could be argued that without this internal voice, we would all just eat too much food and too much 'junk' food all the time. But with the other aspects of intuitive eating in play, a wonderful thing happens: the body and mind reset and food becomes a positive partner. Eating too much (*see principle 5*) doesn't appeal any more and, while some junk food may be pleasurable at times, it won't be desirable a lot of the time.

7 Cope with your emotions with kindness

Food and emotions are linked for most people. Food has long been used for celebration, comfort, expression and pleasure. And everyone experiences emotions from sadness, anger and frustration to anxiety and boredom. Recognising when food or eating is taking place to control, appease or comfort an emotional trigger is an important step. Restrictive eating can be a way of taking control when life or emotions feel uncontrollable – often a time when uncontrolled or binge eating can also happen. Separating food from emotions is really tricky, and, of course, using food as a comfort is not always a negative thing – it can be helpful at times and feel nourishing. What this principle focuses on is creating an awareness of where emotions are creating unhelpful eating behaviours and negative feedback loops. Stepping out of these patterns and focusing on the emotions and their causes with kindness may be more productive and supportive in the long run.

8 Respect your body

All bodies deserve respect. Accepting the genetic blueprint you have been given can feel tough if it doesn't fit the expectations you may hold or fit the desired profile of your sport. Historically, climbing favours the strong, lean aesthetic, although more and more we are seeing a focus on strength, power and athleticism over lightness. Finding a level of acceptance, admiration and respect for your body is liberating. Constantly trying to change your body is exhausting and emotionally draining. It's very difficult to reject a diet mentality or a 'less is more' approach to food and eating if, underneath it all, there is no respect for your current body. Culturally, this is an age where people are often trying to be smaller, take up less space and be lighter. In sports like climbing this can be even more emphasised due to the belief that performance will also be better. This principle urges you to look in the mirror and respect what you see, regardless. Celebrate what your body can do, how it feels and how it looks – even if that doesn't fit a predetermined ideal. Put your energy into climbing itself, rather than into an effort to change your body. Take up space and do it now; don't wait until some future point, where you look a certain way or weigh a certain amount, to respect your body.

9 Movement – feel the difference

While this principle has a broader audience and is not specifically aimed at athletes, it has a lot to offer. Movement is a natural part of being human and feeling good. Humans were not meant to be as sedentary as we often are and this part of the intuitive eating model aims to redefine the relationship with moving our bodies. Exercise is often very prescriptive, goal-orientated and can be unenjoyable for many. For climbers and climbing this is hopefully not true! But there might be an element for some climbers of training for climbing or exercising to alter body composition that is not positive. Recognising this and coming back to the basics of moving the body for the pleasure it brings in that moment and the moments directly afterwards can feel freeing. Move your body not to change your body, hit a target or burn calories. Move your body to feel the difference from the inside.

10 Honour your health with gentle nutrition

This principle is a really interesting one and is where the connection between intuitive eating and sports nutrition can flourish. Honouring your health with gentle nutrition means that it is possible to eat in a way that is attuned to your senses, emotions, satisfaction and culture, while also prioritising health and sporting needs. For example, you mostly eat according to hunger and fullness cues but, after exercise, you know that appetite may be suppressed and that it is in the interests of your body, health and climbing progress to eat despite not feeling hungry. Or, you finish a big climbing day and you really want to eat just lots of carbohydrates (your body is likely craving them because you used a lot of energy that day) but you add some protein to your meal, not because you really want it, but because you know it will help support your muscle recovery. These are examples of mechanical eating and, in the right context, it shows your body respect as much as honouring your hunger does. This principle is about arming yourself with knowledge about nutrition but using it gently. 'Good' nutrition is not built in one meal or one snack, just as it is not derailed so quickly either. This is the same in sport; it is about consistency over time with supportive nutrition. Intuitive eating is an incredibly person-centred, supportive approach to food and eating and, with sports nutrition knowledge overlaid on top, it's a perfect pairing.

Intuitive eating for climbers

There are lots of practicalities to consider with climbing, along with the nutrition recommendations for optimal performance and recovery. So, can climbers fuel and recover optimally, meet all the practical needs of climbing and also eat intuitively?

It's a big ask and maybe in some situations it isn't possible. But rather than disregarding it completely, consider what can be taken from intuitive eating that will have a positive impact. Perhaps on climbing days mechanical eating will need to prevail to ensure that nutritional demands are met, but on rest days food intake can follow more of an intuitive approach laced with some knowledge of recovery needs. When picking foods, consider satisfaction *as well as* nutritional needs for the day. Be flexible in your eating habits to allow for foods where the value is purely enjoyment and pleasure. Pay attention to the signals your body is sending you with a sense of curiosity and give it the respect it deserves.

Research has shown that athletes often wait until after their sporting career is over to recalibrate and nourish their relationship with food, eating and their body, but wouldn't it be wonderful if this could be done while still in the thick of performance?[4] It begs the question of whether some climbers – and athletes in general – might actually perform better if led by their bodies. A tendency to outsource decisions around food is understandable in this age of tracking, measuring and collecting data, but do we really know better than our bodies? Learning to truly listen is the first step to exploring this question.

KEY TAKEAWAYS

- → Intuitive eating is a framework for eating that is centred around self-care, integrating rational thought, emotion and instinct.
- → It was created in 1995 by two American dietitians, Evelyn Tribole and Elyse Resch.
- → It is based on ten principles: reject the diet mentality; honour your hunger; make peace with food; discover the satisfaction factor; feel your fullness; challenge the food police; cope with your emotions with kindness; respect your body; movement - feel the difference; and honour your health with gentle nutrition.
- → Integrating intuitive eating with nutrition to optimally support climbing nutrition is complex and nuanced but can be worthwhile for many climbers.

WHAT CAN I DO?

- → Consider the impact of this chapter: does this framework and approach to eating resonate with you?
- → Are there particular principles that you feel you could work on in more depth?
- → Pick one principle at a time to work on over the next few days and weeks.
- → Focus first on increasing your awareness of thoughts and behaviours that relate to this principle.
- → Create mental space for challenging your thoughts and feelings as they come up and practising the positive aspects within each principle.
- → Think about how you might be able to honour this framework while also optimising your performance in specific scenarios.

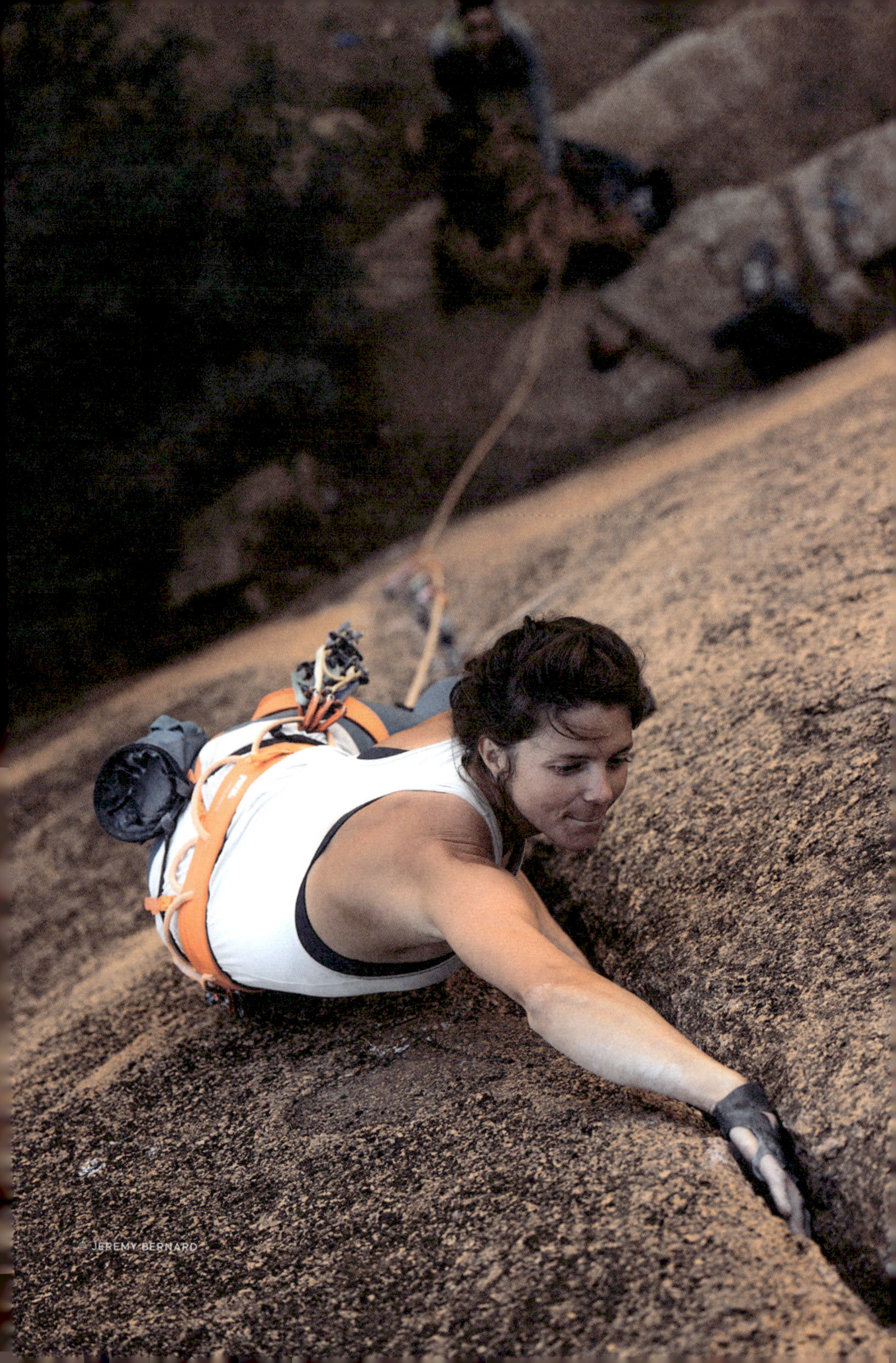

NINA CAPREZ ON THE ROAD WITH ANDREA

After many years as a professional climber pushing her athletic goals on rock, Nina took on a different kind of adventure. Morocco was the destination, the vision was to connect with people and to share the values and enjoyment of climbing. With a new sense of purpose, Nina set off with her family. *Andrea* was their vehicle: for travel, living and spreading the love of climbing. Nina shares their experience with food and nutrition while living on the road.

This trip to Morocco was a different kind of trip to my usual adventures. It was about more than just climbing; it was a chance to make a bigger impact. We set off as a family: me, my partner Jeremy and our then 15-month-old daughter, Lia. The plan was to combine our personal adventures as a family with social projects that brought the joy and values of climbing to the communities we visited.

Andrea is our Unimog truck, an expedition truck that has a four-metre-square climbing wall on it. We worked on it together, combining our skills to build something that allowed us to connect with others through the fun of climbing. We communicated with existing organisations in Morocco to ensure that we could be as useful as possible and take our vision to places it would benefit the most. Alongside this we did some climbing of our own, mostly cragging and some bolting.

Not long after we arrived, on 8 September 2023, a huge earthquake hit Morocco. With a magnitude of 6.9, it was catastrophic. It left in its wake a high death toll, extensive damage and many people without homes. Our focus shifted and we headed to the Atlas Mountains. We wanted to help in any way we could. It was no longer about climbing and had instead become a humanitarian mission. Our aim was to create a friendly space for children and adults whose lives had been turned upside down and to help with the delivery of aid. It was all-consuming; both rewarding and exhausting. To bring some moments of joy to people who had suffered so deeply was a privilege that left us with many emotions to process.

After we left the Atlas Mountains, we returned to our original focus – to connect with

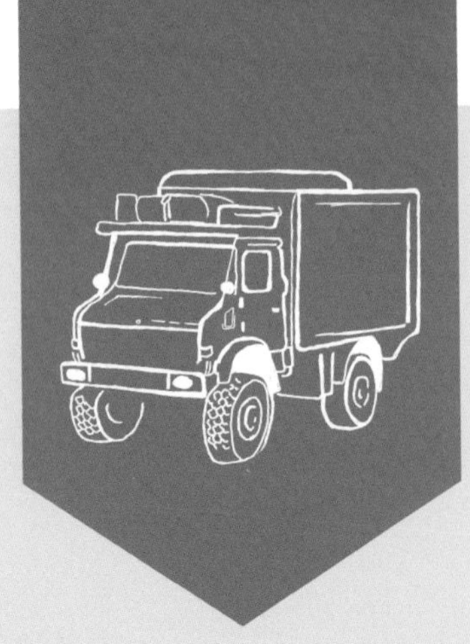

the climbing communities in Morocco, to share skills and to create experiences that bring people together through climbing. It was a pleasure to teach, to climb with new people and to immerse ourselves in a new place. So much of this was possible because of *Andrea*, our truck that was our home away from home.

Andrea needed to be big and sturdy to support a fixed climbing wall, as well as being capable of off-road driving. Not only that, we would be living in *Andrea* for months at a time so we needed a set-up that was practical and made us feel as comfortable and 'at home' as possible. For us, the kitchen and being able to cook and eat together was a huge part of this, especially as the truck was built with longer-term travel in mind. Jeremy and I love cooking, so we wanted to be able to be creative with food. We installed a large workspace made from really durable material so that there was space to prepare things, and we decided to put in an oven as well as a hob. This meant we could cook in similar ways to at home most of the time. One section of the workspace also morphed into a seating area to eat in as a family, which was important for us. We had a sink connected to our water storage and a fridge too. *Andrea* was pretty well equipped.

In many ways food on this trip was easy. We ate simple, fresh food; it was basic, delicious and all that we needed. The local market was full of fresh fruit and vegetables, all grown nearby and not travel-worn. The food quality was so good. Chickens in the market were fresh, killed that morning, so we knew they would be safe to eat. We actually didn't eat much meat other than chicken as we couldn't always guarantee the age and storage time. Dairy products are not a huge part of Moroccan cuisine, so we had very little of that which is unusual for us – at home we love cheese!

Bread is an important part of Moroccan food culture; it's special and revered. To share bread with people we met was a common ritual. We would eat bread in the mornings with an amazing Moroccan spread called amlou – a mix of almond paste, honey and argan oil. Lunches were often picnic style: more bread, some tomatoes, olive oil and La Vache qui rit (aka The Laughing Cow – the only cheese we found!). In the evenings we cooked lots of regional dishes like tagine, a slow-cooked stew with vegetables, meat (in this case chicken) and spices. We would make a fire and cook the tagine for three hours. Not only did this save gas, it gave a beautiful richness to the taste. We both love to discover local foods and cuisines when we travel but we had also brought with us some staple basics – things like good coffee, pasta, rice, quinoa, pulses, beans and pesto. This meant that quick, familiar meals were also an option. We had our baby cooker to prepare some of Lia's meals, along with milk powder for her.

Water was interesting on this trip. We had a 120-litre tank for drinking water in the truck and, although this sounds like a lot, we would need to fill up about once a week. This could be tricky as fountains were sparse; we often knocked on farmers' doors and asked if they might help us out. *Andrea* had an inbuilt filtering system operated by a pump so that by the time it came out of our tap it was safe to drink. Despite this and our best efforts with food hygiene, Jeremy and I both got ill multiple times. I even ended up in hospital one time. It turns out our daughter has the toughest guts of us all – she wasn't sick once!

Even though we had some sickness, overall

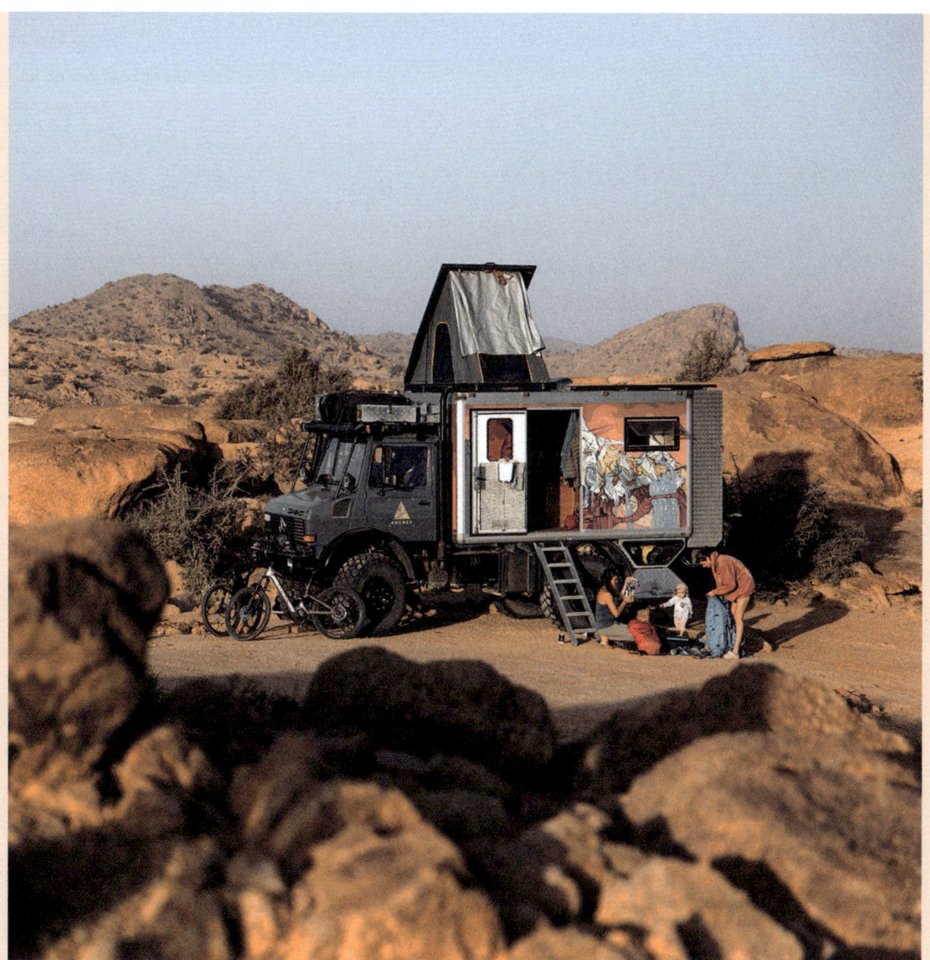

© JEREMY BERNARD

I felt so healthy on this trip and when we got home. I don't usually think about nutrition much when it comes to my climbing, but I can tell when I feel good and when I don't. The food felt nourishing, wholesome and uncomplicated in a way that is harder to do and maintain at home and generally in more Westernised cultures. We ate such unrefined, fresh produce with very little temptation for processed or 'junk' type food. It just wasn't available in rural areas, so we didn't ever have it. We also didn't drink alcohol at all, and both felt good for it. Of course, a nice glass of wine is something we missed, along with good Swiss chocolate. We won't be chocolate free and teetotal forever, but it was an interesting observation.

As we welcome our second child, we will be saying goodbye to *Andrea* but not to trips of this kind. We need more seats and more space so it's time for a new truck. The kitchen will be a priority again; food and eating as a family is a key part of making a truck feel like home. We plan to have many more adventures as a team of four, to continue to spread the joy of climbing and help people when we can.

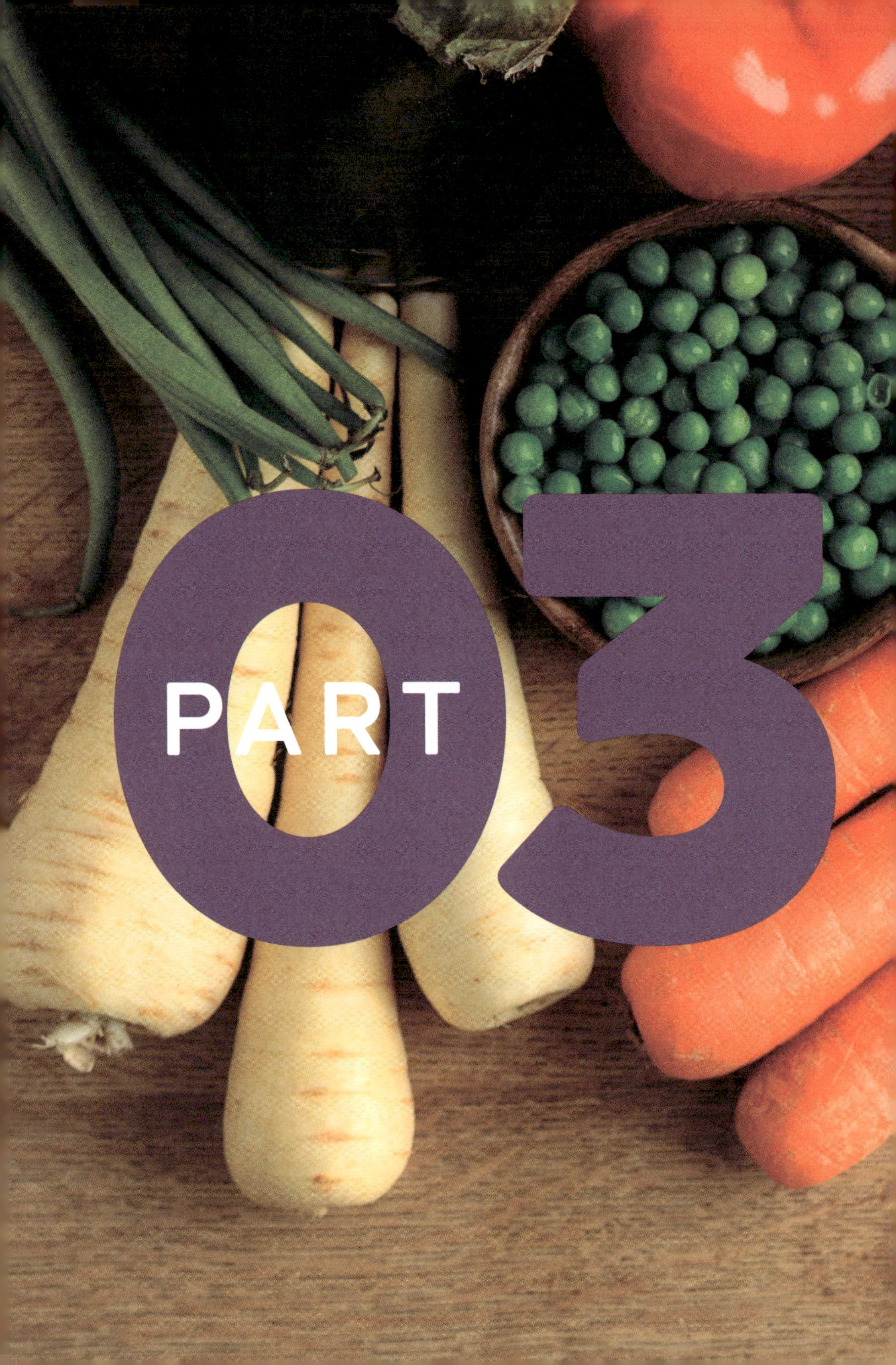
PART 03

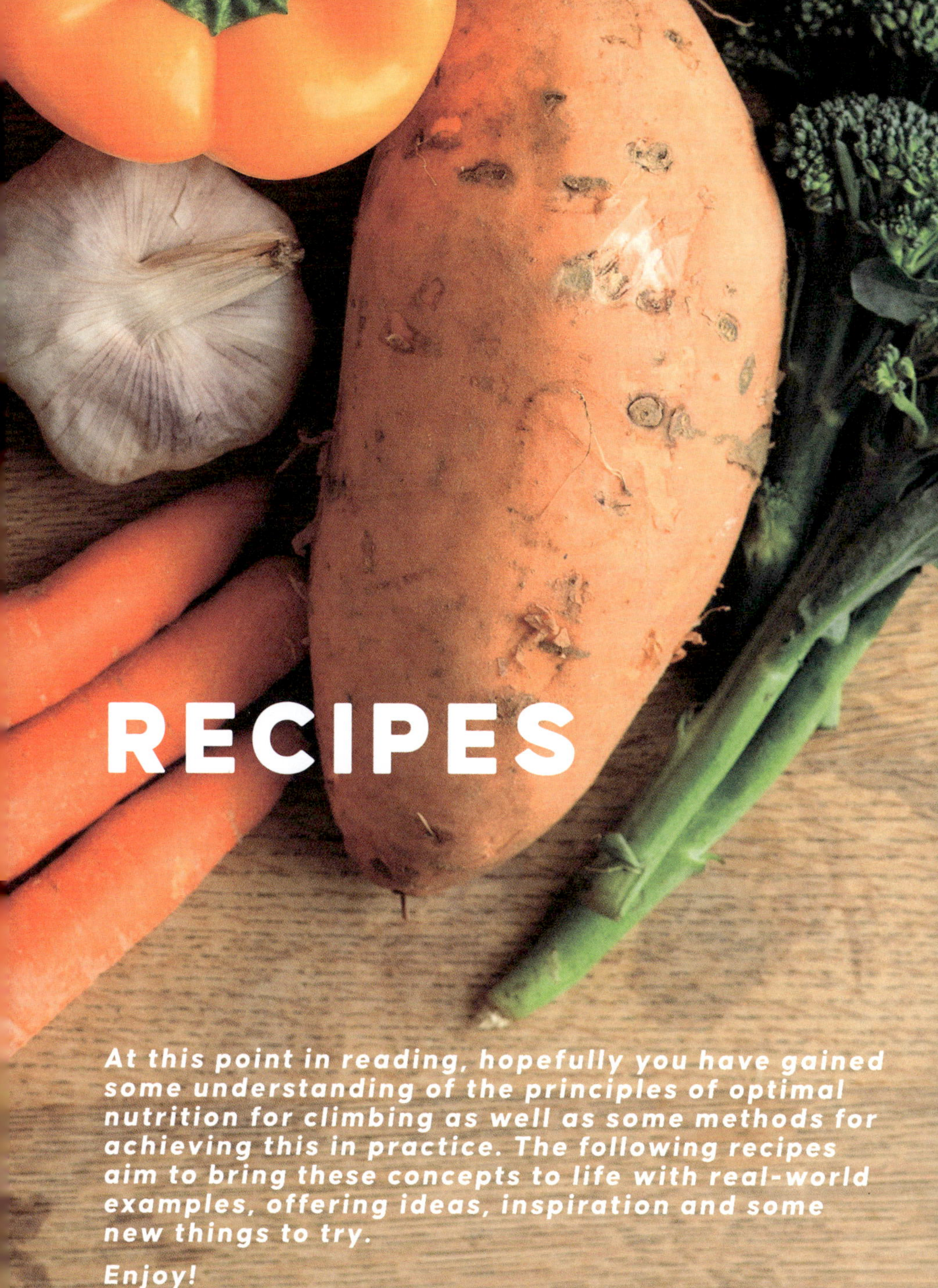

RECIPES

At this point in reading, hopefully you have gained some understanding of the principles of optimal nutrition for climbing as well as some methods for achieving this in practice. The following recipes aim to bring these concepts to life with real-world examples, offering ideas, inspiration and some new things to try.

Enjoy!

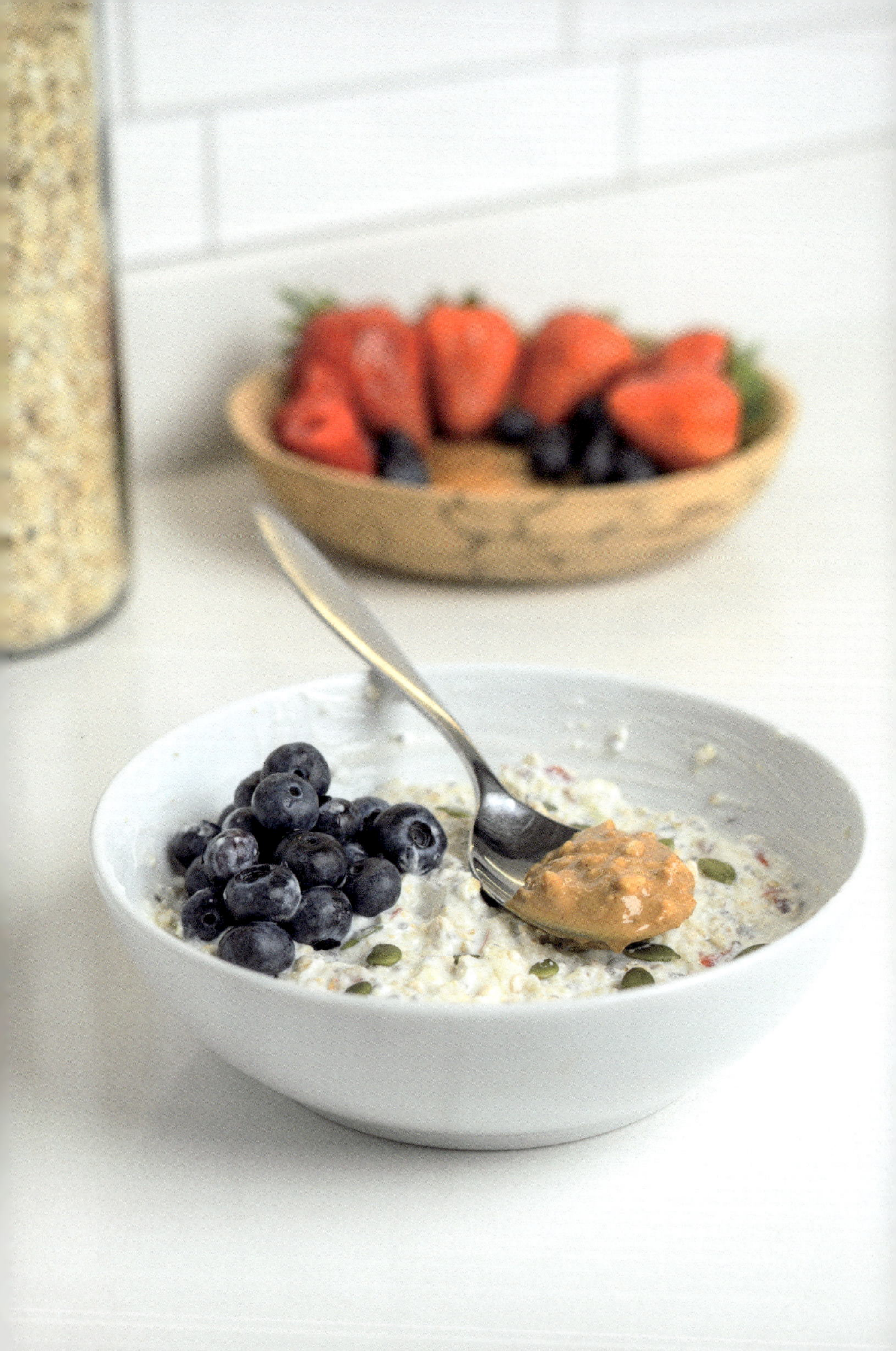

OVERNIGHT OATS

Serves 2

This is a classic breakfast, but it can also double up as crag fuel or a post-training snack. Easy to prepare the night before, it can be a great way to start the day, to drip-feed your system during the day, or to recover. With carbohydrates, protein, healthy fats, fibre and micronutrients, it's a perfect choice for many situations.

Ingredients

80 g oats
1 apple, grated
20 g pumpkin seeds
10 g chia seeds
½ teaspoon cinnamon
300 g 0% fat Greek yoghurt
100 ml whole milk
100 g blueberries
Nut butter of choice to serve

Method

1. Mix the oats, grated apple, pumpkin and chia seeds, cinnamon, yoghurt and milk together in a large bowl.
2. Split into two tubs or bowls and store in the fridge overnight.
3. In the morning, add half the blueberries and a dollop of nut butter to each bowl.

Oats are great, as not only are they carb-rich (about 25 grams per 40-gram serving), they are also a complex carbohydrate which means they release their energy in a steady stream. Oats also contain a decent amount of protein – about 5 grams per 40-gram serving.

Quality Greek yoghurt is high in protein – usually 10 grams per 100-gram serving. Watch out for 'Greek-style' yoghurts as these often contain much less protein so may not help as much with hitting your protein targets.

The pumpkin seeds, chia seeds, blueberries and apple are great sources of vitamins and fibre, while quality nut butters provide healthy fats and some additional protein.

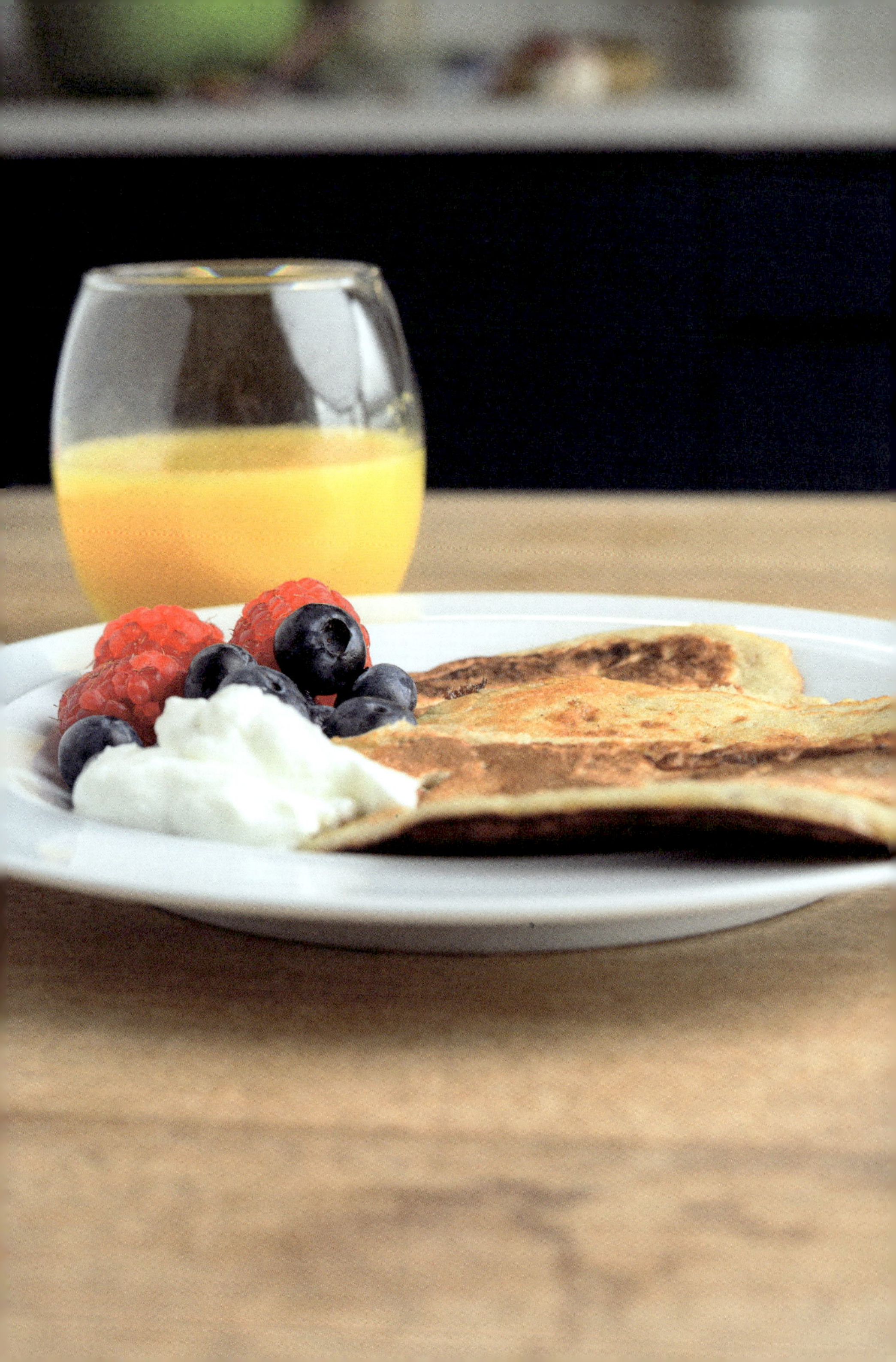

BANANA PANCAKES

Makes 8 pancakes

This is a quick and easy breakfast; with just three base ingredients, it's a must-have on your regular recipe list. Deliciously simple but easy to dress up with extras like yoghurt and berries for added taste. This pancake recipe offers quality protein, carbohydrates, fibre and micronutrients; what a great way to start off your day!

Ingredients

2 ripe bananas
4 eggs
60 g plain flour
Butter
Greek yoghurt and berries to serve

Method

1. Mash the bananas in a bowl.
2. Add the eggs and whisk together with the banana.
3. Sieve in the flour and mix thoroughly.
4. Heat your pan and add a knob of butter.
5. When the pan is very hot, spoon in the batter, leaving 2–3 centimetres around each pancake for expansion.
6. Cook like this for 2–3 minutes and then flip the pancakes to cook the other side.
7. Serve with Greek yoghurt and berries.

Bananas make these pancakes lovely and sweet, but they are also a great source of potassium, vitamin C and fibre. As well as this, they provide a decent dose of carbohydrate – there's about 25–30 grams in a medium-sized banana.

Eggs are very nutrient dense; they are a great protein source (approximately 6 grams per egg) as well as a good source of vitamin D and choline, among other things.

Plain flour serves as a source of calories in the form of carbohydrates (70–80 grams per 100 grams). If you have coeliac disease or a gluten intolerance, make sure to sub this out for a gluten-free flour or gluten-free oats.

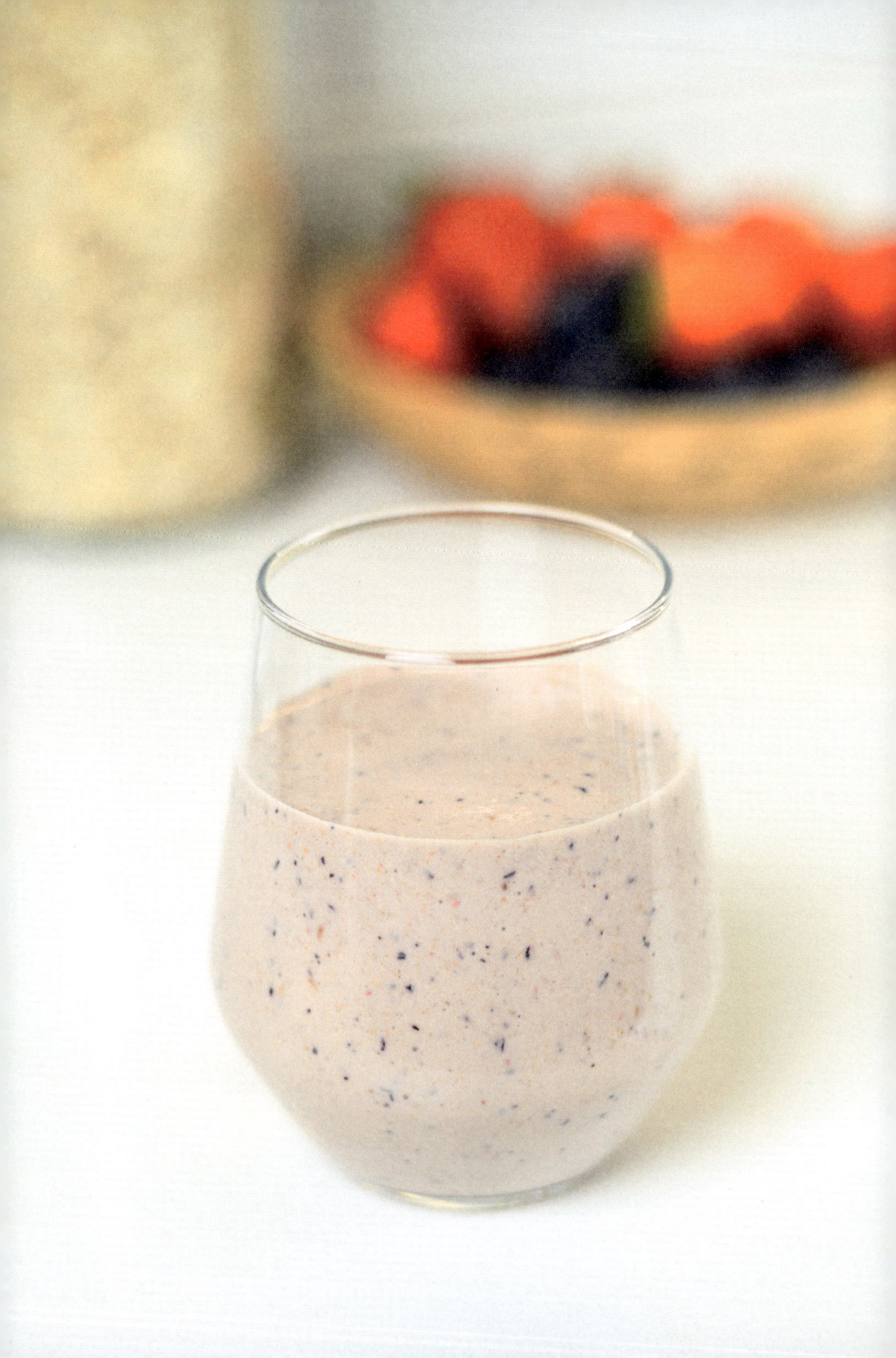

BANANA AND BERRY PROTEIN SMOOTHIE

Serves 1–2

This is a hearty smoothie with more going for it than just the average fruit smoothie. With added whey protein powder, it's a great way to hit your protein targets. The peanut butter adds some healthy fats to keep you feeling full, and the oats mean you also get carbohydrates. It's a brilliant option whether you are fuelling up for adventures ahead or recovering from a session. Oh, and it tastes wonderful.

Ingredients

40 g oats
20 g unflavoured whey protein powder
1 banana
1 cupful of berries
1 tablespoon peanut butter
200 ml whole milk
Water

Method

1. Add all the ingredients to a blender, using water as needed to achieve a consistency that you like.
2. Blend, drink and enjoy!

Oats are great, and here they are again – complex carbohydrates (about 25 grams per 40-gram serving) for long-lasting energy as well as some lovely fibre for your gut microbes to feast on. With 40 grams in this recipe that's also an extra 5 grams of protein.

Whey protein is an efficient and effective way to bolster your protein intake with high-quality amino acids and plenty of our good friend leucine. The gold standard in protein supplements, a serving of whey usually offers about 20 grams of protein.

Whole milk brings even more protein to the party (3–4 grams per 100 millilitres), as well as vitamin D, calcium and phosphorus.

Berries and banana are great sources of vitamins and fibre while also bringing the sweet taste and colourful vibes.

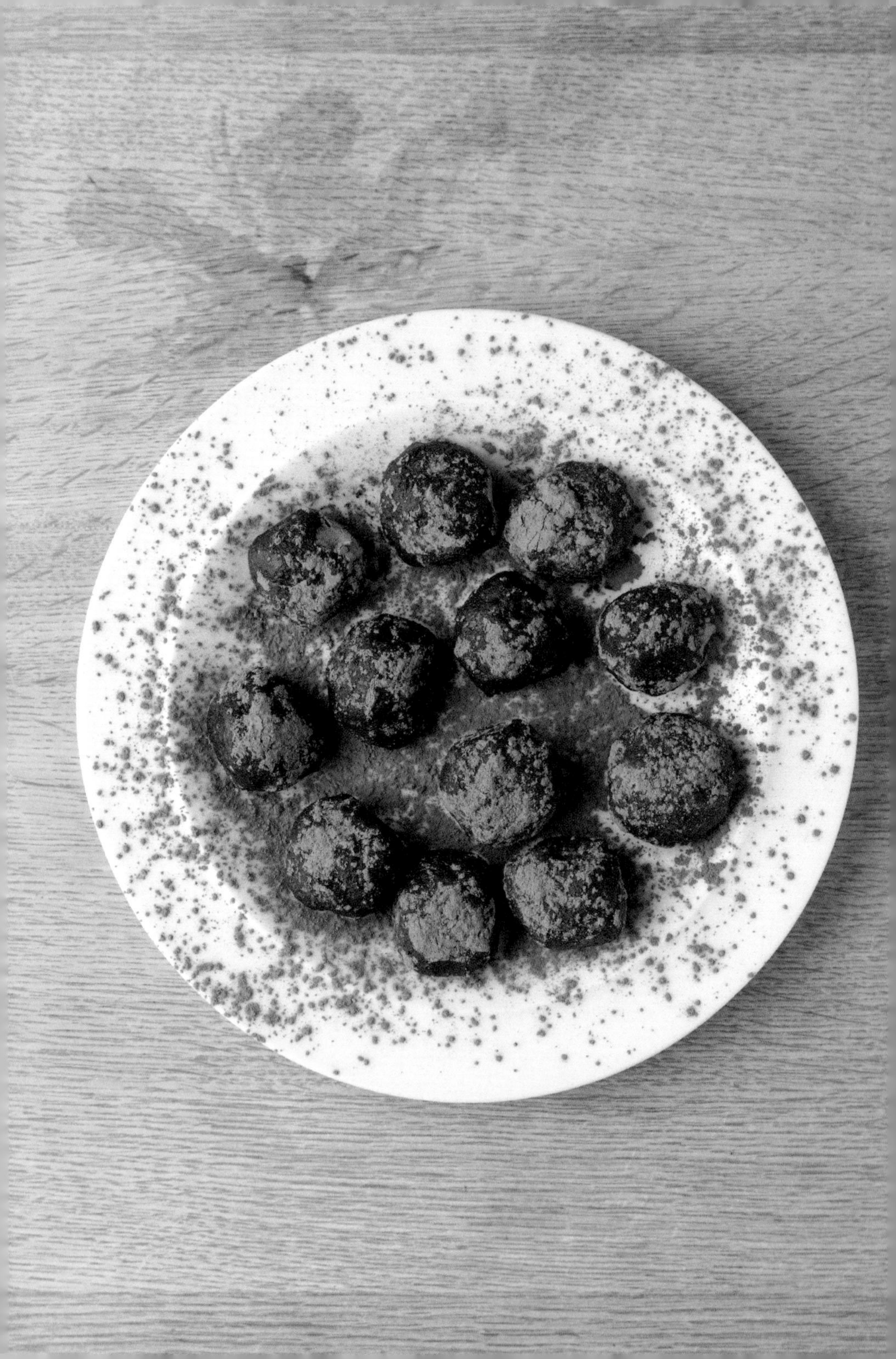

OAT, DATE AND NUT BALLS

Makes 12

These oat, date and nut balls are a perfect addition to your crag bag. With a mix of protein, carbohydrate and fat, these yummy snacks are great to have on a climbing day when you want something to drip-feed your system with much-needed energy. And they taste delicious as well. They can also be made in bigger batches and frozen, ready to be used at your convenience.

Ingredients

50 g ground oats
75 g peanut or almond butter
4 dates, pitted
50 g cashew nuts
2 tablespoons honey
1 tablespoon coconut oil
2 tablespoons ground almonds
Cacao powder

Method

1. Put the oats, nut butter, dates, cashew nuts, honey, coconut oil and ground almonds into a food processor and blend until combined.
2. The mixture needs to be firm enough to hold together. If it's too wet, add more ground almonds.
3. Spread out your cacao powder on a work surface or large plate.
4. Split the mixture into 12 lumps and roll them into balls, then roll each ball in the cacao powder until it is fully coated.
5. Place them on a tray in the fridge and leave to set for at least 2 hours. You can also freeze them if desired.

Oats are extremely versatile and, as they are such a good source of carbohydrate and fibre, they are central to this recipe, adding around 4 grams of carbohydrate to each ball. This is compounded by the quick-release simple carbohydrates that the dates and honey offer (another 1–2 grams and around 3 grams per ball).

The peanut butter, almonds and cashews are high in fat which helps to keep you satiated as well as supporting many important bodily processes. They are also rich in minerals such as iron, zinc, calcium and magnesium.

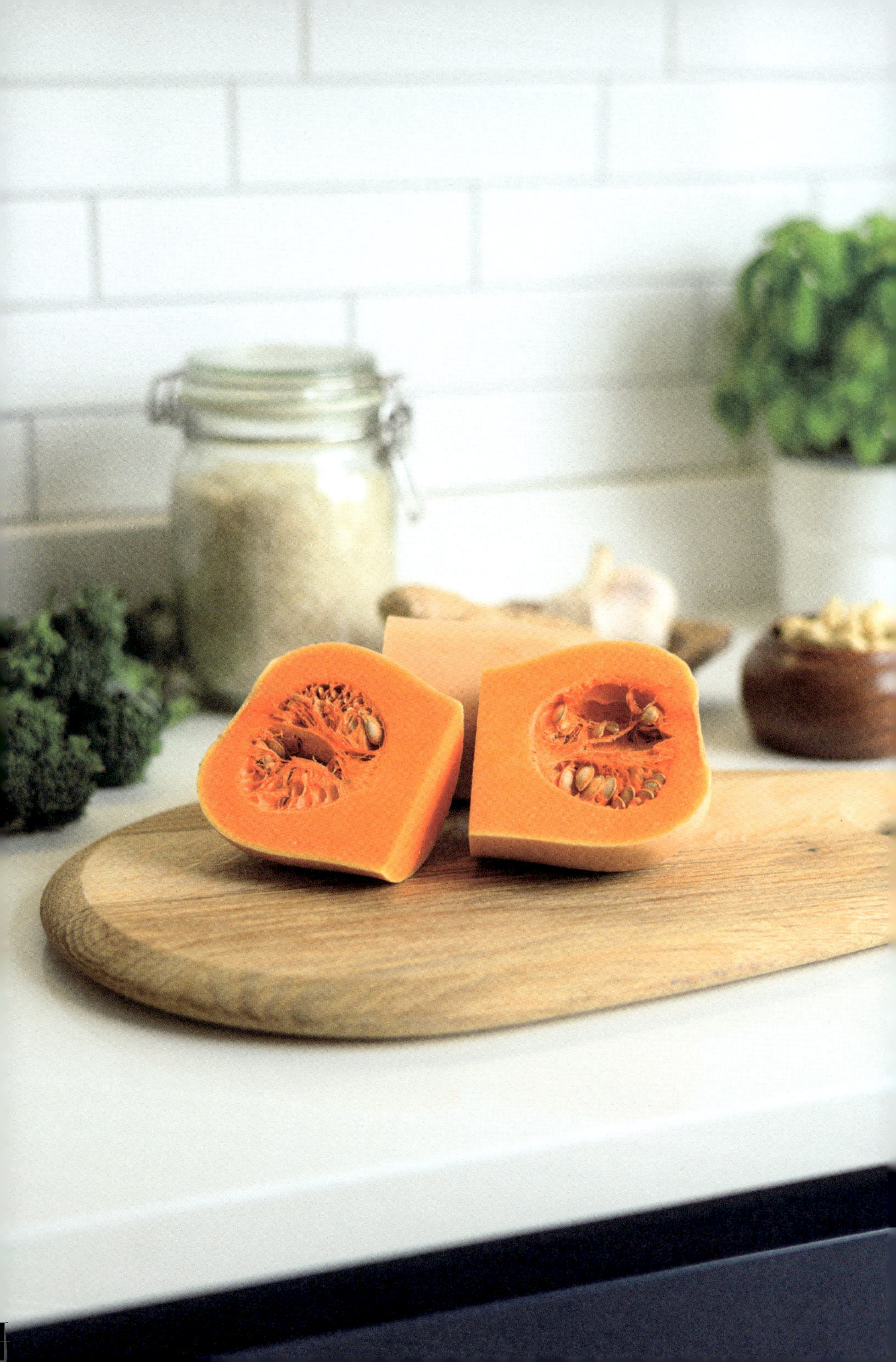

SALMON, BUTTERNUT SQUASH AND ASIAN RICE

Serves 4–6

This dish is a delicious mix of flavours with a bit of spice (you can take out the chilli if you prefer your meals mild). It ticks all the boxes of a great recovery meal, with carbohydrates from the rice and squash, protein and healthy fats from the salmon and cashews, as well as plenty of fibre and micronutrients from the various fresh ingredients.

Ingredients

3 cm chunk of fresh ginger
2 garlic cloves
1 butternut squash
300 g white rice
1 can coconut milk
2 tablespoons soy sauce
300 g tenderstem broccoli
Salmon steaks (one for each person)
30 g toasted cashew nuts

For the dressing

3 cm chunk of fresh ginger
1 red chilli
30 g fresh coriander
4 tablespoons sesame oil
4 tablespoons lemon juice
4 tablespoons soy sauce

Method

1. Preheat the oven to 180 °C.
2. Finely chop the ginger and garlic.
3. Peel and chop the butternut squash into cubes.
4. In a large oven tray, mix the rice, coconut milk, soy sauce, ginger and garlic with 400 ml water.
5. Put the chopped squash on top, cover with foil and place in the oven for 45 minutes.
6. After the 45 minutes, remove the foil and lay the tenderstem broccoli on top of the rice and squash mixture, replace the foil, and return to the oven for 15 minutes.
7. At the same time, put the salmon steaks in the oven in a separate tray.
8. For the dressing, finely chop the ginger, chilli and fresh coriander and then mix all the dressing ingredients together.
9. When the 15 minutes are up, pour the dressing over the rice and squash, add the toasted cashews and mix through.
10. Serve with the salmon steaks.

A typical 100-gram salmon fillet offers in the range of 25 grams of protein with the additional benefit of about 15 grams of fat, primarily omega-3s. Along with eggs, salmon is one of the rare foods that also provides vitamin D.

White rice is the carbohydrate source in this recipe and it offers about 240 grams to the full dish, with an added 30–40 grams from the butternut squash. This means, depending on serving size, you could be looking at 45–70 grams of carbohydrate per portion.

Broccoli is a good source of vitamins (particularly vitamin C), minerals and fibre, and the tenderstem variety works particularly well in this recipe – plenty of stalk but it's all tasty!

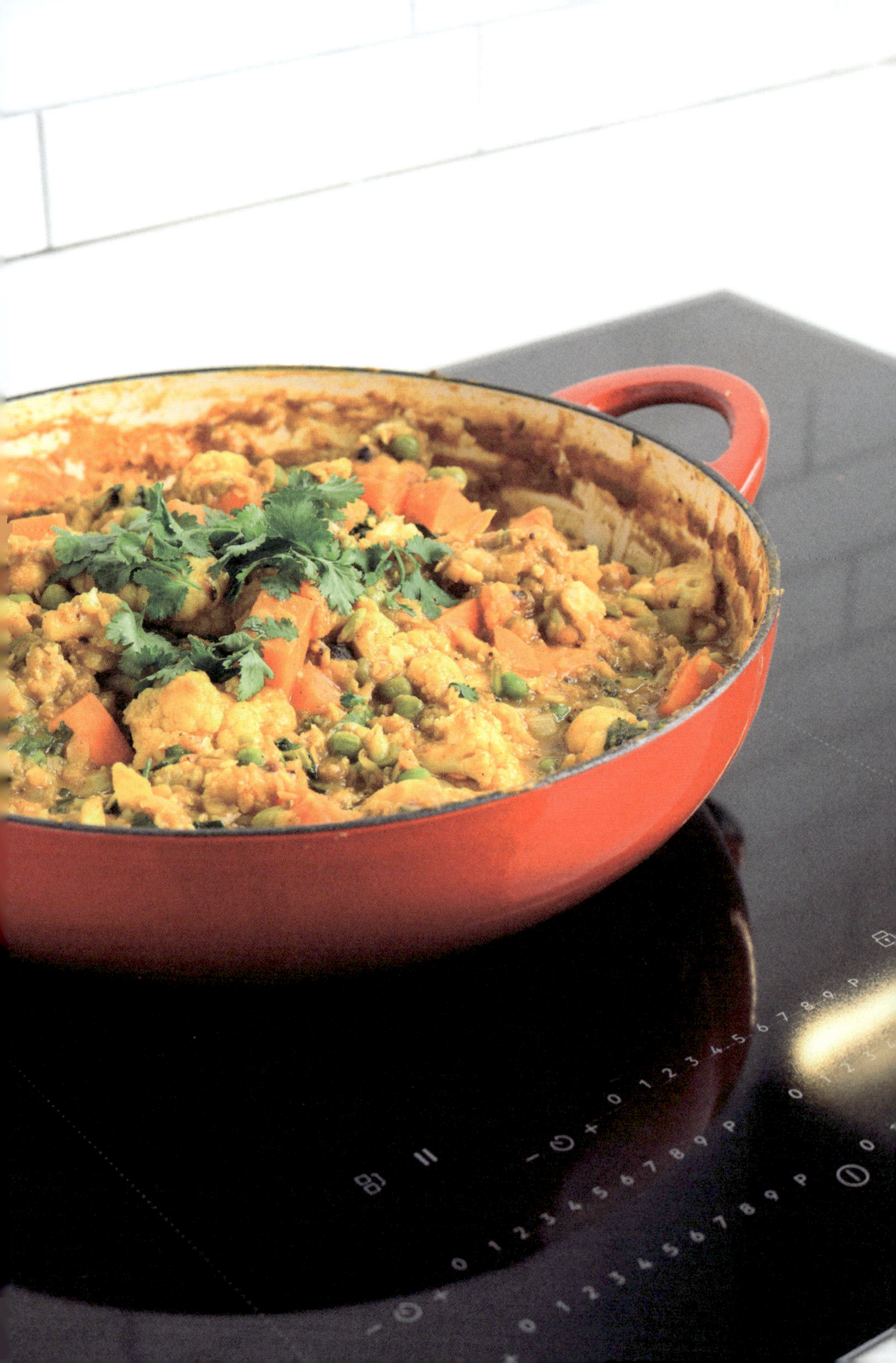

LENTIL, CAULIFLOWER AND PEA DHAL

Serves 4–6

This is a delicious vegan winter warmer. With classic curry spices, cauliflower, sweet potato, lentils and peas, it gives a lot of variety in taste and texture as well as a multitude of vitamins, minerals and gut-friendly fibre. The lentils provide protein and the sweet potato offers carbohydrate, alongside whatever you decide to serve it with, such as bread or rice. If you're not vegan, try adding some Greek yoghurt to serve – it works a treat and boosts the protein content.

Ingredients

2 tablespoons rapeseed oil
1 large onion, chopped
2 garlic cloves, chopped
1 teaspoon turmeric
1 teaspoon ground coriander
2 teaspoons garam masala
1 teaspoon black mustard seeds
50 g curry paste
1 tablespoon tomato puree
200 g red lentils
500 ml vegetable stock
1 can coconut milk
Large cauliflower, chopped into florets
Large sweet potato, peeled and cubed
2 handfuls fresh spinach
100 g frozen peas
30 g fresh coriander, chopped

Method

1. Heat the oil in a large pot and add the onion and garlic. Cook until soft.
2. Add all the spices, mustard seeds, curry paste and tomato puree and stir.
3. Add the lentils with the stock and the coconut milk and stir well.
4. Add the cauliflower and the sweet potato, making sure they are covered by the liquid; add more water if needed. Simmer for 30–40 minutes or until the cauliflower and sweet potato are tender.
5. Stir in the spinach and the frozen peas and cook for a further 5 minutes.
6. Mix in half the fresh coriander and season to taste with salt and pepper.
7. Garnish with the other half of the fresh coriander and serve with bread or rice.

Red lentils are a brilliant source of carbohydrates (around 60 grams per 100 grams) and fibre (around 13 grams per 100 grams), as well as offering a respectable portion of protein (around 25 grams per 100 grams).

Sweet potato is another great source of carbohydrates, offering around 25 grams per medium sweet potato. Not only that, this orange vegetable boasts many vitamins such as vitamins C and A, and potassium. Depending on what you need from this meal, you can bolster the carb content even more by serving with bread or rice.

Herbs and spices like those used in this recipe are packed with antioxidants like polyphenols and flavonoids; some, such as turmeric, are known for their anti-inflammatory properties and they are all great for promoting gut bacteria diversity. Oh, and they make this dish taste delicious.

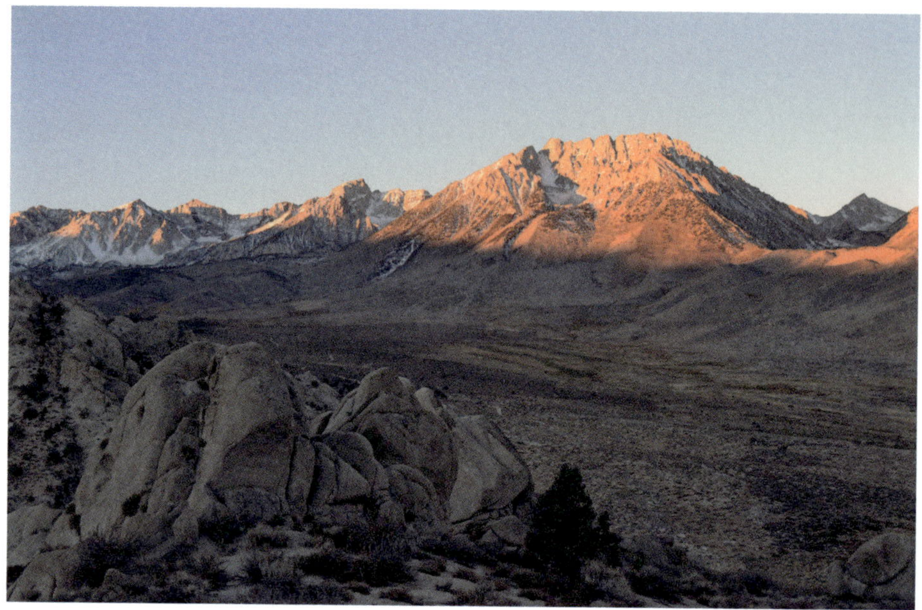

© DAVID MASON

ACKNOWLEDGEMENTS

While all the words in this book are mine, there are many people who influenced my thoughts and learning, supported me, advised me or made space for me to write.

First, I would like to thank the wonderful team at Vertebrate Publishing. Kirsty Reade initially approached me about this book in the summer of 2022. She explained that Vertebrate wanted to add a book about nutrition for climbing to their training books and that they were interested in the idea of me writing it. Honestly, it took me by surprise and, although I liked the idea and felt flattered to be asked, life felt a bit too hectic at that time. I was already spinning plates and the idea of a big project like this felt too much. I said no. Fast forward to autumn of 2023 and Kirsty's name popped up in my inbox again. She said they had parked the idea but planned to pick it up again and wanted to check in with me to see if anything had changed before they asked someone else. This time, despite being busy still and around 18 weeks pregnant with my second child, I jumped at the chance. I love writing and this seemed too good an opportunity to turn down; I had since regretted my initial no. So, thank you Kirsty for believing in me in the first place, accepting my initial 'no' so kindly and for coming back to me on it. Not only that, the process of writing this book was full of kind exchanges with Kirsty as she helped me to build confidence with each chapter I sent her for review.

I would also like to thank John Coefield and the rest of the team from Vertebrate for the attention to detail in the editing process, vision with the images and for bringing the words to life as you see it today in book form. John in particular for his patience with all my references!

Embedded in the book is the concept of *principles* and *methods*: aim to understand the principles of evidence-based nutrition and exercise metabolism, then explore the many methods to find what works for you. This concept is core to the way I think about nutrition for climbing and it played a key role in how I wanted to communicate through this book. I feel it offers individuals the power of knowledge combined with autonomy of choice. I'd like to thank Martin MacDonald for introducing to me this way of framing things when I did my first nutrition course through Mac-Nutrition Uni back in 2018.

Another influential nutrition expert who I would like to thank is performance dietitian Rebecca Dent. Rebecca has helped me in a number of ways over the years. She was the first nutrition professional that I encountered when I was a full-time athlete competing for the GB team. She helped me to optimise my nutrition back then and it piqued my interest in the subject. Rebecca also advised me on where to study when I expressed interest in expanding my knowledge and working in nutrition; she recommended the course I did with Martin MacDonald and also the IOC diploma I undertook after that. Last but not least, Rebecca proofread this book. I feel very appreciative to have had Rebecca's eyes on it and it gives me great confidence to have her approval.

Another person who I was lucky to have as a proofreader was dietitian Renee McGregor. I have also known Renee for some time and, with her expertise in areas such as REDs, it has been great to get her feedback and support. Renee is a powerful voice in athlete health and well-being and I hope that this book can be a contribution to that message.

I would like to thank all the climbers whose stories are told in this book. Shauna Coxsey, Billy Ridal, Maddy Cope, Molly Thompson-Smith, Libby Peter, Kai Lightner, Nina Caprez, Aidan Roberts and Ben Moon. The stories were ghostwritten by me following interviews with each person and I can't thank you all enough for how open, honest and generous you were with your time and your experience. I really feel that these stories bring the book to life by sharing lived experiences with nutrition and climbing. Another thank you goes to all the photographers who contributed images to this book; the imagery really brings it to life. In particular thanks to Colin Perkins – who knew food could look so good?

Lastly, I would like to thank my family and friends for their unwavering support: David for believing in my knowledge and ability to write, my sister Ania for her expertise on the publishing side of things, and the many friends (you know who you are) who counselled me when I had major imposter syndrome about writing a book. And, last but not least, my children: Isaac for being such a joy as always, and Lily for taking some naps so I could write while on maternity leave.

REFERENCES

A word from the author

1. Leslie-Wujastyk, M. & Gibson-Smith, E. (2025). 'Nutritional considerations for female rock climbers'. *Journal of Science in Sport and Exercise*, 7, 28–39. https://doi.org/10.1007/s42978-023-00267-4

Introduction

1. Mora-Fernandez, A., Argüello-Arbe, A., Tojeiro-Iglesias, A. et al. (2024). 'Nutritional assessment, body composition, and low energy availability in sport climbing athletes of different genders and categories: A cross-sectional study'. *Nutrients*, 16(17), 2974. https://doi.org/10.3390/nu16172974;
   Michael, M.K., Joubert, L. & Witard, O.C. (2019). 'Assessment of dietary intake and eating attitudes in recreational and competitive adolescent rock climbers: A pilot study'. *Frontiers in Nutrition*, 6. https://doi.org/10.3389/fnut.2019.00064;
   Chmielewska, A. & Regulska-Ilow, B. (2023). 'The evaluation of energy availability and dietary nutrient intake of sport climbers at different climbing levels'. *International Journal of Environmental Research and Public Health*, 20(6), 5176. https://doi.org/10.3390/ijerph20065176;
   Sas-Nowosielski, K. & Judyta, W. (2019). 'Energy and macronutrient intake of advanced Polish sport climbers'. *Journal of Physical Education and Sport*, 19(3), 829–832. https://doi.org/10.7752/jpes.2019.s3119;
   Monedero, J., Duff, C. & Egan, B. (2023). 'Dietary intakes and the risk of low energy availability in male and female advanced and elite rock climbers'. *Journal of Strength and Conditioning Research*, 37(3), e8–e15. https://doi.org/10.1519/JSC.0000000000004317;
   Gibson-Smith, E., Storey, R. & Ranchordas, M. (2020). 'Dietary intake, body composition and iron status in experienced and elite climbers'. *Frontiers in Nutrition*, 7. https://doi.org/10.3389/fnut.2020.00122;
   Neufeld, E.E. & Meyers, M.C. (2018). 'Nutritional status of rock climbers.' *Medicine & Science in Sports & Exercise*, 50(5S), 303. https://doi.org/10.1249/01.mss.0000536080.40813.28

1 Energy: eat to perform

1. Giles, D., Chidley, J.B., Taylor, N. et al. (2019). 'The determination of finger-flexor critical force in rock climbers'. *International Journal of Sports Physiology and Performance*, 14(7), 972–979. https://doi.org/10.1123/ijspp.2018-0809
2. O'Neill, J.E.R., Corish, C.A. & Horner, K. (2023). 'Accuracy of resting metabolic rate prediction equations in athletes: A systematic review with meta-analysis'. *Sports Medicine* 53, 2373–2398. https://doi.org/10.1007/s40279-023-01896-z;
   ten Haaf, T. & Weijs, P.J.M. (2014). 'Resting energy expenditure prediction in recreational athletes of 18–35 years: Confirmation of cunningham equation and an improved weight-based alternative'. *PLOS ONE* 9(10): e108460. https://doi.org/10.1371/journal.pone.0108460;
   Chmielewska, A., Kujawa, K. & Regulska-Ilow, B. (2023). 'Accuracy of resting metabolic rate prediction equations in sport climbers'. *International Journal of Environmental Research and Public Health*. 20(5), 4216. https://doi.org/10.3390/ijerph20054216;
   De Lorenzo, A., Bertini, I., Candeloro N., et al. (1999). 'A new predictive equation to calculate resting metabolic rate in athletes'. *The Journal of Sports Medicine and Physical Fitness*. 39(3):213–219.
3. Mountjoy, M., Ackerman, K.E., Bailey, D.M. et al. (2023). '2023 International Olympic Committee's (IOC) consensus statement on Relative Energy Deficiency in Sport (REDs)'. *British Journal of Sports Medicine*, 57, 1073–1098. https://doi.org/10.1136/bjsports-2023-106994
4. Chmielewska et al. (2023). 'Accuracy of Resting Metabolic Rate Prediction Equations in Sport Climbers'.
5. Hills, A.P., Mokhtar, N. & Byrne, N.M. (2014). 'Assessment of physical activity and energy expenditure: An overview of objective measures'. *Frontiers in Nutrition*, 1. https://doi.org/10.3389/fnut.2014.00005
6. Michael, M.K., Witard, O.C. & Joubert, L. (2019). 'Physiological demands and nutritional considerations for Olympic-style competitive rock climbing'. *Cogent Medicine*, 6(1). https://doi.org/10.1080/2331205x.2019.1667199
7. Speakman, J.R. & Elmquist, J.K. (2022). 'Obesity: an evolutionary context'. *Life Metabolism*, 1(1), 10–24. https://doi.org/10.1093/lifemeta/loac002;
   Speakman, J.R. & Hall, K.D. (2023). 'Models of body weight and fatness regulation'. *Philosophical Transactions of the Royal Society B: Biological Sciences*, 378(1888). https://doi.org/10.1098/rstb.2022.0231;
   Farias, M.M., Cuevas, A.M. & Rodriguez, F. (2011). 'Set-point theory and obesity'. *Metabolic Syndrome and Related Disorders*, 9(2), 85–89. https://doi.org/10.1089/met.2010.0090;
   Ganipisetti, V.M. & Bollimunta, P. (2023). 'Obesity and set-point theory', in *StatPearls*. StatPearls Publishing, Treasure Island (FL).
8. Kennedy, G.C. (1953). 'The role of depot fat in the hypothalamic control of food intake in the rat'. *Proceedings of the Royal Society B: Biological Sciences*, 140(901), 578–592. https://doi.org/10.1098/rspb.1953.0009
9. Austin, J. & Marks, D. (2009). 'Hormonal regulators of appetite'. *International Journal of Pediatric Endocrinology*, 2009. https://doi.org/10.1155/2009/141753
10. Forde, C.G. & de Graaf, K.C. (2022). '12 – Sensory influences on food choice and energy intake: recent developments and future directions', in *Flavor* (second edition), Woodhead Publishing, Sawston, 329–362. https://doi.org/10.1016/B978-0-323-89903-1.00013-X
11. Schubert, M.M., Sabapathy, S., Leveritt, M. & Desbrow, B. (2014). 'Acute exercise and hormones related to appetite regulation: A meta-analysis'. *Sports Medicine*, 44(3), 387–403. https://doi.org/10.1007/s40279-013-0120-3

2 Macronutrients: carbohydrates

1. Cordain, L., Eades, M.R. & Eades, M.D. (2003). 'Hyperinsulinemic diseases of civilization: More than just Syndrome X'. *Comparative Biochemistry and Physiology Part A: Molecular and Integrative Physiology*, 136(1), 95–112. https://doi.org/10.1016/S1095-6433(03)00011-4

2. Veronese, N., Solmi, M., Caruso, M.G. et al. (2018). 'Dietary fiber and health outcomes: An umbrella review of systematic reviews and meta-analyses'. *The American Journal of Clinical Nutrition*, 107(3), 436–444. https://doi.org/10.1093/ajcn/nqx082

3. British Nutrition Foundation (October 2023). 'Fibre', https://www.nutrition.org.uk/nutritional-information/fibre accessed 22 May 2025.

4. British Dietetic Association (April 2024). 'Fibre', https://www.bda.uk.com/resource/fibre.html accessed 22 May 2025.

5. Michael, M.K., Witard, O.C. & Joubert, L. (2019). 'Physiological demands and nutritional considerations for Olympic-style competitive rock climbing'. *Cogent Medicine*, 6(1). https://doi.org/10.1080/2331205x.2019.1667199;
   Smith, E.J., Storey, R. & Ranchordas, M.K. (2017). 'Nutritional considerations for bouldering'. *International Journal of Sport Nutrition and Exercise Metabolism*, 27(4), 314–324. https://doi.org/10.1123/ijsnem.2017-0043

6. Jeukendrup, A. (2014). 'A step towards personalized sports nutrition: Carbohydrate intake during exercise'. *Sports Medicine*, 44(Suppl.1), 25–33. https://doi.org/10.1007/s40279-014-0148-z

7. Hokken, R., Laugesen, S., Aagaard, P. et al. (2021). 'Subcellular localization- and fibre type-dependent utilization of muscle glycogen during heavy resistance exercise in elite power and Olympic weightlifters'. *Acta Physiologica*, 231(2). https://doi.org/10.1111/apha.13561

8. Foo, W.L., Harrison, J.D., Mhizha, F.T. et al. (2022). 'A short-term low-fiber diet reduces body mass in healthy young men: Implications for weight-sensitive sports'. *International Journal of Sport Nutrition and Exercise Metabolism*, 32(4), 256–264. https://doi.org/10.1123/IJSNEM.2021-0324

9. Gonzalez, J.T. & Wallis, G.A. (2021). 'Carb-conscious: The role of carbohydrate intake in recovery from exercise'. *Current Opinion in Clinical Nutrition and Metabolic Care*, 24(4), 364–371. https://doi.org/10.1097/MCO.0000000000000761;
   Cermak, N.M. & van Loon, L.J.C. (2013). 'The use of carbohydrates during exercise as an ergogenic aid'. *Sports Medicine*, 43(11), 1139–1155. https://doi.org/10.1007/s40279-013-0079-0

10. Paoli, A., Rubini, A., Volek, J.S. & Grimaldi, K.A. (2013). 'Beyond weight loss: A review of the therapeutic uses of very-low-carbohydrate (ketogenic) diets'. *European Journal of Clinical Nutrition*, 67(8), 789–796. https://doi.org/10.1038/ejcn.2013.116

11. Stellingwerff, T., Spriet, L.L., Watt, M.J. et al. (2006). 'Decreased PDH activation and glycogenolysis during exercise following fat adaptation with carbohydrate restoration'. *American Journal of Physiology: Endocrinology and Metabolism*, 290(2), e380–e388. https://doi.org/10.1152/ajpendo.00268.2005

12. Burke, L.M. (2021). 'Ketogenic low-CHO, high-fat diet: the future of elite endurance sport?' *The Journal of Physiology*, 599(3), 819–843. https://doi.org/10.1113/JP278928

13. Burke (2021). 'Ketogenic low-CHO, high-fat diet: the future of elite endurance sport?'

14. Burke, L.M., Ross, M.L., Garvican-Lewis, L.A. et al. (2017). 'Low carbohydrate, high fat diet impairs exercise economy and negates the performance benefit from intensified training in elite race walkers'. *The Journal of Physiology*, 595(9), 2785–2807. https://doi.org/10.1113/JP273230

15. Burke, L.M., Sharma, A.P., Heikura, I.A. et al. (2020). 'Crisis of confidence averted: Impairment of exercise economy and performance in elite race walkers by ketogenic low carbohydrate, high fat (LCHF) diet is reproducible'. *PLOS ONE*, 15(6), e0234027. https://doi.org/10.1371/journal.pone.0234027

16. Chmielewska, A. & Regulska-Ilow, B. (2023). 'The evaluation of energy availability and dietary nutrient intake of sport climbers at different climbing levels'. *International Journal of Environmental Research and Public Health*, 20(6), 5176. https://doi.org/10.3390/ijerph20065176;
   Monedero, J., Duff, C. & Egan, B. (2023). 'Dietary intakes and the risk of low energy availability in male and female advanced and elite rock climbers'. *Journal of Strength and Conditioning Research*, 37(3), e8–e15. https://doi.org/10.1519/JSC.0000000000004317;
   Smith et al. (2017). 'Nutritional considerations for bouldering'.

17. Impey, S.G., Hearris, M.A., Hammond, K.M. et al. (2018). 'Fuel for the work required: A theoretical framework for carbohydrate periodization and the glycogen threshold hypothesis'. *Sports Medicine*, 48(5), 1031–1048. https://doi.org/10.1007/S40279-018-0867-7

18. Creer, A., Gallagher, P., Slivka, D. et al. (2005). 'Influence of muscle glycogen availability on ERK1/2 and Akt signaling after resistance exercise in human skeletal muscle'. *Journal of Applied Physiology*, 99(3), 950–956. https://doi.org/10.1152/japplphysiol.00110.2005;
   Burke, L.M., Hawley, J.A., Wong, S.H.S. & Jeukendrup, A.E. (2011). 'Carbohydrates for training and competition'. *Journal of Sports Sciences*, 29(Suppl.1), S17–S27. https://doi.org/10.1080/02640414.2011.585473

3 Macronutrients: proteins

1. Areta, J.L., Hawley, J.A., Ye, J.-M. et al. (2014). 'Increasing leucine concentration stimulates mechanistic target of rapamycin signaling and cell growth in C2C12 skeletal muscle cells'. *Nutrition Research*, 34(11), 1000–1007. https://doi.org/10.1016/j.nutres.2014.09.011;
   Zaromskyte, G., Prokopidis, K., Ioannidis, T. et al. (2021). 'Evaluating the leucine trigger hypothesis to explain the

post-prandial regulation of muscle protein synthesis in young and older adults: A systematic review'. *Frontiers in Nutrition*, 8. https://doi.org/10.3389/fnut.2021.685165;

Wilkinson, K., Koscien, C.P., Monteyne, A.J. et al. (2023). 'Association of postprandial postexercise muscle protein synthesis rates with dietary leucine: A systematic review'. *Physiological Reports*, 11(15). https://doi.org/10.14814/phy2.15775

2. Rondanelli, M., Nichetti, M., Peroni, G. et al. (2021). 'Where to find leucine in food and how to feed elderly with sarcopenia in order to counteract loss of muscle mass: Practical advice'. *Frontiers in Nutrition*, 7. https://doi.org/10.3389/fnut.2020.622391
3. Fouré, A. & Bendahan, D. (2017). 'Is branched-chain amino acids supplementation an efficient nutritional strategy to alleviate skeletal muscle damage? A systematic review'. *Nutrients*, 9(10), 1047. https://doi.org/10.3390/nu9101047;

   Wolfe, R.R. (2017). 'Branched-chain amino acids and muscle protein synthesis in humans: Myth or reality?' *Journal of the International Society of Sports Nutrition*, 14(1). https://doi.org/10.1186/s12970-017-0184-9;

   Martinho, D.V., Nobari, H., Faria, A. et al. (2022). 'Oral branched-chain amino acids supplementation in athletes: A systematic review'. *Nutrients*, 14(19), 4002. https://doi.org/10.3390/nu14194002
4. Smith, E.J., Storey, R. & Ranchordas, M.K. (2017). 'Nutritional considerations for bouldering'. *International Journal of Sport Nutrition and Exercise Metabolism*, 27(4), 314–324. https://doi.org/10.1123/ijsnem.2017-0043;

   Michael, M.K., Witard, O.C. & Joubert, L. (2019). 'Physiological demands and nutritional considerations for Olympic-style competitive rock climbing'. *Cogent Medicine*, 6(1). https://doi.org/10.1080/2331205x.2019.1667199;

   Thomas, D.T., Erdman, K.A. & Burke, L.M. (2016). 'American College of Sports Medicine Joint Position Statement. Nutrition and Athletic Performance'. *Medicine & Science in Sports & Exercise*, 48(3), 543–568. https://doi.org/10.1249/mss.0000000000000852
5. Papadopoulou, S.K. (2020). 'Rehabilitation nutrition for injury recovery of athletes: The role of macronutrient intake'. *Nutrients*, 12(8), 2449. https://doi.org/10.3390/nu12082449;

   Hector, A.J. & Phillips, S.M. (2018). 'Protein recommendations for weight loss in elite athletes: A focus on body composition and performance'. *International Journal of Sport Nutrition and Exercise Metabolism*, 28(2), 170–177. https://doi.org/10.1123/ijsnem.2017-0273
6. Areta, J.L., Burke, L.M., Ross, M.L. et al. (2013). 'Timing and distribution of protein ingestion during prolonged recovery from resistance exercise alters myofibrillar protein synthesis'. *The Journal of Physiology*, 591(9), 2319–2331. https://doi.org/10.1113/jphysiol.2012.244897;

   Jäger, R., Kerksick, C.M., Campbell, B.I. et al. (2017). 'International Society of Sports Nutrition position stand: Protein and exercise'. *Journal of the International Society of Sports Nutrition*, 14(1), 20. https://doi.org/10.1186/S12970-017-0177-8;

   Moore, D.R., Robinson, M.J., Fry, J.L. et al. (2009). 'Ingested protein dose response of muscle and albumin protein synthesis after resistance exercise in young men'. *The American Journal of Clinical Nutrition*, 89(1), 161–168. https://doi.org/10.3945/ajcn.2008.26401
7. Snijders, T., Trommelen, J., Kouw, I.W.K. et al. (2019). 'The impact of pre-sleep protein ingestion on the skeletal muscle adaptive response to exercise in humans: An update'. *Frontiers in Nutrition*, 6. https://doi.org/10.3389/fnut.2019.00017;

   Jäger et al. (2017). 'International Society of Sports Nutrition position stand: Protein and exercise'.;

   Bagheri, R., Pourabbas, M., Moghadam, B.H. et al. (2021). 'High-protein milk ingestion during a resistance training program improves muscular regulatory markers in trained males'. *Medicine & Science in Sports & Exercise*, 53(8S), 278. http://dx.doi.org/10.1249/01.mss.0000762316.51394.38
8. Rogeri, P.S., Zanella, R., Jr., Martins, G.L. et al. (2022). 'Strategies to prevent sarcopenia in the aging process: Role of protein intake and exercise'. *Nutrients*, 14(1), 52. https://doi.org/10.3390/nu14010052;

   Coelho-Júnior, H.J., Calvani, R., Tosato, M. et al. (2022). 'Protein intake and physical function in older adults: A systematic review and meta-analysis'. *Ageing Research Reviews*, 81. https://doi.org/10.1016/j.arr.2022.101731
9. Moore, D.R., Churchward-Venne, T.A., Witard, O. et al. (2015). 'Protein ingestion to stimulate myofibrillar protein synthesis requires greater relative protein intakes in healthy older versus younger men'. *The Journals of Gerontology: Series A*, 70(1), 57–62. https://doi.org/10.1093/gerona/glu103;

   Churchward-Venne, T.A., Holwerda, A.M., Phillips, S.M. & van Loon, L.J.C. (2016). 'What is the optimal amount of protein to support post-exercise skeletal muscle reconditioning in the older adult?' *Sports Medicine*, 46(9), 1205–1212. https://doi.org/10.1007/s40279-016-0504-2
10. Moore, D.R. (2021). 'Protein requirements for master athletes: Just older versions of their younger selves'. *Sports Medicine*, 51(Suppl.1), 13–30. https://doi.org/10.1007/s40279-021-01510-0

4 Macronutrients: fats

1. Maughan, R.J., Burke, L.M., Dvorak, J. et al. (2018). 'IOC consensus statement: Dietary supplements and the high-performance athlete'. *British Journal of Sports Medicine*, 52(7), 439–455. https://doi.org/10.1136/bjsports-2018-099027;

   Smith, G.I., Atherton, P., Reeds, D.N. et al. (2011). 'Dietary omega-3 fatty acid supplementation increases the rate of muscle protein synthesis in older adults: a randomized controlled trial. *The American Journal of Clinical Nutrition*, 93(2), 402–412. https://doi.org/10.3945/ajcn.110.005611
2. Thielecke, F. & Blannin, A. (2020). 'Omega-3 fatty acids for sport performance - are they equally beneficial for athletes and amateurs? A narrative review'. *Nutrients*, 12(12), 3712. https://doi.org/10.3390/nu12123712;

   Gammone, M.A., Riccioni, G., Parrinello, G. & D'Orazio, N. (2019). 'Omega-3 polyunsaturated fatty acids: Benefits and endpoints in sport'. *Nutrients*, 11(1), 46. https://doi.org/10.3390/nu11010046

3. Maughan et al. (2018). 'IOC consensus statement: Dietary supplements and the high-performance athlete'.; Gammone et al. (2019). 'Omega-3 polyunsaturated fatty acids: Benefits and endpoints in sport'.
4. Astrup, A., Magkos, F., Bier, D.M. et al. (2020). 'Saturated fats and health: A reassessment and proposal for food-based recommendations: *JACC* state-of-the-art review'. *Journal of the American College of Cardiology*, 76(7), 844–857. https://doi.org/10.1016/j.jacc.2020.05.077; Astrup, A., Teicholz, N., Magkos, F. et al. (2021). 'Dietary saturated fats and health: Are the U.S. guidelines evidence-based?' *Nutrients*, 13(10), 3305. https://doi.org/10.3390/nu13103305; Siri-Tarino, P.W., Sun, Q., Hu, F.B. & Krauss, R.M. (2010). 'Meta-analysis of prospective cohort studies evaluating the association of saturated fat with cardiovascular disease'. *The American Journal of Clinical Nutrition*, 91(3), 535–546. https://doi.org/10.3945/ajcn.2009.27725; Teicholz, N. (2023). 'A short history of saturated fat: The making and unmaking of a scientific consensus'. *Current Opinion in Endocrinology, Diabetes and Obesity*, 30(1), 65–71. https://doi.org/10.1097/MED.0000000000000791
5. Givens, D.I. (2023). 'Dairy foods and cardiometabolic diseases: An update and a reassessment of the impact of SFA'. *Proceedings of the Nutrition Society*, 82(3), 329–345. https://doi.org/10.1017/S0029665123000083; Trieu, K., Bhat, S., Dai, Z. et al. (2021). 'Biomarkers of dairy fat intake, incident cardiovascular disease, and all-cause mortality: A cohort study, systematic review, and meta-analysis'. *PLOS Medicine*, 18(9), e1003763. https://doi.org/10.1371/journal.pmed.1003763
6. Hooper, L., Martin, N., Jimoh, O.F. et al. (2020). 'Reduction in saturated fat intake for cardiovascular disease'. *Cochrane Database of Systematic Reviews*, 8. https://doi.org/10.1002/14651858.CD011737.pub3
7. de Souza, R.J., Mente, A., Maroleanu, A. et al. (2015). 'Intake of saturated and trans unsaturated fatty acids and risk of all cause mortality, cardiovascular disease, and type 2 diabetes: Systematic review and meta-analysis of observational studies'. *BMJ*, 351, h3978. https://doi.org/10.1136/bmj.h3978
8. World Health Organization (24 January 2024). 'Trans fat'. https://www.who.int/news-room/fact-sheets/detail/trans-fat#:~:text=Trans%20fat%2C%20or%20trans%2Dfatty,of%20heart%20attacks%20and%20deaths accessed 22 May 2025.
9. Carson, J.A.S., Lichtenstein, A.H., Anderson, C.A.M. et al. (2020). 'Dietary cholesterol and cardiovascular risk: A science advisory from the American Heart Association'. *Circulation*, 141(3), e39–e53. https://doi.org/10.1161/CIR.0000000000000743
10. Antoni, R. (2023). 'Dietary saturated fat and cholesterol: Cracking the myths around eggs and cardiovascular disease'. *Journal of Nutritional Science*, 12, e97. https://doi.org/10.1017/jns.2023.82
11. Griffin, B.A. (2016). 'Eggs: Good or bad?' *Proceedings of the Nutrition Society*, 75(3), 259–264. https://doi.org/10.1017/S0029665116000215
12. Krittanawong, C., Narasimhan, B., Wang, Z. et al. (2021). 'Association between egg consumption and risk of cardiovascular outcomes: A systematic review and meta-analysis'. *The American Journal of Medicine*, 134(1), 76–83. https://doi.org/10.1016/j.amjmed.2020.05.046
13. Michael, M.K., Witard, O.C. & Joubert, L. (2019). 'Physiological demands and nutritional considerations for Olympic-style competitive rock climbing'. *Cogent Medicine*, 6(1). https://doi.org/10.1080/2331205x.2019.1667199
14. Melin, A. (2014). 'Energy availability and reproductive function in female endurance athletes' (PhD thesis). Department of Nutrition, Exercise and Sports, Faculty of Science, University of Copenhagen.

5 Micronutrients: vitamins and minerals

1. Thomas, D.T., Erdman, K.A. & Burke, L.M. (2016). 'American College of Sports Medicine Joint Position Statement. Nutrition and Athletic Performance'. *Medicine & Science in Sports & Exercise*, 48(3), 543–568. https://doi.org/10.1249/mss.0000000000000852
2. Angeline, M.E., Gee, A.O., Shindle, M. et al. (2013). 'The effects of vitamin D deficiency in athletes'. *The American Journal of Sports Medicine*, 41(2), 461–464. https://doi.org/10.1177/0363546513475787
3. Ogan, D. & Pritchett, K. (2013). 'Vitamin D and the athlete: Risks, recommendations, and benefits'. *Nutrients*, 5(6), 1856–1868. https://doi.org/10.3390/nu5061856
4. Harju, T., Gray, B., Mavroedi, A. et al. (2022). 'Prevalence and novel risk factors for vitamin D insufficiency in elite athletes: Systematic review and meta-analysis'. *European Journal of Nutrition*, 61(8), 3857–3871. https://doi.org/10.1007/s00394-022-02967-z; Monedero, J., Duff, C. & Egan, B. (2023). 'Dietary intakes and the risk of low energy availability in male and female advanced and elite rock climbers'. *Journal of Strength and Conditioning Research*, 37(3), e8–e15. https://doi.org/10.1519/JSC.0000000000004317
5. Ogan & Pritchett (2013). 'Vitamin D and the athlete: Risks, recommendations, and benefits'.
6. de la Puente Yagüe, M., Collado Yurrita, L., Ciudad Cabañas, M.J. & Cuadrado Cenzual, M.A. (2020). 'Role of vitamin D in athletes and their performance: Current concepts and new trends'. *Nutrients*, 12(2), 579. https://doi.org/10.3390/nu12020579
7. Owens, D.J., Allison, R. & Close, G.L. (2018). 'Vitamin D and the athlete: Current perspectives and new challenges'. *Sports Medicine*, 48(1), 3–16. https://doi.org/10.1007/s40279-017-0841-9
8. Sim, M., Garvican-Lewis, L.A., Cox, G.R. et al. (2019). 'Iron considerations for the athlete: A narrative review'. *European Journal of Applied Physiology*, 119(7), 1463–1478. https://doi.org/10.1007/s00421-019-04157-y
9. Sim et al. (2019). 'Iron considerations for the athlete: A narrative review'.
10. Gibson-Smith, E., Storey, R. & Ranchordas, M. (2020). 'Dietary intake, body composition and iron status in experienced and elite climbers'. *Frontiers in Nutrition*, 7. https://doi.org/10.3389/fnut.2020.00122

11. Sim et al. (2019). 'Iron considerations for the athlete: A narrative review'.

12. Piskin, E., Cianciosi, D., Gulec, S. et al. (2022). 'Iron absorption: Factors, limitations, and improvement methods'. *ACS Omega*, 7(24), 20441–20456. https://doi.org/10.1021/acsomega.2c01833

13. Piskin et al. (2022). 'Iron absorption: Factors, limitations, and improvement methods'.;
Hinton, P. (2013). 'Trace minerals of concern for female athletes: Iron and zinc', in *Nutrition and the Female Athlete*. Ed. K.A. Beals. CRC Press, Boca Raton (FL). https://doi.org/10.1201/b13743;
Mountjoy, M., Sundgot-Borgen, J., Burke, L. et al. (2015). 'Authors' 2015 additions to the IOC consensus statement: Relative Energy Deficiency in Sport (RED-S)'. *British Journal of Sports Medicine*, 49(7), 417–420. https://doi.org/10.1136/bjsports-2014-094371;
Sim et al. (2019). 'Iron considerations for the athlete: A narrative review'.

14. Troutt, J.S., Rudling, M., Persson, L. et al. (2012). 'Circulating human hepcidin-25 concentrations display a diurnal rhythm, increase with prolonged fasting, and are reduced by growth hormone administration'. *Clinical Chemistry*, 58(8), 1225–1232. https://doi.org/10.1373/clinchem.2012.186866;
Sim et al. (2019). 'Iron considerations for the athlete: A narrative review'.

15. Monedero et al. (2023). 'Dietary intakes and the risk of low energy availability in male and female advanced and elite rock climbers'.

16. British Dietetic Association (March 2021). 'Calcium', https://www.bda.uk.com/resource/calcium.html accessed 22 May 2025.

17. British Dietetic Association (2024). 'Nutritional considerations for dietitians', https://www.bda.uk.com/news-campaigns/campaigns/sustainable-september/nutritional-considerations-for-dietitians.html accessed 22 May 2025;
Goolsby, M.A. & Boniquit, N. (2017). 'Bone health in athletes: The role of exercise, nutrition, and hormones. *Sports Health*, 9(2), 108–117. https://doi.org/10.1177/1941738116677732

18. Krzywański, J., Mikulski, T., Pokrywka, A. et al. (2020). 'Vitamin B12 status and optimal range for hemoglobin formation in elite athletes'. *Nutrients*, 12(4), 1038. https://doi.org/10.3390/nu12041038

19. Krzywański et al. (2020). 'Vitamin B12 status and optimal range for hemoglobin formation in elite athletes'.

20. Niklewicz, A., Smith, A.D., Smith, A. et al. (2023). 'The importance of vitamin B12 for individuals choosing plant-based diets'. *European Journal of Nutrition*, 62(3), 1551–1559. https://doi.org/10.1007/s00394-022-03025-4

21. Gilsing, A.M.J., Crowe, F.L., Lloyd-Wright, Z. et al. (2010). 'Serum concentrations of vitamin B12 and folate in British male omnivores, vegetarians and vegans: Results from a cross-sectional analysis of the EPIC-Oxford cohort study'. *European Journal of Clinical Nutrition*, 64(9), 933–939. https://doi.org/10.1038/ejcn.2010.142

22. British Dietetic Association (2024). 'Nutritional considerations for dietitians'.

23. Milton Keynes University Hospital NHS Foundation Trust. 'Iron (good sources of)', https://www.mkuh.nhs.uk/patient-information-leaflet/good-sources-of-iron accessed 22 May 2025.

24. British Nutrition Foundation (2021). 'Calcium counts!' https://www.nutrition.org.uk/media/xjtlxtfo/calcium-counts.pdf accessed 22 May 2025.

25. University Hospitals Plymouth NHS Trust (2022). 'Vitamin B12 diet sheet', www.plymouthhospitals.nhs.uk/display-pil/pil-vitamin-b12-diet-sheet-5865 accessed 16 June 2025.

Gut health

1. Ley, R.E., Peterson, D.A. & Gordon, J.I. (2006). 'Ecological and evolutionary forces shaping microbial diversity in the human intestine'. *Cell*, 124(4), 837–848. https://doi.org/10.1016/j.cell.2006.02.017

2. Miranda-Comas, G., Petering, R.C., Zaman, N. & Chang, R. (2022). 'Implications of the gut microbiome in sports'. *Sports Health*, 14(6), 894–898. https://doi.org/10.1177/19417381211060006

3. Tan, J., McKenzie, C., Potamitis, M. et al. (2014). 'Chapter three – The role of short-chain fatty acids in health and disease'. *Advances in Immunology*, 121, 91–119. https://doi.org/10.1016/B978-0-12-800100-4.00003-9

4. Wegierska, A.E., Charitos, I.A., Topi, S. et al. (2022). 'The connection between physical exercise and gut microbiota: Implications for competitive sports athletes'. *Sports Medicine*, 52(10), 2355–2369. https://doi.org/10.1007/s40279-022-01696-x

5. Pane, M., Amoruso, A., Deidda, F. et al. (2018). 'Gut microbiota, probiotics, and sport: From clinical evidence to agonistic performance'. *Journal of Clinical Gastroenterology*, 52, S46–S49. https://doi.org/10.1097/MCG.0000000000001058

6. Wegierska et al. (2022). 'The connection between physical exercise and gut microbiota: Implications for competitive sports athletes'.;
Clauss, M., Gérard, P., Mosca, A. & Leclerc, M. (2021). 'Interplay between exercise and gut microbiome in the context of human health and performance'. *Frontiers in Nutrition*, 8. https://doi.org/10.3389/fnut.2021.637010

7. McDonald, D., Hyde, E., Debelius, J.W. et al. (2018). 'American gut: An open platform for citizen science microbiome research'. *mSystems*, 3(3), e00031-18. https://doi.org/10.1128/msystems.00031-18

8. Kim, S.-K., Guevarra, R.B., Kim, Y.-T. et al. (2019). 'Role of probiotics in human gut microbiome-associated diseases'. *Journal of Microbiology and Biotechnology*, 29(9), 1335–1340. https://doi.org/10.4014/jmb.1906.06064;
Suez, J., Zmora, N., Segal, E. & Elinav, E. (2019). 'The pros, cons, and many unknowns of probiotics'. *Nature Medicine*, 25(5), 716–729. https://doi.org/10.1038/s41591-019-0439-x;

Merenstein, D., Pot, B., Leyer, G. et al. (2023). 'Emerging issues in probiotic safety: 2023 perspectives'. *Gut Microbes*, 15(1). https://doi.org/10.1080/19490976.2023.2185034

9. Pane et al. (2018). 'Gut microbiota, probiotics, and sport: From clinical evidence to agonistic performance'.

6 Hydration

1. British Dietetic Association (19 August 2019). 'The importance of hydration', https://www.bda.uk.com/resource/the-importance-of-hydration.html accessed 22 May 2025.
2. Armstrong, L.E. (2021). 'Rehydration during endurance exercise: Challenges, research, options, methods'. *Nutrients*, 13(3), 887. https://doi.org/10.3390/nu13030887
3. Singer, P., Berger, M.M., Van den Berghe, G. et al. (2009). 'ESPEN guidelines on parenteral nutrition: Intensive care'. *Clinical Nutrition*, 28(4), 387–400. https://doi.org/10.1016/j.clnu.2009.04.024
4. Belval, L.N., Hosokawa, Y., Casa, D.J. et al. (2019). 'Practical hydration solutions for sports'. *Nutrients*, 11(7), 1550. https://doi.org/10.3390/nu11071550
5. Barley, O.R., Chapman, D.W. & Abbiss, C.R. (2020). 'Reviewing the current methods of assessing hydration in athletes'. *Journal of the International Society of Sports Nutrition*, 17(1), 52. https://doi.org/10.1186/s12970-020-00381-6
6. Armstrong (2021). 'Rehydration during endurance exercise: Challenges, research, options, methods'.
7. Smith, E.J., Storey, R. & Ranchordas, M.K. (2017). 'Nutritional considerations for bouldering'. *International Journal of Sport Nutrition and Exercise Metabolism*, 27(4), 314–324. https://doi.org/10.1123/ijsnem.2017-0043
8. Armstrong (2021). 'Rehydration during endurance exercise: Challenges, research, options, methods'.
9. Michael, M.K., Witard, O.C. & Joubert, L. (2019). 'Physiological demands and nutritional considerations for Olympic-style competitive rock climbing'. *Cogent Medicine*, 6(1). https://doi.org/10.1080/2331205x.2019.1667199;
   Thomas, D.T., Erdman, K.A. & Burke, L.M. (2016). 'American College of Sports Medicine Joint Position Statement. Nutrition and Athletic Performance'. *Medicine & Science in Sports & Exercise*, 48(3), 543–568. https://doi.org/10.1249/mss.0000000000000852
10. Barley et al. (2020). 'Reviewing the current methods of assessing hydration in athletes'.
11. Belval et al. (2019). 'Practical hydration solutions for sports'.
12. Kenefick, R.W. (2018). 'Drinking strategies: Planned drinking versus drinking to thirst'. *Sports Medicine*, 48, 31–37. https://doi.org/10.1007/s40279-017-0844-6
13. Armstrong (2021). 'Rehydration during endurance exercise: Challenges, research, options, methods'.
14. Kostelnik, S.B., Davy, K.P., Hedrick, V.E. et al. (2020). 'The validity of urine color as a hydration biomarker within the general adult population and athletes: A systematic review'. *Journal of the American College of Nutrition*, 40(2), 172–179. https://doi.org/10.1080/07315724.2020.1750073
15. Barley et al. (2020). 'Reviewing the current methods of assessing hydration in athletes'.
16. Gunawan, A.A.S., Brandon, D., Puspa, V.D. & Wiweko, B. (2018). 'Development of urine hydration system based on urine color and support vector machine'. *Procedia Computer Science*, 135, 481–489. https://doi.org/10.1016/j.procs.2018.08.200
17. Armstrong, L.E. & Casa, D.J. (2009). 'Methods to evaluate electrolyte and water turnover of athletes'. *Athletic Training & Sports Health Care*, 1(4), 169–179. https://doi.org/10.3928/19425864-20090625-06
18. Racinais, S., Hosokawa, Y., Akama, T. et al. (2023). 'IOC consensus statement on recommendations and regulations for sport events in the heat'. *British Journal of Sports Medicine*, 57(1), 8–25. https://doi.org/10.1136/bjsports-2022-105942
19. Racinais et al. (2023). 'IOC consensus statement on recommendations and regulations for sport events in the heat'.
20. Racinais et al. (2023). 'IOC consensus statement on recommendations and regulations for sport events in the heat'.
21. Viscor, G., Corominas, J. & Carceller, A. (2023). 'Nutrition and hydration for high-altitude alpinism: A narrative review'. *International Journal of Environmental Research and Public Health*, 20(4), 3186. https://doi.org/10.3390/ijerph20043186

7 Sports supplements

1. Maughan, R.J., Burke, L.M., Dvorak, J. et al. (2018). 'IOC consensus statement: Dietary supplements and the high-performance athlete'. *British Journal of Sports Medicine*, 52(7), 439–455. https://doi.org/10.1136/bjsports-2018-099027
2. Maughan et al. (2018). 'IOC consensus statement: Dietary supplements and the high-performance athlete'.
3. Forbes, S.C., Cordingley, D.M., Cornish, S.M. et al. (2022). 'Effects of creatine supplementation on brain function and health'. *Nutrients*, 14(5), 921. https://doi.org/10.3390/nu14050921;
   Roschel, H., Gualano, B., Ostojic, S.M. & Rawson, E.S. (2021). 'Creatine supplementation and brain health'. *Nutrients*, 13(2), 586. https://doi.org/10.3390/nu13020586;
   Kreider, R.B., Kalman, D.S., Antonio, J. et al. (2017). 'International Society of Sports Nutrition position stand: Safety and efficacy of creatine supplementation in exercise, sport, and medicine'. *Journal of the International Society of Sports Nutrition*, 14(1). https://doi.org/10.1186/s12970-017-0173-z
4. Maughan et al. (2018). 'IOC consensus statement: Dietary supplements and the high-performance athlete'.
5. Doran, D.A. & Godfrey, A. (2001). 'Effects of creatine supplementation on upper body power output in elite rock climbers'. *Biology of Sport*, 18(1), 55–69.

6. Smith, E.J., Storey, R. & Ranchordas, M.K. (2017). 'Nutritional considerations for bouldering'. *International Journal of Sport Nutrition and Exercise Metabolism*, 27(4), 314–324. https://doi.org/10.1123/ijsnem.2017-0043
7. Forbes et al. (2022). 'Effects of creatine supplementation on brain function and health'.;
   Roschel et al. (2021). 'Creatine supplementation and brain health'.
8. Michael, M.K., Witard, O.C. & Joubert, L. (2019). 'Physiological demands and nutritional considerations for Olympic-style competitive rock climbing'. *Cogent Medicine*, 6(1). https://doi.org/10.1080/2331205x.2019.1667199
9. Antonio, J., Candow, D.G., Forbes, S.C. et al. (2021). 'Common questions and misconceptions about creatine supplementation: What does the scientific evidence really show?' *Journal of the International Society of Sports Nutrition*, 18(1). https://doi.org/10.1186/s12970-021-00412-w
10. Antonio et al. (2021). 'Common questions and misconceptions about creatine supplementation: What does the scientific evidence really show?'.
11. Saunders, B., Elliott-Sale, K., Artioli, G.G. et al. (2017). 'β-Alanine supplementation to improve exercise capacity and performance: A systematic review and meta-analysis.' *British Journal of Sports Medicine*, 51(8), 658–669. https://doi.org/10.1136/bjsports-2016-096396;
   Maughan et al. (2018). 'IOC consensus statement: Dietary supplements and the high-performance athlete'.
12. Sas-Nowosielski, K., Wyciślik, J. & Kaczka, P. (2021). 'Beta-alanine supplementation and sport climbing performance'. *International Journal of Environmental Research and Public Health*, 18(10), 5370. https://doi.org/10.3390/ijerph18105370
13. Sas-Nowosielski, K. & Kaczka, P. (2022). 'A pilot study to examine the effects of beta-alanine and sodium citrate (CarnoRushTM, Olimp®) supplementation on climbing-specific performance'. *Baltic Journal of Health and Physical Activity*, 14(1). https://doi.org/10.29359/BJHPA.14.1.04
14. Blancquaert, L., Everaert, I. & Derave, W. (2015). 'Beta-alanine supplementation, muscle carnosine and exercise performance'. *Current Opinion in Clinical Nutrition and Metabolic Care*, 18(1), 63–70. https://doi.org/10.1097/MCO.0000000000000127;
   Hobson, R. M., Saunders, B., Ball, G. et al. (2012). 'Effects of β-alanine supplementation on exercise performance: A meta-analysis'. *Amino Acids*, 43(1), 25–37. https://doi.org/10.1007/s00726-011-1200-z
15. Maughan et al. (2018). 'IOC consensus statement: Dietary supplements and the high-performance athlete'.
16. Maughan et al. (2018). 'IOC consensus statement: Dietary supplements and the high-performance athlete'.;
   Guest, N.S., VanDusseldorp, T.A., Nelson, M.T. et al. (2021). 'International Society of Sports Nutrition position stand: Caffeine and exercise performance'. *Journal of the International Society of Sports Nutrition*, 18(1). https://doi.org/10.1186/s12970-020-00383-4
17. Cabañes, A., Salinero, J. & Del Coso, J. (2013). 'The ingestion of a caffeine-containing energy drink improves resistance capacity and sport rock climbing performance'. *Archivos de Medicina del Deporte*, 30, 215–220.
18. Gardiner, C., Weakley, J., Burke, L.M. et al. (2023). 'The effect of caffeine on subsequent sleep: A systematic review and meta-analysis'. *Sleep Medicine Reviews*, 69. https://doi.org/10.1016/j.smrv.2023.101764
19. de Souza, J.G., Del Coso, J., de Souza Fonseca, F. et al. (2022). 'Risk or benefit? Side effects of caffeine supplementation in sport: A systematic review'. *European Journal of Nutrition*, 61(8), 3823–3834. https://doi.org/10.1007/s00394-022-02874-3
20. Maughan et al. (2018). 'IOC consensus statement: Dietary supplements and the high-performance athlete'.
21. Jones, L., Bailey, S.J., Rowland, S.N. et al. (2021). 'The effect of nitrate-rich beetroot juice on markers of exercise-induced muscle damage: A systematic review and meta-analysis of human intervention trials'. *Journal of Dietary Supplements*, 19(6), 749–771. https://doi.org/10.1080/19390211.2021.1939472
22. Senefeld, J.W., Wiggins, C.C., Regimbal, R.J. et al. (2020). 'Ergogenic effect of nitrate supplementation: A systematic review and meta-analysis'. *Medicine & Science in Sports & Exercise*, 52(10), 2250–2261. https://doi.org/10.1249/MSS.0000000000002363
23. Berlanga, L.A., Lopez-Samanes, A., Martin-Lopez, J. et al. (2023). 'Dietary nitrate ingestion does not improve neuromuscular performance in male sport climbers'. *Journal of Human Kinetics*, 87, 47–57. https://doi.org/10.5114/jhk/161812
24. Maughan et al. (2018). 'IOC consensus statement: Dietary supplements and the high-performance athlete'.;
   Hunt, J.E.A., Coelho, M.O.C., Buxton, S. et al. (2021). 'Consumption of New Zealand blackcurrant extract improves recovery from exercise-induced muscle damage in non-resistance trained men and women: A double-blind randomised trial'. *Nutrients*, 13(8), 2875. https://doi.org/10.3390/nu13082875;
   Li, S., Fasipe, B. & Laher, I. (2022). 'Potential harms of supplementation with high doses of antioxidants in athletes'. *Journal of Exercise Science & Fitness*, 20(4), 269–275. https://doi.org/10.1016/j.jesf.2022.06.001;
   Clemente-Suárez, V.J., Bustamante-Sanchez, Á., Mielgo-Ayuso, J. et al. (2023). 'Antioxidants and sports performance'. *Nutrients*, 15(10), 2371. https://doi.org/10.3390/nu15102371;
   Braakhuis, A.J. & Hopkins, W.G. (2015). 'Impact of dietary antioxidants on sport performance: A review'. *Sports Medicine*, 45(7), 939–955. https://doi.org/10.1007/s40279-015-0323-x
25. Bowtell, J. & Kelly, V. (2019). 'Fruit-derived polyphenol supplementation for athlete recovery and performance'. *Sports Medicine*, 49(Suppl.1), 3–23. https://doi.org/10.1007/s40279-018-0998-x
26. Cook, M.D., Myers, S.D., Blacker, S.D. & Willems, M.E.T. (2015). 'New Zealand blackcurrant extract improves cycling performance and fat oxidation in cyclists'.

European Journal of Applied Physiology, 115(11), 2357–2365. https://doi.org/10.1007/s00421-015-3215-8;
Perkins, I.C., Vine, S.A., Blacker, S.D. & Willems, M.E.T. (2015). 'New Zealand blackcurrant extract improves high-intensity intermittent running'. *International Journal of Sport Nutrition and Exercise Metabolism*, 25(5), 487–493. https://doi.org/10.1123/ijsnem.2015-0020;
Murphy, C.A., Cook, M.D. & Willems, M.E.T. (2017). 'Effect of New Zealand blackcurrant extract on repeated cycling time trial performance'. *Sports*, 5(2), 25. https://doi.org/10.3390/sports5020025;
Godwin, C., Cook, M.D. & Willems, M.E.T. (2017). 'Effect of New Zealand blackcurrant extract on performance during the running based anaerobic sprint test in trained youth and recreationally active male football players'. *Sports*, 5(3), 69. https://doi.org/10.3390/sports5030069;
Willems, M.E.T., Cousins, L., Williams, D. & Blacker, S.D. (2016). 'Beneficial effects of New Zealand blackcurrant extract on maximal sprint speed during the Loughborough intermittent shuttle test'. *Sports*, 4(3), 42. https://doi.org/10.3390/sports4030042;
Willems, M.E.T., Bradley, M., Blacker, S.D. & Perkins, I.C. (2020). 'Effect of New Zealand blackcurrant extract on isometric contraction-induced fatigue and recovery: Potential muscle-fiber specific effects'. *Sports*, 8(10), 135. https://doi.org/10.3390/sports8100135;
Hunt et al. (2021). 'Consumption of New Zealand blackcurrant extract improves recovery from exercise-induced muscle damage in non-resistance trained men and women: A double-blind randomised trial'.

27. Potter, J.A., Hodgson, C.I., Broadhurst, M. et al. (2020). 'Effects of New Zealand blackcurrant extract on sport climbing performance'. *European Journal of Applied Physiology*, 120(1), 67–75. https://doi.org/10.1007/s00421-019-04226-2;
Potter, J.A., Hodgson, C.I., Broadhurst, M. et al. (2020). 'Correction to: Effects of New Zealand blackcurrant extract on sport climbing performance'. *European Journal of Applied Physiology*, 120(1), 77. https://doi.org/10.1007/s00421-019-04268-6

28. Fryer, S., Paterson, C., Perkins, I.C. et al. (2020). 'New Zealand blackcurrant extract enhances muscle oxygenation during forearm exercise in intermediate-level rock climbers'. *International Journal of Sport Nutrition and Exercise Metabolism*, 30(4), 258–263. https://doi.org/10.1123/ijsnem.2019-0365;
Fryer, S., Giles, D., Bird, E. et al. (2021). 'New Zealand blackcurrant extract enhances muscle oxygenation during repeated intermittent forearm muscle contractions in advanced and elite rock climbers'. *European Journal of Sport Science*, 21(9), 1290–1298. https://doi.org/10.1080/17461391.2020.1827048

29. Couppé, C., Kongsgaard, M., Aagaard, P. et al. (2008). 'Habitual loading results in tendon hypertrophy and increased stiffness of the human patellar tendon'. *Journal of Applied Physiology*, 105(3), 805–810. https://doi.org/10.1152/japplphysiol.90361.2008

30. Shaw, G., Lee-Barthel, A., Ross, M.L.R. et al. (2017). 'Vitamin C-enriched gelatin supplementation before intermittent activity augments collagen synthesis'. *The American Journal of Clinical Nutrition*, 105(1), 136–143. https://doi.org/10.3945/ajcn.116.138594;
Clark, K.L., Sebastianelli, W., Flechsenhar, K.R. et al. (2008). '24-Week study on the use of collagen hydrolysate as a dietary supplement in athletes with activity-related joint pain'. *Current Medical Research and Opinion*, 24(5), 1485–1496. https://doi.org/10.1185/030079908X291967;
Zdzieblik, D., Oesser, S., Gollhofer, A. & König, D. (2017). 'Improvement of activity-related knee joint discomfort following supplementation of specific collagen peptides'. *Applied Physiology, Nutrition, and Metabolism*, 42(6), 588–595. https://doi.org/10.1139/apnm-2016-0390;
Khatri, M., Naughton, R.J., Clifford, T. et al. (2021). 'The effects of collagen peptide supplementation on body composition, collagen synthesis, and recovery from joint injury and exercise: A systematic review'. *Amino Acids*, 53(10), 1493–1506. https://doi.org/10.1007/s00726-021-03072-x;
Hijlkema, A., Roozenboom, C., Mensink, M. & Zwerver, J. (2022). 'The impact of nutrition on tendon health and tendinopathy: A systematic review'. *Journal of the International Society of Sports Nutrition*, 19(1), 474–504. https://doi.org/10.1080/15502783.2022.2104130

31. Lis, D.M., Jordan, M., Lipuma, T. et al. (2022). 'Collagen and vitamin C supplementation increases lower limb rate of force development'. *International Journal of Sport Nutrition and Exercise Metabolism*, 32(2), 65–73. https://doi.org/10.1123/ijsnem.2020-0313

32. Maughan et al. (2018). 'IOC consensus statement: Dietary supplements and the high-performance athlete'.;
Rawson, E.S., Miles, M.P. & Larson-Meyer, D.E. (2018). 'Dietary supplements for health, adaptation, and recovery in athletes'. *International Journal of Sport Nutrition and Exercise Metabolism* 28 (2), 188–199. https://doi.org/10.1123/ijsnem.2017-0340
Aussieker, T., Kaiser, J., Hendriks, F.K. et al. (2025). 'The effects of ingesting a single bolus of hydrolyzed collagen versus free amino acids on muscle connective protein synthesis rates'. *Medicine and Science in Sports and Exercise*, advance online publication. https://doi.org/10.1249/MSS.0000000000003788 accessed 25 June 2025.

33. Khatri et al. (2021). 'The effects of collagen peptide supplementation on body composition, collagen synthesis, and recovery from joint injury and exercise: A systematic review'.

34. Khatri et al. (2021). 'The effects of collagen peptide supplementation on body composition, collagen synthesis, and recovery from joint injury and exercise: A systematic review'.

35. Shaw et al. (2017). 'Vitamin C-enriched gelatin supplementation before intermittent activity augments collagen synthesis'.
Khatri et al. (2021). 'The effects of collagen peptide supplementation on body composition, collagen synthesis, and recovery from joint injury and exercise: A systematic review'

8 Crag nutrition

1. Smith, E.J., Storey, R. & Ranchordas, M.K. (2017). 'Nutritional considerations for bouldering'. *International Journal of Sport Nutrition and Exercise Metabolism*, 27(4), 314–324. https://doi.org/10.1123/ijsnem.2017-0043
2. Michael, M.K., Witard, O.C. & Joubert, L. (2019). 'Physiological demands and nutritional considerations for Olympic-style competitive rock climbing'. *Cogent Medicine*, 6(1). https://doi.org/10.1080/2331205x.2019.1667199
3. Viscor, G., Corominas, J. & Carceller, A. (2023). 'Nutrition and hydration for high-altitude alpinism: A narrative review'. *International Journal of Environmental Research and Public Health*, 20(4), 3186. https://doi.org/10.3390/ijerph20043186
4. Stellingwerff, T., Peeling, P., Garvican-Lewis, L.A. et al. (2019). 'Nutrition and altitude: Strategies to enhance adaptation, improve performance and maintain health: A narrative review'. *Sports Medicine*, 49(Suppl.2), 169–184. https://doi.org/10.1007/s40279-019-01159-w
5. Stellingwerff et al. (2019). 'Nutrition and altitude: Strategies to enhance adaptation, improve performance and maintain health: A narrative review'.;
   Viscor et al. (2023). 'Nutrition and hydration for high-altitude alpinism: A narrative review'.
6. Viscor et al. (2023). 'Nutrition and hydration for high-altitude alpinism: A narrative review'.
7. Viscor et al. (2023). 'Nutrition and hydration for high-altitude alpinism: A narrative review'.;
   Watts, P.B., Martin, D.T., Schmeling, M.H. et al. (1990). 'Exertional intensities and energy requirements of technical mountaineering at moderate altitude'. *Journal of Sports Medicine and Physical Fitness*, 30(4), 265–376.
8. Stellingwerf et al. (2019). 'Nutrition and altitude: Strategies to enhance adaptation, improve performance and maintain health: A narrative review'.

9 The female climber

1. Moore, D.R., Sygo, J. & Morton, J.P. (2022). 'Fuelling the female athlete: Carbohydrate and protein recommendations'. *European Journal of Sport Science*, 22(5), 684–696. https://doi.org/10.1080/17461391.2021.1922508;
   Wohlgemuth, K.J., Arieta, L.R., Brewer, G.J. et al. (2021). 'Sex differences and considerations for female specific nutritional strategies: a narrative review'. *Journal of the International Society of Sports Nutrition*, 18(1). https://doi.org/10.1186/s12970-021-00422-8;
   Holtzman, B. & Ackerman, K.E. (2021). 'Recommendations and nutritional considerations for female athletes: Health and performance'. *Sports Medicine*, 51(Suppl.1), 43–57. https://doi.org/10.1007/s40279-021-01508-8;
   Stachenfeld, N.S. (2018). 'Including women in research. It's necessary, and really not so hard to do'. *Experimental Physiology*, 103(10), 1296–1297. https://doi.org/10.1113/EP087261
2. Roepstorff, C., Steffensen, C.H., Madsen, M. et al. (2002). 'Gender differences in substrate utilization during submaximal exercise in endurance-trained subjects'. *American Journal of Physiology - Endocrinology and Metabolism*, 282(2), E435–E447. https://doi.org/10.1152/ajpendo.00266.2001;
   Pivarnik, J.M., Marichal, C.J., Spillman, T. & Morrow, J.R. (1992). 'Menstrual cycle phase affects temperature regulation during endurance exercise'. *Journal of Applied Physiology*, 72(2), 543–548. https://doi.org/10.1152/jappl.1992.72.2.543;
   Bredella, M.A. (2017). 'Sex differences in body composition', in *Sex and Gender Factors Affecting Metabolic Homeostasis, Diabetes and Obesity*. (Advances in Experimental Medicine and Biology 1043). Ed. F. Mauvais-Jarvis. Springer, Cham, 9–27. https://doi.org/10.1007/978-3-319-70178-3_2;
   Hunter, S.K. (2016). 'Sex differences in fatigability of dynamic contractions'. *Experimental Physiology*, 101(2), 250–255. https://doi.org/10.1113/EP085370;
   Hackney, A.C., Kallman, A.L. & Ağgön, E. (2019). 'Female sex hormones and the recovery from exercise: Menstrual cycle phase affects responses'. *Biomedical Human Kinetics*, 11(1), 87–89. https://doi.org/10.2478/bhk-2019-0011
3. Kemmler, W., Roloff, I., Baumann, H. et al. (2006). 'Effect of exercise, body composition, and nutritional intake on bone parameters in male elite rock climbers'. *International Journal of Sports Medicine*, 27(8), 653–659. https://doi.org/10.1055/s-2005-872828;
   Zapf, J., Fichtl, B., Wielgoss, S. & Schmidt, W. (2001). 'Macronutrient intake and eating habits in elite rock climbers'. *Medicine & Science in Sports & Exercise*, 33(5), S72. https://doi.org/10.1097/00005768-200105001-00407
4. Monedero, J., Duff, C. & Egan, B. (2023). 'Dietary intakes and the risk of low energy availability in male and female advanced and elite rock climbers'. *Journal of Strength and Conditioning Research*, 37(3), e8–e15. https://doi.org/10.1519/JSC.0000000000004317;
   Gibson-Smith, E., Storey, R. & Ranchordas, M. (2020). 'Dietary intake, body composition and iron status in experienced and elite climbers'. *Frontiers in Nutrition*, 7. https://doi.org/10.3389/fnut.2020.00122;
   Giles, D., Barnes, K., Taylor, N., et al. (2021). 'Anthropometry and performance characteristics of recreational advanced to elite female rock climbers'. *Journal of Sports Sciences*, 39(1), 48–56. https://doi.org/10.1080/02640414.2020.1804784
5. Smith, E.J., Storey, R. & Ranchordas, M.K. (2017). 'Nutritional considerations for bouldering'. *International Journal of Sport Nutrition and Exercise Metabolism*, 27(4), 314–324. https://doi.org/10.1123/ijsnem.2017-0043;
   Michael, M.K., Witard, O.C. & Joubert, L. (2019). 'Physiological demands and nutritional considerations for Olympic-style competitive rock climbing'. *Cogent Medicine*, 6(1). https://doi.org/10.1080/2331205x.2019.1667199
6. Leslie-Wujastyk, M. & Gibson-Smith, E. (2025). 'Nutritional considerations for female rock climbers'. *Journal of Science in Sport and Exercise*, 7, 28–39. https://doi.org/10.1007/s42978-023-00267-4

7. Sims, S.T., Kerksick, C.M., Smith-Ryan, A.E. et al. (2023). 'International Society of Sports Nutrition position stand: Nutritional concerns of the female athlete'. *Journal of the International Society of Sports Nutrition*, 20(1). https://doi.org/10.1080/15502783.2023.2204066

8. Chmielewska, A. & Regulska-Ilow, B. (2023). 'The evaluation of energy availability and dietary nutrient intake of sport climbers at different climbing levels'. *International Journal of Environmental Research and Public Health*, 20(6), 5176. https://doi.org/10.3390/ijerph20065176;
Monedero et al. (2023). 'Dietary intakes and the risk of low energy availability in male and female advanced and elite rock climbers'.

9. Gibson-Smith et al. (2020). 'Dietary intake, body composition and iron status in experienced and elite climbers'.;
Monedero et al. (2023). 'Dietary intakes and the risk of low energy availability in male and female advanced and elite rock climbers'.

10. Chmielewska & Regulska-Ilow (2023). 'The evaluation of energy availability and dietary nutrient intake of sport climbers at different climbing levels'.;
Monedero et al. (2023). 'Dietary intakes and the risk of low energy availability in male and female advanced and elite rock climbers'.

11. Spence, K. (2013). 'Nutrients needed for optimal bone health in the female athlete', in *Nutrition and the Female Athlete*. Ed. K.A. Beals. CRC Press, Boca Raton (FL). https://doi.org/10.1201/b13743

12. Leslie-Wujastyk & Gibson-Smith (2025). 'Nutritional considerations for female rock climbers'.;
Moore et al. (2022). 'Fuelling the female athlete: Carbohydrate and protein recommendations'.;
Rossi, K.A. (2017). 'Nutritional aspects of the female athlete'. *Clinics in Sports Medicine*, 36(4), 627–653. https://doi.org/10.1016/j.csm.2017.05.007

13. Hackney et al. (2019). 'Female sex hormones and the recovery from exercise: Menstrual cycle phase affects responses'.

14. Benton, M.J., Hutchins, A.M. & Dawes, J.J. (2020). 'Effect of menstrual cycle on resting metabolism: A systematic review and meta-analysis'. *PLOS ONE*, 15(7), e0236025. https://doi.org/10.1371/journal.pone.0236025

15. Barr, S.I., Janelle, K.C. & Prior, J.C. (1995). 'Energy intakes are higher during the luteal phase of ovulatory menstrual cycles'. *The American Journal of Clinical Nutrition*, 61(1), 39–43. https://doi.org/10.1093/ajcn/61.1.39

16. Desbrow, B., Burd, N.A., Tarnopolsky, M. et al. (2019). 'Nutrition for special populations: Young, female, and masters athletes'. *International Journal of Sport Nutrition and Exercise Metabolism*, 29(2), 220–227. https://doi.org/10.1123/ijsnem.2018-0269

17. Rodriguez-Giustiniani, P., Rodriguez-Sanchez, N. & Galloway, S.D.R. (2022). 'Fluid and electrolyte balance considerations for female athletes'. *European Journal of Sport Science*, 22(5), 697–708. https://doi.org/10.1080/17461391.2021.1939428

18. Giersch, G.E.W., Charkoudian, N., Stearns, R.L. & Casa, D.J. (2020). 'Fluid balance and hydration considerations for women: Review and future directions'. *Sports Medicine*, 50(2), 253–261. https://doi.org/10.1007/s40279-019-01206-6;
Rodriguez-Giustiniani et al. (2022). 'Fluid and electrolyte balance considerations for female athletes'.

19. Holtzman & Ackerman (2021). 'Recommendations and nutritional considerations for female athletes: Health and performance'.;
Rehrer, N.J., McLay-Cooke, R.T. & Sims, S.T. (2023). 'Nutritional strategies and sex hormone interactions in women', in *Sex Hormones, Exercise and Women*. Ed. A.C. Hackney, second edition. Springer, Cham. https://doi.org/10.1007/978-3-031-21881-1_12;
Rossi (2017). 'Nutritional aspects of the female athlete'.

20. Moore et al. (2022). 'Fuelling the female athlete: Carbohydrate and protein recommendations'.;
Wohlgemuth et al. (2021). 'Sex differences and considerations for female specific nutritional strategies: a narrative review'.;
Mercer, D., Convit, L., Condo, D. et al. (2020). 'Protein requirements of pre-menopausal female athletes: Systematic literature review'. *Nutrients*, 12(11), 3527. https://doi.org/10.3390/nu12113527;
Rehrer et al. (2023). 'Nutritional strategies and sex hormone interactions in women'.

21. Aguilar-Aguilar, E. (2020). 'Menstrual disorders: What we know about dietary-nutritional therapy.' *Nutricion Hospitalaria*, 37(Ext2), 52–56. https://doi.org/10.20960/nh.03358

22. Siminiuc, R. & Ţurcanu, D. (2023). 'Impact of nutritional diet therapy on premenstrual syndrome'. *Frontiers in Nutrition*, 10. https://doi.org/10.3389/fnut.2023.1079417;
Abdi, F., Ozgoli, G. & Rahnemaie, F.S. (2019). 'A systematic review of the role of vitamin D and calcium in premenstrual syndrome'. *Obstetrics and Gynecology Science*, 62(2), 73–86. https://doi.org/10.5468/ogs.2019.62.2.73

23. Arab, A., Rafie, N., Askari, G. & Taghiabadi, M. (2020). 'Beneficial role of calcium in premenstrual syndrome: A systematic review of current literature'. *International Journal of Preventive Medicine*, 11(1), 156. https://doi.org/10.4103/ijpvm.ijpvm_243_19

24. Pallante, P.I., Vega, A.C., Escobar, A. et al. (2023). 'Micronutrient intake and premenstrual syndrome in female collegiate athletes'. *The Journal of Sports Medicine and Physical Fitness*, 63(3), 444–451. https://doi.org/10.23736/S0022-4707.22.13829-6;
Abdi et al. (2019). 'A systematic review of the role of vitamin D and calcium in premenstrual syndrome'.;
Bahrami, A., Avan, A., Sadeghnia, H.R. et al. (2018). 'High dose vitamin D supplementation can improve menstrual problems, dysmenorrhea, and premenstrual syndrome in adolescents'. *Gynecological Endocrinology*, 34(8), 659–663. https://doi.org/10.1080/09513590.2017.1423466

25. Jafari, F., Amani, R. & Tarrahi, M.J. (2020). 'Effect of zinc supplementation on physical and psychological symptoms, biomarkers of inflammation, oxidative stress, and brain-derived neurotrophic factor in young

women with premenstrual syndrome: A randomized, double-blind, placebo-controlled trial'. *Biological Trace Element Research*, 194(1), 89–95. https://doi.org/10.1007/s12011-019-01757-9;
Retallick-Brown, H., Blampied, N. & and Rucklidge, J.J. (2020). 'A pilot randomized treatment-controlled trial comparing vitamin B6 with broad-spectrum micronutrients for premenstrual syndrome'. *The Journal of Alternative and Complementary Medicine*, 26(2), 88–97. https://doi.org/10.1089/acm.2019.0305;
Parazzini, F., Di Martino, M. & Pellegrino, P. (2017). 'Magnesium in the gynecological practice: A literature review'. *Magnesium Research*, 30(1):1–7. https://doi.org/10.1684/mrh.2017.0419

26. Elliott-Sale, K.J., McNulty, K.L., Ansdell, P. et al. (2020). 'The effects of oral contraceptives on exercise performance in women: A systematic review and meta-analysis. *Sports Medicine*, 50(10), 1785–1812. https://doi.org/10.1007/s40279-020-01317-5
27. Thompson, B., Almarjawi, A., Sculley, D. & Janse de Jonge, X. (2020). 'The effect of the menstrual cycle and oral contraceptives on acute responses and chronic adaptations to resistance training: A systematic review of the literature'. *Sports Medicine*, 50(1), 171–185. https://doi.org/10.1007/s40279-019-01219-1
28. Glenner-Frandsen, A., With, C., Gunnarsson, T.P. & Hostrup, M. (2022). 'The effect of monophasic oral contraceptives on muscle strength and markers of recovery after exercise-induced muscle damage: A systematic review'. *Sports Health*, 15(3), 318–327. https://doi.org/10.1177/19417381221121653;
Larsen, B., Cox, A., Colbey, C. et al. (2020). 'Inflammation and oral contraceptive use in female athletes before the Rio Olympic Games'. *Frontiers in Physiology*, 11. https://doi.org/10.3389/fphys.2020.00497
29. Wohlgemuth et al. (2021). 'Sex differences and considerations for female specific nutritional strategies: a narrative review'.
30. Sims et al. (2023). 'International Society of Sports Nutrition position stand: Nutritional concerns of the female athlete'.;
Glenner-Frandsen et al, (2022). 'The effect of monophasic oral contraceptives on muscle strength and markers of recovery after exercise-induced muscle damage: A systematic review'.
31. American College of Obstetricians and Gynecologists (2020). 'Physical activity and exercise during pregnancy and the postpartum period: ACOG committee opinion summary, number 804.' *Obstetrics & Gynecology*, 135(4), 991–993. https://doi.org/10.1097/aog.0000000000003773
32. Elliott-Sale, K.J., Graham, A., Hanley, S.J. et al. (2019). 'Modern dietary guidelines for healthy pregnancy; maximising maternal and foetal outcomes and limiting excessive gestational weight gain'. *European Journal of Sport Science*, 19(1), 62–70. https://doi.org/10.1080/17461391.2018.1476591
33. Artal, R. & O'Toole, M. (2003). 'Guidelines of the American College of Obstetricians and Gynecologists for exercise during pregnancy and the postpartum period'. *British Journal of Sports Medicine*, 37(1), 6–12. https://doi.org/10.1136/bjsm.37.1.6
34. McGregor, R. (2022). *More Fuel You*. Vertebrate Publishing, Sheffield.
35. Desbrow et al. (2019). 'Nutrition for special populations: Young, female, and masters athletes'.
36. Sims et al. (2023). 'International Society of Sports Nutrition position stand: Nutritional concerns of the female athlete'.
37. Smith-Ryan, A.E., Cabre, H.E., Eckerson, J.M. & Candow, D.G. (2021). 'Creatine supplementation in women's health: A lifespan perspective'. *Nutrients*, 13(3), 877. https://doi.org/10.3390/nu13030877

10 Nutrition for injury

1. Puga, T.B., Mazumder, R.M., Ruan, T. et al. (2023). 'Sleep, nutrition, hydration and rest: The equal importance of external factors outside of training and practice for sports injury prevention'. *Scientific Journal of Sport and Performance*, 2(4), 428–438. https://doi.org/10.55860/LZNO4932
2. Giraldo-Vallejo, J.E., Cardona-Guzmán, M.Á, Rodríguez-Alcivar, E.J. et al. (2023). 'Nutritional strategies in the rehabilitation of musculoskeletal injuries in athletes: A systematic integrative review'. *Nutrients*, 15(4), 819. https://doi.org/10.3390/nu15040819
3. Close, G.L., Sale, C., Baar, K. & Bermon, S. (2019). 'Nutrition for the prevention and treatment of injuries in track and field athletes'. *International Journal of Sport Nutrition and Exercise Metabolism*, 29(2), 189–197. https://doi.org/10.1123/ijsnem.2018-0290
4. Giraldo-Vallejo et al. (2023). 'Nutritional strategies in the rehabilitation of musculoskeletal injuries in athletes: A systematic integrative review'.;
Papadopoulou, S.K. (2020). 'Rehabilitation nutrition for injury recovery of athletes: The role of macronutrient intake'. *Nutrients*, 12(8), 2449. https://doi.org/10.3390/nu12082449
5. Smith-Ryan, A.E., Hirsch, K.R., Saylor, H.E. et al. (2020). 'Nutritional considerations and strategies to facilitate injury recovery and rehabilitation'. *Journal of Athletic Training*, 55(9) 918–930. https://doi.org/10.4085/1062-6050-550-19;
Frankenfield, D. (2006). 'Energy expenditure and protein requirements after traumatic injury'. *Nutrition in Clinical Practice*, 21(5), 430–437. https://doi.org/10.1177/0115426506021005430;
Wolfe, R.R. (2006). 'The underappreciated role of muscle in health and disease'. *The American Journal of Clinical Nutrition*, 84(3), 475–482. https://doi.org/10.1093/ajcn/84.3.475
6. Biolo, G., Agostini, F., Simunic, B. et al. (2008). 'Positive energy balance is associated with accelerated muscle atrophy and increased erythrocyte glutathione turnover during 5 wk of bed rest'. *The American Journal of Clinical Nutrition*, 88(4), 950–958. https://doi.org/10.1093/ajcn/88.4.950

7. Giraldo-Vallejo et al. (2023). 'Nutritional strategies in the rehabilitation of musculoskeletal injuries in athletes: A systematic integrative review'.;
Wall, B.T. & van Loon, L.J.C. (2013). 'Nutritional strategies to attenuate muscle disuse atrophy'. *Nutrition Reviews*, 71(4), 195–208. https://doi.org/10.1111/nure.12019;
Seki, K., Taniguchi, Y. & Narusawa, M. (2001). 'Alterations in contractile properties of human skeletal muscle induced by joint immobilization.' *The Journal of Physiology*, 530(3), 521–532. https://doi.org/10.1111/j.1469-7793.2001.0521k.x

8. Giraldo-Vallejo et al. (2023). 'Nutritional strategies in the rehabilitation of musculoskeletal injuries in athletes: A systematic integrative review'.;
Close et al. (2019). 'Nutrition for the prevention and treatment of injuries in track and field athletes'.

9. Giraldo-Vallejo et al. (2023). 'Nutritional strategies in the rehabilitation of musculoskeletal injuries in athletes: A systematic integrative review'.;
Tipton, K.D. (2017). 'Nutritional support for injuries requiring reduced activity'. *Sports Science Exchange*, 30(169), 1–6;
Papadopoulou (2020). 'Rehabilitation nutrition for injury recovery of athletes: The role of macronutrient intake'.

10. Smith-Ryan et al. (2020). 'Nutritional considerations and strategies to facilitate injury recovery and rehabilitation'.

11. Giraldo-Vallejo et al. (2023). 'Nutritional strategies in the rehabilitation of musculoskeletal injuries in athletes: A systematic integrative review'.;
Trommelen, J. & van Loon, L.J.C. (2016). 'Pre-sleep protein ingestion to improve the skeletal muscle adaptive response to exercise training'. *Nutrients*, 8(12), 763. https://doi.org/10.3390/nu8120763;
Papadopoulou (2020). 'Rehabilitation nutrition for injury recovery of athletes: The role of macronutrient intake'.

12. Papadopoulou (2020). 'Rehabilitation nutrition for injury recovery of athletes: The role of macronutrient intake'.;
Smith-Ryan et al. (2020). 'Nutritional considerations and strategies to facilitate injury recovery and rehabilitation'.

13. Shaw, G., Lee-Barthel, A., Ross, M.L.R. et al. (2017). 'Vitamin C-enriched gelatin supplementation before intermittent activity augments collagen synthesis'. *The American Journal of Clinical Nutrition*, 105(1), 136–143. https://doi.org/10.3945/ajcn.116.138594

14. Khatri, M., Naughton, R.J., Clifford, T. et al. (2021). 'The effects of collagen peptide supplementation on body composition, collagen synthesis, and recovery from joint injury and exercise: A systematic review'. *Amino Acids*, 53(10), 1493–1506. https://doi.org/10.1007/s00726-021-03072-x;
Close et al. (2019). 'Nutrition for the prevention and treatment of injuries in track and field athletes'.

15. Shaw et al. (2017). 'Vitamin C-enriched gelatin supplementation before intermittent activity augments collagen synthesis'.;
Khatri et al. (2021). 'The effects of collagen peptide supplementation on body composition, collagen synthesis, and recovery from joint injury and exercise: A systematic review'.

16. Close et al. (2019). 'Nutrition for the prevention and treatment of injuries in track and field athletes'.;
Turnagöl, H.H., Koşar, Ş.N., Güzel, Y. et al. (2022). 'Nutritional considerations for injury prevention and recovery in combat sports'. *Nutrients*, 14(1), 53. https://doi.org/10.3390/nu14010053

17. MacDougall, J.D., Ward, G.R., Sale, D.G. & Sutton, J.R. (1977). 'Biochemical adaptation of human skeletal muscle to heavy resistance training and immobilization'. *Journal of Applied Physiology*, 43(4), 700–703. https://doi.org/10.1152/jappl.1977.43.4.700

18. Giraldo-Vallejo et al. (2023). 'Nutritional strategies in the rehabilitation of musculoskeletal injuries in athletes: A systematic integrative review'.;
Rawson, E.S., Miles, M.P. & Larson-Meyer, D.E. (2018). 'Dietary supplements for health, adaptation, and recovery in athletes'. *International Journal of Sport Nutrition and Exercise Metabolism*, 28(2), 188–199. https://doi.org/10.1123/ijsnem.2017-0340;
Harmon, K.K., Stout, J.R., Fukuda, D.H. et al. (2021). 'The application of creatine supplementation in medical rehabilitation'. *Nutrients*, 13(6), 1825. https://doi.org/10.3390/nu13061825

19. Turnagöl et al. (2022). 'Nutritional considerations for injury prevention and recovery in combat sports'.;
Smith-Ryan et al. (2020). 'Nutritional considerations and strategies to facilitate injury recovery and rehabilitation'.

20. Gammone, M.A., Riccioni, G., Parrinello, G. & D'Orazio, N. (2019). 'Omega-3 polyunsaturated fatty acids: Benefits and endpoints in sport'. *Nutrients*, 11(1), 46. https://doi.org/10.3390/nu11010046

21. McGlory, C., Calder, P.C. & Nunes, E.A. (2019). 'The influence of omega-3 fatty acids on skeletal muscle protein turnover in health, disuse, and disease'. *Frontiers in Nutrition*, 6. https://doi.org/10.3389/fnut.2019.00144

22. Smith-Ryan et al. (2020). 'Nutritional considerations and strategies to facilitate injury recovery and rehabilitation'.;
Giraldo-Vallejo et al. (2023). 'Nutritional strategies in the rehabilitation of musculoskeletal injuries in athletes: A systematic integrative review'.

23. Giraldo-Vallejo et al. (2023). 'Nutritional strategies in the rehabilitation of musculoskeletal injuries in athletes: A systematic integrative review'.;
Turnagöl et al. (2022). 'Nutritional considerations for injury prevention and recovery in combat sports'.

24. Papadopoulou (2020). 'Rehabilitation nutrition for injury recovery of athletes: The role of macronutrient intake'.;
Turnagöl et al. (2022). 'Nutritional considerations for injury prevention and recovery in combat sports'.

25. Giraldo-Vallejo et al. (2023). 'Nutritional strategies in the rehabilitation of musculoskeletal injuries in athletes: A systematic integrative review'.

26. Giraldo-Vallejo et al. (2023). 'Nutritional strategies in the rehabilitation of musculoskeletal injuries in athletes: A systematic integrative review'.;
Sikora-Klak, J., Narvy, S.J., Yang, J. et al. (2018). 'The effect of abnormal vitamin D levels in athletes'. *The Permanente Journal*, 22(3), 17–216. https://doi.org/10.7812/TPP/17-216

27. Barker, T., Henriksen, V.T., Martins, T.B. et al. (2013). 'Higher serum 25-hydroxyvitamin D concentrations associate with a faster recovery of skeletal muscle strength after muscular injury'. *Nutrients*, 5(4), 1253–1275. https://doi.org/10.3390/nu5041253;
Smith-Ryan et al. (2020). 'Nutritional considerations and strategies to facilitate injury recovery and rehabilitation'.

28. Minshull, C., Biant, L.C., Ralston, S.H. & Gleeson, N. (2016). 'A systematic review of the role of vitamin D on neuromuscular remodelling following exercise and injury'. *Calcified Tissue International*, 98(5), 426–437. https://doi.org/10.1007/s00223-015-0099-x

29. Peeling, P., Binnie, M.J., Goods, P.S.R. et al. (2018). 'Evidence-based supplements for the enhancement of athletic performance'. *International Journal of Sport Nutrition and Exercise Metabolism*, 28(2), 178–187. https://doi.org/10.1123/ijsnem.2017-0343

30. Giraldo-Vallejo et al. (2023). 'Nutritional strategies in the rehabilitation of musculoskeletal injuries in athletes: A systematic integrative review'.

11 Weight loss and climbing

1. Gibson-Smith, E., Storey, R., Michael, M. & Ranchordas, M. (2024). 'Nutrition knowledge, weight loss practices, and supplement use in senior competition climbers'. *Frontiers in Nutrition*, 10. https://doi.org/10.3389/fnut.2023.1277623

2. Jeukendrup, A.E. (2017). 'Periodized nutrition for athletes'. *Sports Medicine*, 47(Suppl.1), 51–63. https://doi.org/10.1007/s40279-017-0694-2

3. Burke, L.M., Slater, G.J., Matthews, J.J. et al. (2021). 'ACSM expert consensus statement on weight loss in weight-category sports'. *Current Sports Medicine Reports*, 20(4), 199–217. https://doi.org/10.1249/JSR.0000000000000831

4. Helms, E.R., Aragon, A.A. & Fitschen, P.J. (2014). 'Evidence-based recommendations for natural bodybuilding contest preparation: Nutrition and supplementation'. *Journal of the International Society of Sports Nutrition*, 11(1). https://doi.org/10.1186/1550-2783-11-20

5. Mettler, S., Mitchell, N. & Tipton, K.D. (2010). 'Increased protein intake reduces lean body mass loss during weight loss in athletes'. *Medicine & Science in Sports & Exercise*, 42(2), 326–337. https://doi.org/10.1249/MSS.0b013e3181b2ef8e;
Hector, A.J. & Phillips, S.M. (2018). 'Protein recommendations for weight loss in elite athletes: A focus on body composition and performance'. *International Journal of Sport Nutrition and Exercise Metabolism*, 28(2), 170–177. https://doi.org/10.1123/ijsnem.2017-0273

6. Mountjoy, M., Ackerman, K.E., Bailey, D.M. et al. (2023). '2023 International Olympic Committee's (IOC) consensus statement on Relative Energy Deficiency in Sport (REDs)'. *British Journal of Sports Medicine*, 57, 1073–1098. https://doi.org/10.1136/bjsports-2023-106994

7. Melin, A. (2014). 'Energy availability and reproductive function in female endurance athletes' (PhD thesis). Department of Nutrition, Exercise and Sports, Faculty of Science, University of Copenhagen.

8. Mountjoy et al. (2023). '2023 International Olympic Committee's (IOC) consensus statement on Relative Energy Deficiency in Sport (REDs)'.

9. Nazem, T.G. & Ackerman, K.E. (2012). 'The female athlete triad'. *Sports Health*, 4(4), 302–311. https://doi.org/10.1177/1941738112439685

10. Mountjoy, M., Sundgot-Borgen, J., Burke, L. et al. (2014). 'The IOC consensus statement: Beyond the female athlete triad–Relative Energy Deficiency in Sport (RED-S)'. *British Journal of Sports Medicine*, 48(7), 491-497. https://doi.org/10.1136/bjsports-2014-093502

11. Mountjoy, M., Sundgot-Borgen, J.K., Burke, L.M. et al. (2018). 'IOC consensus statement on Relative Energy Deficiency in Sport (RED-S): 2018 update'. *British Journal of Sports Medicine*, 52(11), 687–697. https://doi.org/10.1136/bjsports-2018-099193;
Mountjoy et al. (2023). '2023 International Olympic Committee's (IOC) consensus statement on Relative Energy Deficiency in Sport (REDs)'.

12. Mountjoy et al. (2023). '2023 International Olympic Committee's (IOC) consensus statement on Relative Energy Deficiency in Sport (REDs)'.

12 Can climbers eat intuitively?

1. Tribole, E. & Resch, E. (2012). *Intuitive Eating* (third edition). St Martin's Press, New York.

2. Linardon, J., Tylka, T.L. & Fuller-Tyszkiewicz, M. (2021). 'Intuitive eating and its psychological correlates: A meta-analysis'. *International Journal of Eating Disorders*, 54(7), 1073–1098. https://doi.org/10.1002/eat.23509;
Bruce, L.J. & Ricciardelli, L.A. (2016). 'A systematic review of the psychosocial correlates of intuitive eating among adult women'. *Appetite*, 96, 454–472. https://doi.org/10.1016/j.appet.2015.10.012;
Hensley-Hackett, K., Bosker, J., Keefe, A. et al. (2022). 'Intuitive eating intervention and diet quality in adults: A systematic literature review'. *Journal of Nutrition Education and Behavior*, 54(12), 1099–1115. https://doi.org/10.1016/j.jneb.2022.08.008;
Babbott, K.M., Cavadino, A., Brenton-Peters, J. et al. (2022). 'Outcomes of intuitive eating interventions: A systematic review and meta-analysis'. *Eating Disorders*, 31(1), 33–63. https://doi.org/10.1080/10640266.2022.2030124

3. Galvin, M., Eck, K., Tullio, K. et al. (2023). 'Sports dietitians' use of intuitive eating when working with athletes'. *Journal of the Academy of Nutrition and Dietetics*, 123(10), A23. https://doi.org/10.1016/j.jand.2023.08.060

4. Plateau, C.R., Petrie, T.A. & Papathomas, A. (2016). 'Learning to eat again: Intuitive eating practices among retired female collegiate athletes'. *Eating Disorders*, 25(1), 92–98. https://doi.org/10.1080/10640266.2016.1219185